Psychoneurobiology Research and Personalized Treatment of Schizophrenia

Psychoneurobiology Research and Personalized Treatment of Schizophrenia

Editor

Tomiki Sumiyoshi

MDPI • Basel • Beijing • Wuhan • Barcelona • Belgrade • Manchester • Tokyo • Cluj • Tianjin

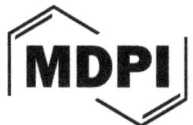

Editor
Tomiki Sumiyoshi
Department of Preventive
Intervention for Psychiatric
Disorders
National Center of Neurology
and Psychiatry
Tokyo
Japan

Editorial Office
MDPI
St. Alban-Anlage 66
4052 Basel, Switzerland

This is a reprint of articles from the Special Issue published online in the open access journal *Journal of Personalized Medicine* (ISSN 2075-4426) (available at: www.mdpi.com/journal/jpm/special_issues/Psychoneurobiolog_Personalized_Schizophrenia).

For citation purposes, cite each article independently as indicated on the article page online and as indicated below:

LastName, A.A.; LastName, B.B.; LastName, C.C. Article Title. *Journal Name* **Year**, *Volume Number*, Page Range.

ISBN 978-3-0365-2859-5 (Hbk)
ISBN 978-3-0365-2858-8 (PDF)

© 2022 by the authors. Articles in this book are Open Access and distributed under the Creative Commons Attribution (CC BY) license, which allows users to download, copy and build upon published articles, as long as the author and publisher are properly credited, which ensures maximum dissemination and a wider impact of our publications.

The book as a whole is distributed by MDPI under the terms and conditions of the Creative Commons license CC BY-NC-ND.

Contents

About the Editor vii

Preface to "Psychoneurobiology Research and Personalized Treatment of Schizophrenia" ix

Tomiki Sumiyoshi
Psychoneurobiology Research and Personalized Treatment of Schizophrenia
Reprinted from: *J. Pers. Med.* **2021**, *11*, 1319, doi:10.3390/jpm11121319 1

Tsutomu Takahashi, Daiki Sasabayashi, Yoichiro Takayanagi, Atsushi Furuichi, Mikio Kido, Tien Viet Pham, Haruko Kobayashi, Kyo Noguchi and Michio Suzuki
Increased Heschl's Gyrus Duplication in Schizophrenia Spectrum Disorders: A Cross-Sectional MRI Study
Reprinted from: *J. Pers. Med.* **2021**, *11*, 40, doi:10.3390/jpm11010040 5

Yuko Higuchi, Tomiki Sumiyoshi, Takahiro Tateno, Suguru Nakajima, Daiki Sasabayashi, Shimako Nishiyama, Yuko Mizukami, Tsutomu Takahashi and Michio Suzuki
Prolonged P300 Latency in Antipsychotic-Free Subjects with At-Risk Mental States Who Later Developed Schizophrenia
Reprinted from: *J. Pers. Med.* **2021**, *11*, 327, doi:10.3390/jpm11050327 17

Marta Barrera-Conde, Karina Ausin, Mercedes Lachén-Montes, Joaquín Fernández-Irigoyen, Liliana Galindo, Aida Cuenca-Royo, Cristina Fernández-Avilés, Víctor Pérez, Rafael de la Torre, Enrique Santamaría and Patricia Robledo
Cannabis Use Induces Distinctive Proteomic Alterations in Olfactory Neuroepithelial Cells of Schizophrenia Patients
Reprinted from: *J. Pers. Med.* **2021**, *11*, 160, doi:10.3390/jpm11030160 31

Diana Z. Paderina, Anastasiia S. Boiko, Ivan V. Pozhidaev, Anna V. Bocharova, Irina A. Mednova, Olga Yu. Fedorenko, Elena G. Kornetova, Anton J.M. Loonen, Arkadiy V. Semke, Nikolay A. Bokhan and Svetlana A. Ivanova
Genetic Polymorphisms of 5-HT Receptors and Antipsychotic-Induced Metabolic Dysfunction in Patients with Schizophrenia
Reprinted from: *J. Pers. Med.* **2021**, *11*, 181, doi:10.3390/jpm11030181 47

Atsumi Nitta, Naotaka Izuo, Kohei Hamatani, Ryo Inagaki, Yuka Kusui, Kequan Fu, Takashi Asano, Youta Torii, Chikako Habuchi, Hirotaka Sekiguchi, Shuji Iritani, Shin-ichi Muramatsu, Norio Ozaki and Yoshiaki Miyamoto
Schizophrenia-Like Behavioral Impairments in Mice with Suppressed Expression of Piccolo in the Medial Prefrontal Cortex
Reprinted from: *J. Pers. Med.* **2021**, *11*, 607, doi:10.3390/jpm11070607 57

Naotaka Izuo and Atsumi Nitta
New Insights Regarding Diagnosis and Medication for Schizophrenia Based on Neuronal Synapse–Microglia Interaction
Reprinted from: *J. Pers. Med.* **2021**, *11*, 371, doi:10.3390/jpm11050371 75

Irene Birulés, Raquel López-Carrilero, Daniel Cuadras, Esther Pousa, Maria Luisa Barrigón, Ana Barajas, Ester Lorente-Rovira, Fermín González-Higueras, Eva Grasa, Isabel Ruiz-Delgado, Jordi Cid, Ana de Apraiz, Roger Montserrat, Trinidad Pélaez, Steffen Moritz, the Spanish Metacognition Study Group and Susana Ochoa
Cognitive Insight in First-Episode Psychosis: Changes during Metacognitive Training
Reprinted from: *J. Pers. Med.* **2020**, *10*, 253, doi:10.3390/jpm10040253 91

Hiroki Okano, Ryotaro Kubota, Ryo Okubo, Naoki Hashimoto, Satoru Ikezawa, Atsuhito Toyomaki, Akane Miyazaki, Yohei Sasaki, Yuji Yamada, Takahiro Nemoto and Masafumi Mizuno
Evaluation of Social Cognition Measures for Japanese Patients with Schizophrenia Using an Expert Panel and Modified Delphi Method
Reprinted from: *J. Pers. Med.* **2021**, *11*, 275, doi:10.3390/jpm11040275 . . . . **105**

Ryotaro Kubota, Ryo Okubo, Hisashi Akiyama, Hiroki Okano, Satoru Ikezawa, Akane Miyazaki, Atsuhito Toyomaki, Yohei Sasaki, Yuji Yamada, Takashi Uchino, Takahiro Nemoto, Tomiki Sumiyoshi, Naoki Yoshimura and Naoki Hashimoto
Study Protocol: The Evaluation Study for Social Cognition Measures in Japan (ESCoM)
Reprinted from: *J. Pers. Med.* **2021**, *11*, 667, doi:10.3390/jpm11070667 . . . . **117**

Yuji Yamada, Takuma Inagawa, Yuma Yokoi, Aya Shirama, Kazuki Sueyoshi, Ayumu Wada, Naotsugu Hirabayashi, Hideki Oi and Tomiki Sumiyoshi
Efficacy and Safety of Multi-Session Transcranial Direct Current Stimulation on Social Cognition in Schizophrenia: A Study Protocol for an Open-Label, Single-Arm Trial
Reprinted from: *J. Pers. Med.* **2021**, *11*, 317, doi:10.3390/jpm11040317 . . . . **131**

About the Editor

Tomiki Sumiyoshi

Dr. Tomiki Sumiyoshi, MD, PhD, obtained his MD in Medicine and PhD in Medical Science in Kanazawa University, and was trained at the Department of Psychiatry Case Western Reserve University as Research Associate. He was appointed Visiting Professor in the Department of Psychiatry, Vanderbilt University from 2000 to 2002. Dr. Sumiyoshi is currently Director of the Department of Preventive Intervention for Psychiatric Disorders, National Institute of Mental Health, National Center of Neurology and Psychiatry.

His research interests include investigating neurobiological substrates responsible for cognitive impairment, implementing methods for early intervention and discovering effective therapeutics to facilitate social outcomes in patients with psychosis, mood disorders or neurodevelopmental disorders.

As Chairman of Section on Psychoneurobiology of World Psychiatric Association, Dr. Sumiyoshi is promoting worldwide interactions among researchers and clinicians on cognitive sciences, psychopharmacology, neurophysiology, neuromodulation, and related fields.

Preface to "Psychoneurobiology Research and Personalized Treatment of Schizophrenia"

Schizophrenia is a common disease characterized by psychotic symptoms (e.g., delusions, hallucinations, blunted affect) and disturbances of cognitive function (e.g., memory, abstraction, attention). If not treated properly, patients may experience serious consequences in terms of social function.

Much endeavor in several disciplines of medical science has been made to overcome the paucity of effective treatments for unmet needs, including cognitive impairment associated with schizophrenia. Accordingly, psycho-neuro-biological approaches have been attempted, leading to the development of innovative compounds, as well as non-pharmacological therapeutics, including cognitive rehabilitation and neuromodulation (e.g., non-invasive brain stimulation). These endeavors should bear individualized medicine in mind to optimize the risk/benefit ratios of pharmacotherapy and other modalities of intervention.

This Book, contributed to by experts from various regions of the globe, provides up-to-date information on the phenomenology, underlying mechanisms, and treatment of schizophrenia, and especially facilitates the development of personal therapeutics for this enigmatic illness.

Tomiki Sumiyoshi
Editor

Editorial
Psychoneurobiology Research and Personalized Treatment of Schizophrenia

Tomiki Sumiyoshi

Department of Preventive Intervention for Psychiatric Disorders, National Institute of Mental Health, National Center of Neurology and Psychiatry, 4-1-1-Ogawahigashi-cho, Kodaira, Tokyo 187-8551, Japan; sumiyot@ncnp.go.jp

Psychoneurobiological approaches have been used to develop effective treatments for unmet needs in schizophrenia, e.g., some types of cognitive disturbances. To overcome the paucity of breakthrough therapeutics, observations from molecular biology, brain sciences, and their combinations need to be integrated. Besides the development of innovative compounds, there has been a trend towards non-pharmacological therapeutics, including cognitive rehabilitation and neuromodulation (e.g., non-invasive brain stimulation), targeting schizophrenia. These endeavors should bear individualized medicine in mind to optimize the risk/benefit ratios of pharmacotherapy and other modalities of intervention. This Special Issue, consisting of 10 articles, provides a forum for researchers interested in the phenomenology, underlying mechanisms, and treatment of schizophrenia.

Structural and functional anomalies in the brains of individuals with schizophrenia have been identified to promote more effective intervention strategies for the illness. Accordingly, Takahashi et al. [1] observed derangement of temporal lobe structures (e.g., Heschl's gyrus) in subjects with schizotypal disorder. As similar anatomical findings have been noted in patients with schizophrenia, the finding suggests a common neural substrate across these schizophrenia-spectrum disorders. These lines of morphological changes that are characteristic of schizophrenia are often reflected in neurophysiological observations. Thus, Higuchi et al. [2] examined the P300 component of event-related potentials derived from EEG in people with vulnerability to developing schizophrenia, or in those in an "at-risk mental state (ARMS)". At baseline, the P300 latencies in ARMS subjects who later converted to schizophrenia were longer compared to those in ARMS non-converters, providing a feasible electrical marker to facilitate early intervention into psychosis.

The search for objective markers to predict a variety of clinical manifestations associated with schizophrenia is enriched by the use of biochemical and genetic findings; for example, Barrera-Conde et al. [3] report the relationship between cannabis use and expressions of RNA-related proteins in olfactory neuroepithelium (ON) cells from clinical samples. This approach is expected to help understand the link between specific proteomic alterations and the increased risk of substance abuse in patients with the illness. Reducing the chance of metabolic syndrome (MetS) caused by antipsychotic drugs has been a major concern from the standpoint of precision medicine. Among several subtypes of serotonin (5-HT) receptors, Paderina et al. [4] found that allelic variants of genes encoding $5HT_{2C}$ receptors (*HTR2C*) were associated with the incidence of MetS in patients with schizophrenia, highlighting the importance of genetic examinations before starting medications.

It is noteworthy that neurobiological findings in preclinical research have frequently advanced the knowledge in this field, to improve clinical studies. Accordingly, Nitta et al. [5] present animal data on single-nucleotide polymorphisms (SNPs) of genes encoding Piccolo, a presynaptic cytomatrix protein. Specifically, mutant mice with reduced expression of Piccolo in their prefrontal cortex exhibited behavioral and neurochemical abnormalities reminiscent of schizophrenia. The same group of investigators also provide a review of the dysregulated immune system implicated in the pathophysiology of the disease [6].

In particular, the role of the overactivation of synaptic pruning (elimination) by microglia is discussed, suggesting that modulation of the interaction between microglia and synapses may provide an avenue to novel therapeutics.

In addition to psychotic symptoms, some of the key areas of cognitive function, e.g., neurocognition, social cognition, and metacognition, have attracted growing interest to improve social outcomes, or functionality, in schizophrenia patients. Here, Birules et al. [7] examined the time course of the effect of metacognitive training (MCT) on cognitive insight in patients with schizophrenia. The results indicate the benefits of MCT for reducing self-certainty, a component of mega-cognition, which became evident after repeated administrations. On the other hand, Okano et al. [8] report an expert consensus on which assessment tools are to be used to evaluate social cognition in Japanese populations. Considerations were placed on reliability and validity, as well as international comparability and clinical usefulness. This initiative to develop a comprehensive set of social cognition tests is embodied by the Evaluation Study of Social Cognition Measures in Japan (ESCoM), as reported by Kubota et al. [9]. As a novel treatment approach, Yamada et al. [10] are conducting a clinical trial to determine if transcranial direct current stimulation on the temporal lobe sulcus regions alleviates social cognition impairment in schizophrenia.

Overall, the information provided by the authors contributing to this Special Issue will facilitate the development of personal therapeutics of greater clinical value.

Funding: Not applicable.

Institutional Review Board Statement: Not applicable.

Informed Consent Statement: Not applicable.

Data Availability Statement: Not applicable.

Acknowledgments: The author thanks all the authors who contributed their work. Technical assistance of Yumi Hasegawa is greatly appreciated. The author also wishes to thank the staff of *JPM* for their excellent support throughout the editorial process.

Conflicts of Interest: The author declares no conflict of interest.

References

1. Takahashi, T.; Sasabayashi, D.; Takayanagi, Y.; Furuichi, A.; Kido, M.; Pham, T.V.; Kobayashi, H.; Noguchi, K.; Suzuki, M. Increased Heschl's Gyrus Duplication in Schizophrenia Spectrum Disorders: A Cross-Sectional MRI Study. *J. Pers. Med.* **2021**, *11*, 40. [CrossRef] [PubMed]
2. Higuchi, Y.; Sumiyoshi, T.; Tateno, T.; Nakajima, S.; Sasabayashi, D.; Nishiyama, S.; Mizukami, Y.; Takahashi, T.; Suzuki, M. Prolonged P300 Latency in Antipsychotic-Free Subjects with At-Risk Mental States Who Later Developed Schizophrenia. *J. Pers. Med.* **2021**, *11*, 327. [CrossRef] [PubMed]
3. Barrera-Conde, M.; Ausin, K.; Lachén-Montes, M.; Fernández-Irigoyen, J.; Galindo, L.; Cuenca-Royo, A.; Fernández-Avilés, C.; Pérez, V.; de la Torre, R.; Santamaría, E.; et al. Cannabis Use Induces Distinctive Proteomic Alterations in Olfactory Neuroepithelial Cells of Schizophrenia Patients. *J. Pers. Med.* **2021**, *11*, 160. [CrossRef] [PubMed]
4. Paderina, D.Z.; Boiko, A.S.; Pozhidaev, I.V.; Bocharova, A.V.; Mednova, I.A.; Fedorenko, O.Y.; Kornetova, E.G.; Loonen, A.J.M.; Semke, A.V.; Bokhan, N.A.; et al. Genetic Polymorphisms of 5-HT Receptors and Antipsychotic-Induced Metabolic Dysfunction in Patients with Schizophrenia. *J. Pers. Med.* **2021**, *11*, 181. [CrossRef]
5. Nitta, A.; Izuo, N.; Hamatani, K.; Inagaki, R.; Kusui, Y.; Fu, K.; Asano, T.; Torii, Y.; Habuchi, C.; Sekiguchi, H.; et al. Schizophrenia-Like Behavioral Impairments in Mice with Suppressed Expression of Piccolo in the Medial Prefrontal Cortex. *J. Pers. Med.* **2021**, *11*, 607. [CrossRef] [PubMed]
6. Izuo, N.; Nitta, A. New Insights Regarding Diagnosis and Medication for Schizophrenia Based on Neuronal Synapse–Microglia Interaction. *J. Pers. Med.* **2021**, *11*, 371. [CrossRef]
7. Birulés, I.; López-Carrilero, R.; Cuadras, D.; Pousa, E.; Barrigón, M.L.; Barajas, A.; Lorente-Rovira, E.; González-Higueras, F.; Grasa, E.; Ruiz-Delgado, I.; et al. Cognitive Insight in First-Episode Psychosis: Changes during Metacognitive Training. *J. Pers. Med.* **2020**, *10*, 253. [CrossRef] [PubMed]
8. Okano, H.; Kubota, R.; Okubo, R.; Hashimoto, N.; Ikezawa, S.; Toyomaki, A.; Miyazaki, A.; Sasaki, Y.; Yamada, Y.; Nemoto, T.; et al. Evaluation of Social Cognition Measures for Japanese Patients with Schizophrenia Using an Expert Panel and Modified Delphi Method. *J. Pers. Med.* **2021**, *11*, 275. [CrossRef]

9. Kubota, R.; Okubo, R.; Akiyama, H.; Okano, H.; Ikezawa, S.; Miyazaki, A.; Toyomaki, A.; Sasaki, Y.; Yamada, Y.; Uchino, T.; et al. Study Protocol: The Evaluation Study for Social Cognition Measures in Japan (ESCoM). *J. Pers. Med.* **2021**, *11*, 667. [CrossRef] [PubMed]
10. Yamada, Y.; Inagawa, T.; Yokoi, Y.; Shirama, A.; Sueyoshi, K.; Wada, A.; Hirabayashi, N.; Oi, H.; Sumiyoshi, T. Efficacy and Safety of Multi-Session Transcranial Direct Current Stimulation on Social Cognition in Schizophrenia: A Study Protocol for an Open-Label, Single-Arm Trial. *J. Pers. Med.* **2021**, *11*, 317. [CrossRef] [PubMed]

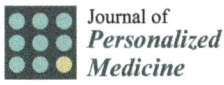

Article

Increased Heschl's Gyrus Duplication in Schizophrenia Spectrum Disorders: A Cross-Sectional MRI Study

Tsutomu Takahashi [1,2,*], Daiki Sasabayashi [1,2], Yoichiro Takayanagi [1,3], Atsushi Furuichi [1,2], Mikio Kido [1,2], Tien Viet Pham [1,2], Haruko Kobayashi [1,2], Kyo Noguchi [4] and Michio Suzuki [1,2]

1 Department of Neuropsychiatry, Graduate School of Medicine and Pharmaceutical Sciences, University of Toyama, Toyama 930-0194, Japan; ds179@med.u-toyama.ac.jp (D.S.); takayanagi-matsu@umin.net (Y.T.); ichi1031@med.u-toyama.ac.jp (A.F.); mikiokid@med.u-toyama.ac.jp (M.K.); tienke93@gmail.com (T.V.P.); harukodayoo@gmail.com (H.K.); suzukim@med.u-toyama.ac.jp (M.S.)
2 Research Center for Idling Brain Science, University of Toyama, Toyama 930-0194, Japan
3 Arisawabashi Hospital, Toyama 939-2704, Japan
4 Department of Radiology, Graduate School of Medicine and Pharmaceutical Sciences, University of Toyama, Toyama 930-0194, Japan; kyo@med.u-toyama.ac.jp
* Correspondence: tsutomu@med.u-toyama.ac.jp; Tel.: +81-76-434-7323

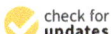

Citation: Takahashi, T.; Sasabayashi, D.; Takayanagi, Y.; Furuichi, A.; Kido, M.; Pham, T.V.; Kobayashi, H.; Noguchi, K.; Suzuki, M. Increased Heschl's Gyrus Duplication in Schizophrenia Spectrum Disorders: A Cross-Sectional MRI Study. *J. Pers. Med.* **2021**, *11*, 40. https://doi.org/10.3390/jpm11010040

Received: 14 December 2020
Accepted: 9 January 2021
Published: 12 January 2021

Publisher's Note: MDPI stays neutral with regard to jurisdictional claims in published maps and institutional affiliations.

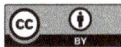

Copyright: © 2021 by the authors. Licensee MDPI, Basel, Switzerland. This article is an open access article distributed under the terms and conditions of the Creative Commons Attribution (CC BY) license (https://creativecommons.org/licenses/by/4.0/).

Abstract: Duplicated Heschl's gyrus (HG) is prevalent in patients with schizophrenia and may reflect early neurodevelopmental anomalies. However, it currently remains unclear whether patients with schizotypal disorder, a prototypic disorder within the schizophrenia spectrum, exhibit a similar HG gyrification pattern. In this magnetic resonance imaging study, HG gyrification patterns were examined in 47 patients with schizotypal disorder, 111 with schizophrenia, and 88 age- and sex-matched healthy subjects. HG gyrification patterns were classified as single, common stem duplication (CSD), or complete posterior duplication (CPD). The prevalence of the duplicated HG patterns (CSD or CPD) bilaterally was higher in the schizophrenia and schizotypal groups than in healthy controls, whereas no significant difference was observed between the schizophrenia and schizotypal groups. Schizophrenia patients with the right CPD pattern had less severe positive symptoms, whereas the right single HG pattern was associated with higher doses of antipsychotic medication in schizotypal patients. The present study demonstrated shared HG gyrification patterns in schizophrenia spectrum disorders, which may reflect a common biological vulnerability factor. HG patterns may also be associated with susceptibility to psychopathology.

Keywords: magnetic resonance imaging; schizophrenia; schizotypal disorder; gyrification; superior temporal gyrus; neurodevelopment

1. Introduction

Heschl's gyrus (HG), which is also termed as transverse temporal gyrus, is a convolution on the superior temporal plane that hosts the primary auditory cortex (Brodmann area (BA) 41) [1,2]. Its gyral pattern markedly varies across individuals, with approximately 30% to 50% of healthy subjects having HG duplication, particularly on the right hemisphere [3–5]. In cases of HG duplication, cytoarchitectonic evidence suggests that the auditory koniocortex (BA41) is restricted to the anterior HG, whereas the posterior HG may correspond to BA42/22 as part of the associative auditory cortex [1–5]. This anatomical variant may reflect differences in cytoarchitectonic development during the gestational period [6,7], with duplicated HG potentially reducing HG functional activity during auditory processing [8]. However, it currently remains unclear whether patients with schizophrenia, who have an early neurodevelopmental pathology [9,10] and are characterized by altered volume/thickness and functional connectivity of HG [11–13], exhibit an altered HG gyrification pattern. In a recent magnetic resonance imaging (MRI) study, we demonstrated that HG duplication was prevalent in first-episode schizophrenia [14], whereas another MRI study in which HG duplication patterns in chronic schizophrenia were specifically examined failed to find significant differences [15]. Although gyrification patterns generally remain stable after birth in healthy subjects [6], this discrepancy may be partly explained by the potential impact of illness chronicity and/or antipsychotic medication on the morphology of the superior temporal plane [16].

Schizotypal disorder [17] or schizotypal personality disorder [18], a prototypical schizophrenia spectrum disorder without overt/sustained psychosis, may have biological, neurocognitive, and phenomenological similarities with schizophrenia as a common vulnerability factor [19,20]. Our recent whole brain analyses revealed that schizophrenia and schizotypal patients both exhibit increased cortical folding, which may be related to neural dysconnectivity due to aberrant neurodevelopmental processes [21], in diverse cortical regions [22,23]. Furthermore, schizotypal patients share decreased functional connectivity in the HG, which may reflect vulnerability to psychopathology [24,25], with patients with overt schizophrenia [26,27]. These previous findings suggest an altered HG gyrification pattern in schizotypal subjects, but no MRI studies to date have specifically examined it. Therefore, it currently remains unclear whether an altered HG gyrification pattern, if present, is specific to schizophrenia or is commonly observed in schizophrenia spectrum disorders.

The present MRI study compared HG gyrification patterns (single convolution, partially duplicated, or fully duplicated) between an expanded sample of schizophrenia patients of different illness stages (i.e., first-episode [14] and chronic), schizotypal disorder, and healthy controls. Based on biological commonalities among schizophrenia spectrum disorders as a vulnerability factor [16,19,20] and our previous findings of first-episode schizophrenia [14], we predicted that HG duplication will be more prevalent in the schizophrenia and schizotypal groups than in healthy controls. Based on the potential early neurodevelopmental pathology of schizophrenia [9,10] and the notion that the gyrification pattern generally remains stable after birth [6,7], we also predicted no influence of illness chronicity on the HG pattern in schizophrenia. Furthermore, we examined the relationship between HG patterns and other clinical variables (e.g., symptom severity and medication) in the patient groups.

2. Materials and Methods

2.1. Subjects

Subjects in the present cross-sectional study consisted of 47 patients with schizotypal disorder (or schizotypal personality disorder), 111 with schizophrenia, and 88 age- and sex-matched healthy subjects (Table 1). The patients were from our observational study (i.e., not from randomized clinical trials), whereas the controls were selected from our MRI database of healthy subjects on the basis of age and sex. They were all physically healthy at MRI and had no previous history of severe obstetric complications, serious head trauma, serious medical diseases (e.g., neurological illness, thyroid dysfunction, diabetes, and hypertension), steroid use, or substance abuse. All subjects were right-handed, Japanese (aged 14 to 46 years), and were screened for gross brain abnormalities by neuroradiologists at the time of scanning. Among 246 subjects, HG patterns in 64 schizophrenia and 64 control subjects were reported in our previous study [14], which demonstrated that HG duplication was more prevalent in first-episode schizophrenia. The study was conducted in accordance with the Declaration of Helsinki. The Committee on Medical Ethics of Toyama University approved the present study (No. I2013006) on 5 February 2014. After the purpose and procedures of the present study were fully explained, written informed consent was received individually from each study participant. When participants were <20 years old, written consent was also received from a parent/guardian.

Table 1. Demographic/clinical parameters and brain measurements of subjects.

	C	SzTypal	Sz	Group Comparisons
Male/female	49/39	29/18	59/52	Chi squared = 0.98, p = 0.613
Age (years)	24.1 ± 6.0	25.0 ± 5.4	25.8 ± 5.4	$F_{(2, 243)}$ = 2.38, p = 0.095
Height (cm)	166.3 ± 7.8	165.9 ± 8.7	164.5 ± 8.0	$F_{(2, 243)}$ = 1.34, p = 0.264
Education (years)	15.7 ± 3.0	13.1 ± 2.0	13.5 ± 2.0	$F_{(2, 243)}$ = 26.23, p < 0.001; Sz, SzTypal < C
Parental education (years) [1]	13.0 ± 2.3	12.3 ± 1.7	12.5 ± 2.0	$F_{(2, 234)}$ = 1.81, p = 0.166
Age of onset (years)	-	-	22.2 ± 4.7	-
Duration of illness (years)	-	-	3.6 ± 4.1	-
Dose of medication (HPD equivalent, mg/day)	-	4.8 ± 5.7	10.1 ± 8.8	$F_{(1, 156)}$ = 14.64, p < 0.001; SzTypal < Sz
Duration of medication (years)	-	1.5 ± 3.0	2.7 ± 3.6	$F_{(1, 156)}$ = 3.70, p = 0.056
Medication type (typical/atypical/mixed) [2]	-	14/26/0	40/65/4	Fisher's exact test, p = 0.636
Total SAPS scores [3]	-	16.0 ± 9.2	27.2 ± 20.9	$F_{(1, 147)}$ = 11.86, p < 0.001; SzTypal < Sz
Total SANS scores [3]	-	41.9 ± 21.7	49.8 ± 22.8	$F_{(1, 147)}$ = 3.93, p = 0.049; SzTypal < Sz

Values represent means ± standard deviations (SDs) unless otherwise stated. C, controls; HPD, haloperidol; SANS, scale for the assessment of negative symptoms; SAPS, scale for the assessment of positive symptoms; Sz, schizophrenia; SzTypal, schizotypal disorder. [1] Data missing for one control, four SzTypal, and four Sz subjects. [2] Seven SzTypal patients were antipsychotic-naïve. Two Sz patients were antipsychotic-free at scanning. [3] Data missing for two SzTypal and seven Sz patients.

Patients with schizotypal disorder and schizophrenia who met the ICD-10 research criteria [28] were recruited from the outpatient and inpatient clinics of the Department of Neuropsychiatry, Toyama University Hospital. Patients were diagnosed by experienced psychiatrists (M.K., T.T. and M.S.) in a structured interview (the Japanese version of Comprehensive Assessment of Symptoms and History [29]), in addition to clinical symptoms scored using the Japanese version of Scale for the Assessment of Negative and Positive Symptoms (SANS/SAPS [30,31]) and a detailed chart review. Cognitive and social functions were not systematically evaluated. The recruitment strategy and sample characteristics of our clinic-based schizotypal group who required clinical care for distress/issues stemming from their schizotypal features were described in detail previously [32,33]. All schizotypal patients fulfilled the DSM-IV criteria of the schizotypal personality disorder on Axis II, whereas 13 had previously experienced transient quasipsychotic episodes fulfilling a DSM Axis I diagnosis of brief psychotic disorder [18]. Although the risk of developing psychosis was previously reported to be higher in schizotypal patients than in the general population [34], none in the present study developed overt schizophrenia during the clinical follow-up period (mean = 3.0 ± 2.6 years). The schizophrenia group was divided into first-episode (illness duration $\leq$ 1 year (N = 48) or first psychiatric hospitalization (N = 16)) and chronic (illness duration $\geq$ 3 years (N = 41)) subgroups to examine the effects of illness chronicity. The medication status and other clinical data are summarized in Table 1.

Control subjects were recruited from the community (N = 29), hospital staff (N = 27), and university students (N = 32). They were screened using a questionnaire consisting of 15 items regarding their present/previous medical history and family histories of illness [35] and were excluded if they had any personal or family history of psychiatric illness among their first-degree relatives.

2.2. MRI Procedure

Brain MRI was performed using the 1.5-T Magnetom Vision (Siemens Medical System, Inc, Erlangen, Germany) at Toyama University Hospital. Three-dimensional gradient-echo sequence FLASH yielded a sagittal series of 160–180 contiguous T1-weighted slices with a thickness of 1.0 mm. Imaging parameters were as follows: time to echo = 5 ms, time repetition = 24 ms, flip angle = 40°, field of view = 256 mm, matrix size = 256 × 256, and voxel dimension = 1.0 × 1.0 × 1.0 mm.

2.3. Assessment of HG Gyrification Patterns

As described in detail previously [14], HG patterns on each hemisphere were classified as follows: single HG, common stem duplication (CSD), and complete posterior duplication (CPD) [2–5]. Anatomical landmarks for this classification were facilely identified on coronal, axial, and sagittal views simultaneously displayed using Dr. View software (Infocom,

Tokyo, Japan) (Figure 1). Briefly, a single HG pattern had no duplication (i.e., one HG per hemisphere), whereas the CPD pattern was defined by completely separate gyri (two (N = 134) or three (N = 6) gyri per hemisphere in this study). The CSD pattern was characterized by a gyrus that was partially split by the sulcus intermedius (SI), which forms a "heart-shaped" HG. Eight subjects (6.5%) in the present study who had a separate HG posterior to the HG with partial duplication were considered to have the CSD pattern.

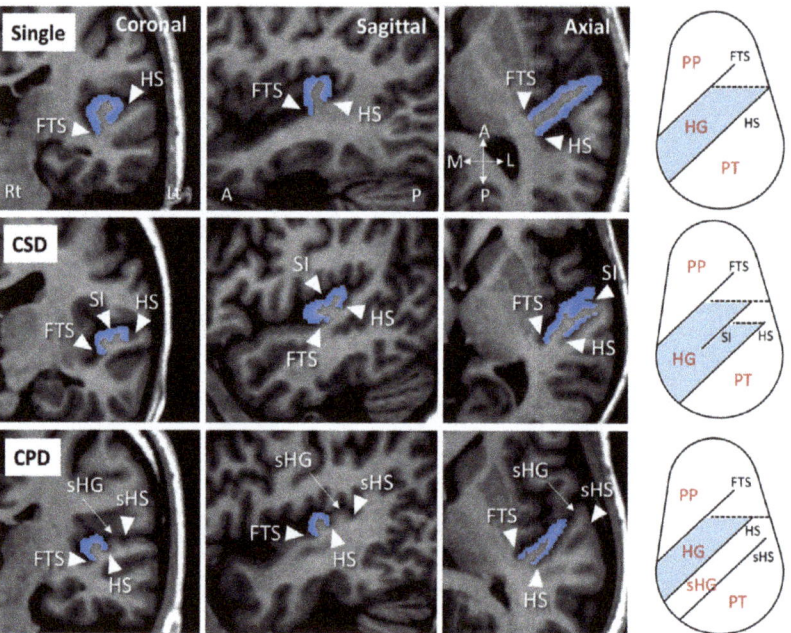

Figure 1. Coronal, sagittal, and axial views of sample MRI of Heschl's gyrus (HG; colored in blue) and schematic drawings of the superior temporal surface on an axial view (right) of different gyrification patterns. A, anterior; CPD, complete posterior duplication; CSD, common stem duplication; FTS, first transverse sulcus; HS, Heschl's sulcus; L, lateral; P, posterior; M, medial; PT, planum temporale; PP, planum polare; sHG, second Heschl's gyrus; sHS, second Heschl's sulcus; SI, sulcus intermedius.

All pattern classifications were performed by one rater (T.T.) without knowledge of the subjects' identity (e.g., sex and diagnosis). The HG pattern in a subset of 15 randomly selected brains (30 hemispheres) was assessed independently by two raters (T.T. and D.S.), and each HG pattern was then reclassified after at least 4 weeks by T.T., who was blinded to the first HG classification; inter- (T.T. and D.S.) and intrarater reliabilities (Cronbach's α) were 0.83 and 1.00, respectively.

2.4. Statistical Analysis

A one-way analysis of variance (ANOVA) or the χ^2 test was performed to assess the significance of group differences in clinical/demographic data.

The HG pattern distribution on each hemisphere was compared across the groups by the χ^2 test. As the HG duplication was more prevalent in the patient groups regardless of its subtype, the odds ratio was calculated to estimate the association between HG duplication (CSD or CPD) and relative risk of developing schizophrenia/schizotypal disorder. Analysis of covariate (ANCOVA) was used to examine the potential contribution of HG pattern to total SANS/SAPS scores, with the HG type as an independent variable and the medication dose/duration as covariates. Significant effects yielded in ANCOVA were then analyzed using post hoc Newman–Keuls tests. The relationship between the HG gyrification pattern and other clinical variables (i.e., onset age and duration of illness (only for the schizophrenia group), and medication status (dose and duration)) was assessed by nonparametric Kruskal–Wallis tests due to the non-normal distribution of these variables (tested by Kolmogorov–Smirnov test). The relationship between the HG type and SAPS score in schizophrenia was also tested by the Kruskal–Wallis test because of the skewed distribution of the score (Kolmogorov–Smirnov test, $p = 0.018$). In order to estimate potential interaction effects of illness stages (first-episode vs. chronic) and other factors (e.g., medication), each subgroup was also tested independently. To test for potential sampling bias, an independent contribution of demographic variables (age, sex, height, education, and parental education) on HG pattern was investigated using stepwise regression analysis. The significance of differences was defined as $p < 0.05$.

3. Results

3.1. Demographic and Clinical Data

Groups were matched for age, sex, and parental education, but control subjects had a higher education level than patients with either disorder (Table 1). As expected, schizophrenia patients had significantly more severe symptom ratings (SANS/SAPS) and higher medication doses than schizotypal patients.

3.2. HG Pattern Distributions

The schizophrenia (left, $\chi^2 = 20.56$, $p < 0.001$; right, $\chi^2 = 11.84$, $p = 0.003$) and schizotypal (left, $\chi^2 = 4.20$, $p = 0.040$; right, $\chi^2 = 4.09$, $p = 0.043$) groups had a significantly higher prevalence of duplicated HG patterns bilaterally (i.e., CSD or CPD) than healthy controls, whereas no significant differences were observed in the HG pattern between the schizophrenia and schizotypal groups ($\chi^2 < 2.73$, $p > 0.098$) (Table 2, Figure 2). When we examined subjects with HG duplication only, no group difference was noted in HG patterns (CSD vs. CPD; $\chi^2 < 0.66$, $p > 0.416$). The odds ratio of HG duplication was 3.90 (left, 95% confidence interval (CI) = 2.14 to 7.12) and 2.91 (right, 95% CI = 1.56 to 5.42) for schizophrenia, and 2.12 (left, 95% CI = 1.03 to 4.37) and 2.22 (right, 95% CI = 1.02 to 4.83) for schizotypal disorder.

HG patterns were also compared between the first-episode and chronic subgroups of schizophrenia, but no significant differences were observed (left, $\chi^2 = 0.00$, $p = 0.998$; right, $\chi^2 = 2.23$, $p = 0.328$).

Sex did not significantly affect HG patterns ($\chi^2 < 2.61$, $p > 0.112$), whereas HG duplication (i.e., CSD or CPD) was more frequent in the right hemisphere ($\chi^2 = 4.77$, $p = 0.029$) when all diagnostic groups were combined.

Stepwise analysis of demographic variables using the entire sample revealed that the HG pattern was predicted by height (beta = 0.160, t = 2.45, $p = 0.015$) and education (beta = -0.152, t = -2.32, $p = 0.021$) only for the right hemisphere (adjusted $R^2 = 0.031$). For validation purposes, we then assessed the relationship between these variables and right HG pattern using the Kruskal–Wallis test; however, only the education level had a trend-level relationship with the HG pattern ($H = 5.878$, $p = 0.053$).

Table 2. Gyrification pattern of Heschl's gyrus (HG) in subjects.

Healthy Controls					
		\multicolumn{4}{c}{Right HG pattern (N (%))}
		Single	CSD	CPD	Total
Left HG pattern (N (%))	Single	25 (28.4)	13 (14.8)	12 (13.6)	50 (56.8)
	CSD	8 (9.1)	9 (10.2)	6 (6.8)	23 (26.1)
	CPD	5 (5.7)	5 (5.7)	5 (5.7)	15 (17.0)
	Total	38 (43.2)	27 (30.7)	23 (26.1)	88 (100.0)
Schizotypal Disorder					
		\multicolumn{4}{c}{Right HG pattern (N (%))}
		Single	CSD	CPD	Total
Left HG pattern (N (%))	Single	7 (14.9)	5 (10.6)	6 (12.8)	18 (38.3)
	CSD	2 (4.3)	10 (21.3)	3 (6.4)	15 (31.9)
	CPD	3 (6.4)	7 (14.9)	4 (8.5)	14 (29.8)
	Total	12 (25.5)	22 (46.8)	13 (27.7)	47 (100.0)
Schizophrenia					
		\multicolumn{4}{c}{Right HG pattern (N (%))}
		Single	CSD	CPD	Total
Left HG pattern (N (%))	Single	11 (9.9)	11 (9.9)	6 (5.4)	28 (25.2)
	CSD	8 (7.2)	25 (22.5)	12 (10.8)	45 (40.5)
	CPD	4 (3.6)	15 (13.5)	19 (17.1)	38 (34.2)
	Total	23 (20.7)	51 (45.9)	37 (33.3)	111 (100.0)

CSD, common stem duplication; CPD, complete posterior duplication.

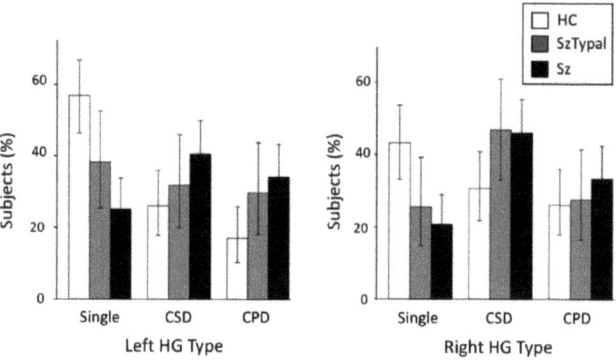

Figure 2. Distribution of Heschl's gyrus (HG) gyrification patterns in schizophrenia (Sz), schizotypal (SzTypal), and healthy control (HC) groups. Error bars show 95% confidence intervals. CPD, complete posterior duplication; CSD, common stem duplication.

3.3. Relationship between the HG Pattern and Clinical Variables

The right HG pattern significantly affected the total SAPS score in the schizophrenia group (ANCOVA, $F (2, 99) = 4.47$, $p = 0.014$), with a lower score being observed in patients with the CPD pattern (mean = 19.8, SD = 15.9) than in those with the CSD (mean = 30.0, SD = 22.6; $p = 0.038$) or single (mean = 32.5, SD = 21.9; $p = 0.027$) pattern. This relationship was replicated using a nonparametric Kruskal–Wallis test ($H = 6.61$, $p = 0.037$) and post hoc pairwise comparisons (CPD < CSD ($p = 0.033$) or single ($p = 0.022$)). Furthermore, subgroup analysis demonstrated that this relationship was specific to first-episode schizophrenia (ANCOVA, $F (2, 60) = 3.78$, $p = 0.028$; Kruskal–Wallis test, $H = 7.78$, $p = 0.020$). The chronic schizophrenia patients with left single HG (mean = 37.9, SD = 13.2) had a higher SAPS score than those with left CSD (mean = 26.4, SD = 26.0; $p = 0.011$) or left CPD (mean = 24.7,

SD = 13.1; p = 0.053) (Kruskal–Wallis test, H = 6.70, p = 0.035), but this relationship was not observed using ANCOVA with medication dose and duration as covariates (F (2, 34) = 0.66, p = 0.526).

Onset age, illness duration, and medication were not related to the HG pattern in the schizophrenia group as a whole (H < 4.81, p > 0.090). However, based on subgroup analyses, patients with left CPD received a lower medication dose (mean = 4.9 mg/day, SD = 3.1) than those with single HG (mean = 15.1 mg/day, SD = 10.0; p = 0.005) or CSD (mean = 11.4 mg/day, SD = 10.1; p = 0.064) only in the chronic subgroup (Kruskal–Wallis test, H = 8.31, p = 0.016).

No relationship was observed between the HG pattern and symptom severity in the schizotypal group (F (2, 40) < 1.46, p > 0.244). However, the right HG pattern significantly affected the medication dose (H = 5.71, p = 0.017). Schizotypal patients with the single HG pattern (mean = 8.4 mg/day, SD = 8.3) were characterized by a higher medication dose than in those with the CSD (mean = 3.6 mg/day, SD = 4.1) or CPD (mean = 3.4 mg/day, SD = 4.0) pattern.

4. Discussion

The present study of HG gyrification patterns in the schizophrenia spectrum demonstrated that the prevalence of HG duplication was higher in schizophrenia patients regardless of the illness stage and that schizotypal disorder patients share a similar HG gyrification pattern. Furthermore, the HG pattern was associated with the severity of psychotic symptoms in schizophrenia patients and with the necessity for a high dose of antipsychotics in both patient groups. The present study supports the gross morphology of the HG reflecting a neurobiological basis for vulnerability factors commonly observed in the schizophrenia spectrum.

As predicted, HG duplication (CSD or CPD) was more prevalent in schizophrenia patients in both the first-episode and chronic stages, and was not related to illness duration. However, previous longitudinal MRI studies demonstrated active gray matter atrophy in the superior temporal region, particularly during the early illness stages of schizophrenia [36,37]. These previous and present studies support the altered sulcogyral pattern in schizophrenia being a stable trait marker associated with neurodevelopmental anomalies [38,39], and the altered HG pattern and atrophy of superior temporal structures having independent mechanisms [14]. Although Hubl et al. [15] reported that the prevalence of duplicated HG was only slightly higher in hallucinating schizophrenia patients than in healthy controls, this negative result may be partly attributed to the small sample size (13 patients and 13 controls) and their anatomical definition that treated the CSD pattern as a variant of single HG. As we demonstrated that HG duplication was more prevalent in schizophrenia regardless of its subtype (CSD or CPD), the schizophrenia cohort by Hubl et al. [15] must have had a higher prevalence of HG duplication according to the traditional HG classification (single vs. duplicated (CSD or CPD)).

One of the main results of the present study was that schizotypal patients considered to share vulnerability-associated biological characteristics with schizophrenia [20] exhibited an altered HG pattern similar to that in patients with schizophrenia. The HG gyrification pattern is thought to reflect neurodevelopmental processes during gestation [7]. Thus, the present results are consistent with previous studies demonstrating shared alterations in neurodevelopmental markers, such as malformation of the adhesio interthalamica [40,41] and widespread cortical hypergyria [23], in schizophrenia spectrum disorders. Conversely, an altered orbitofrontal sulcogyral pattern was specific to schizophrenia and not observed in schizotypal patients [42]. This may support the emergence of overt/sustained psychosis being mitigated by a less deviant frontal neurodevelopmental change in the milder form of schizophrenia spectrum disorders, which may explain the less severe prefrontal atrophy [33,43] and frontal–striatal–temporal dysconnectivity [44] in schizotypal patients than in schizophrenia patients. Collectively, these findings and the present study support the hypothesis that temporal changes underlie vulnerability to schizophrenia, whereas latent dysfunction becomes clinically apparent as the emergence of psychotic symptoms due to additional frontal pathology [45].

The present study replicated the findings of our first-episode schizophrenia study [14] in an expanded schizophrenia group with differing illness stages in that a relationship was observed between the CPD pattern and less susceptibility to psychotic symptoms. Furthermore, our study suggested that the single HG pattern in schizophrenia is associated with poor treatment response (i.e., prolonged positive psychotic symptoms and need for higher doses of antipsychotics) at chronic stages. We also suggested that schizotypal patients with the single HG pattern need higher doses of antipsychotics than those with other HG patterns to control their severe symptoms (e.g., distress and/or transient quasipsychotic symptoms). As the brain gyrification pattern may reflect underlying neural connectivity [21], our study is partly consistent with functional neuroimaging studies in which schizophrenia [26] and schizotypal [27] patients both exhibited abnormal connectivity involving the superior temporal plane, which may underlie the vulnerability to psychopathology [24,25,46]. However, the functional role of the HG gyrification pattern remains controversial; duplicated HG is associated with reduced HG activity during word-listening tasks [8] and learning disabilities [4,47], whereas individuals with HG duplications exhibited advanced auditory skills with an expanded activation area [48,49]. Therefore, further studies are needed to elucidate the functional significance of gross HG gyrification patterns under both normal and pathological conditions.

Several limitations need to be addressed. First, it was not possible to reliably assess group differences in the prevalence of HG multiplications (i.e., ≥3 gyri or CSD with independent second HG) because only 14/246 (5.7%) subjects (eight schizophrenia, three schizotypal, and three control subjects) had these patterns. As HG multiplications function in advanced auditory processing [48,49], further studies are needed using a larger cohort to establish whether this rare HG pattern is associated with the pathophysiology of schizophrenia spectrum disorders. Regarding the sample issue, the smaller sample size of healthy controls ($N = 88$) compared with schizophrenia ($N = 111$) and their high education level may have biased our findings. The lower prevalence of the single HG pattern in our control subjects (left, 56.8%; right, 43.2%) than in previous post mortem or MRI studies (up to 75%) [3] may be partly due to these sampling problems. Multiplicity of statistical analyses should be also noted. Second, as described above, the functional significance of HG gyrification patterns was not directly demonstrated in the present morphological MRI study. Moreover, cognitive functioning was not systematically evaluated in schizophrenia spectrum patients. The HG corresponds to the primary auditory cortex, but also plays a role in the processing of other cognitive domains, including memory and emotion [50,51]. Therefore, future multimodal neuroimaging studies are needed to investigate the function/connectivity of the brain in different HG patterns and its role, particularly in cognitive functioning, in the schizophrenia spectrum. Lastly, atypical sulcogyral patterns in other brain regions (e.g., the orbitofrontal cortex) have also been demonstrated in neuropsychiatric disorders, such as bipolar [52] and autism spectrum [53] disorders, suggesting that the sulcogyral phenotype represents a transdiagnostic trait marker. Therefore, the disease specificity of the present results on HG gyrification patterns warrants further study.

5. Conclusions

This MRI study demonstrated that the prevalence of HG duplications bilaterally was significantly higher in schizotypal patients than in healthy controls. This was similarly observed in patients with overt schizophrenia. In contrast to active gray matter changes in the superior temporal plane during the early stages of schizophrenia [12], the HG gyrification pattern was independent of the illness stage of schizophrenia, but it was partly associated with susceptibility to psychotic symptoms in schizophrenia spectrum disorders. Therefore, the HG gyrification pattern may be a trait marker commonly observed in schizophrenia spectrum disorders, which represents vulnerability to psychopathology due to early neurodevelopmental abnormalities. The present cross-sectional study should be interpreted with caution due to the limitations described above, in addition to the hypothesis that brain gyrification can change over time during the course of schizophrenia [54]. However, our study supports the notion that gross brain morphologic features (e.g., cortical folding) can aid in the classification of neuropsychiatric diseases (e.g., diagnosis and prediction of treatment response) in combination with multimodal neuroimaging data [16]. Furthermore, as clinical high-risk individuals with later psychosis onset may be characterized by more prominent gross brain characteristics [16], the HG pattern in a high-risk cohort in future studies should be assessed to test its possible role as a predictive marker of psychosis, which may lead to the development of specific and targeted preventive strategies [55].

Author Contributions: Conceptualization, M.S. and T.T.; methodology, T.T.; validation, D.S.; formal analysis, T.T.; investigation, T.T., D.S., and T.V.P.; resources, D.S., Y.T., M.K., and H.K.; data curation, A.F.; writing—original draft preparation, T.T.; writing—review and editing, Y.T. and M.S.; supervision, K.N.; project administration, M.S. and K.N.; funding acquisition, T.T., D.S., and M.S. All authors have read and agreed to the published version of the manuscript.

Funding: This study was supported by JSPS KAKENHI Grant Numbers JP18K07550 to T.T., JP18K15509 to D.S., and JP20H03598 to M.S., and by the Health and Labour Sciences Research Grants for Comprehensive Research on Persons with Disabilities from the Japan Agency for Medical Research and Development (AMED) Grant Number JP19dk0307029 to M.S. The APC was funded by JSPS KAKENHI Grant Number JP18K07550.

Institutional Review Board Statement: The study was conducted in accordance with the Declaration of Helsinki. The Committee on Medical Ethics of Toyama University approved the present study (No. I2013006) on 5 February 2014.

Informed Consent Statement: Informed consent was obtained from all subjects involved in the study.

Data Availability Statement: The data presented in this study are available on request from the corresponding author. The data are not publicly available since we do not have permission to share the data.

Acknowledgments: We would like to thank the radiology technologists, particularly Koichi Mori, who assisted in MRI data collection at Toyama University Hospital.

Conflicts of Interest: The authors declare no conflict of interest. The funders had no role in the design of the study; in the collection, analyses, or interpretation of data; in the writing of the manuscript, or in the decision to publish the results.

References

1. Da Costa, S.; van der Zwaag, W.; Marques, J.P.; Frackowiak, R.S.; Clarke, S.; Saenz, M. Human primary auditory cortex follows the shape of Heschl's gyrus. *J. Neurosci.* **2011**, *31*, 14067–14075. [CrossRef]
2. Rademacher, J.; Morosan, P.; Schormann, T.; A Schleicher, A.; Werner, C.; Freund, H.J.; Zilles, K. Probabilistic mapping and volume measurement of human primary auditory cortex. *Neuroimage* **2001**, *13*, 669–683. [CrossRef] [PubMed]
3. Abdul-Kareem, I.A.; Sluming, V. Heschl gyrus and its included primary auditory cortex: Structural MRI studies in healthy and diseased subjects. *J. Magn. Reson. Imaging* **2008**, *28*, 287–299. [CrossRef] [PubMed]
4. Leonard, C.M.; Puranik, C.; Kuldau, J.M.; Lombardino, L.J. Normal variation in the frequency and location of human auditory cortex landmarks. Heschl's gyrus: Where is it? *Cereb. Cortex* **1998**, *8*, 397–406. [CrossRef] [PubMed]
5. Marie, D.; Jobard, G.; Crivello, F.; Perchey, G.; Petit, L.; Mellet, E.; Joliot, M.; Zago, L.; Mazoyer, B.; Tzourio-Mazoyer, N. Descriptive anatomy of Heschl's gyri in 430 healthy volunteers, including 198 left-handers. *Brain Struct. Funct.* **2015**, *220*, 729–743. [CrossRef] [PubMed]
6. Armstrong, E.; Schleicher, A.; Omran, H.; Curtis, M.; Zilles, K. The ontogeny of human gyrification. *Cereb. Cortex* **1995**, *5*, 56–63. [CrossRef]
7. Chi, J.G.; Dooling, E.C.; Gilles, F.H. Gyral development of the human brain. *Ann. Neurol.* **1977**, *1*, 86–93. [CrossRef]
8. Tzourio-Mazoyer, N.; Marie, D.; Zago, L.; Jobard, G.; Perchey, G.; Leroux, G.; Mellet, E.; Joliot, M.; Crivello, F.; Petit, L.; et al. Heschl's gyrification pattern is related to speech-listening hemispheric lateralization: FMRI investigation in 281 healthy volunteers. *Brain Struct. Funct.* **2015**, *220*, 1585–1599. [CrossRef]
9. Insel, T.R. Rethinking schizophrenia. *Nature* **2010**, *468*, 187–193. [CrossRef]
10. Weinberger, D.R. Implications of normal brain development for the pathogenesis of schizophrenia. *Arch. Gen. Psychiatry* **1987**, *44*, 660–669. [CrossRef]

11. Mwansisya, T.E.; Hu, A.; Li, Y.; Chen, X.; Wu, G.; Huang, X.; Lv, D.; Li, Z.; Liu, C.; Xue, Z.; et al. Task and resting-state fMRI studies in first-episode schizophrenia: A systematic review. *Schizophr. Res.* **2017**, *189*, 9–18. [CrossRef] [PubMed]
12. Guo, Q.; Tang, Y.; Li, H.; Zhang, T.; Li, J.; Sheng, J.; Liu, D.; Li, C.; Wang, J. Both volumetry and functional connectivity of Heschl's gyrus are associated with auditory P300 in first episode schizophrenia. *Schizophr. Res.* **2014**, *160*, 57–66. [CrossRef] [PubMed]
13. Chen, X.; Liang, S.; Pu, W.; Song, Y.; Mwansisya, T.E.; Yang, Q.; Liu, H.; Shan, B.; Xue, Z. Reduced cortical thickness in right Heschl's gyrus associated with auditory verbal hallucinations severity in first-episode schizophrenia. *BMC Psychiatry* **2015**, *15*, 152. [CrossRef] [PubMed]
14. Takahashi, T.; Sasabayashi, D.; Takayanagi, Y.; Furuichi, A.; Kido, M.; Nakamura, M.; Pham, T.V.; Kobayashi, H.; Noguchi, K.; Suzuki, M. Altered Heschl's gyrus duplication pattern in first-episode schizophrenia. *Schizophr Res.* **2021**. under review.
15. Hubl, D.; Dougoud-Chauvin, V.; Zeller, M.; Federspiel, A.; Boesch, C.; Strik, W.; Dierks, T.; Koenig, T. Structural analysis of Heschl's gyrus in schizophrenia patients with auditory hallucinations. *Neuropsychobiology* **2010**, *61*, 1–9. [CrossRef] [PubMed]
16. Takahashi, T.; Suzuki, M. Brain morphologic changes in early stages of psychosis: Implications for clinical application and early intervention. *Psychiatry Clin. Neurosci.* **2018**, *72*, 556–571. [CrossRef] [PubMed]
17. World Health Organization. *The ICD-10 Classification of Mental and Behavioural Disorders: Clinical Descriptions and Diagnostic Guidelines*; World Health Organization: Geneva, Switzerland, 1992.
18. American Psychiatric Association. *Diagnostic and Statistical Manual of Mental Disorders*, 4th ed.; American Psychiatric Association Press: Washington, DC, USA, 1994.
19. Siever, L.J.; Kalus, O.F.; Keefe, R.S.E. The boundaries of schizophrenia. *Psychiatr. Clin. N. Am.* **1993**, *16*, 217–244. [CrossRef]
20. Siever, L.J.; Davis, K.L. The pathophysiology of schizophrenia disorders: Perspective from the spectrum. *Am. J. Psychiatry* **2004**, *161*, 398–413. [CrossRef]
21. Zilles, K.; Palomero-Gallagher, N.; Amunts, K. Development of cortical folding during evolution and ontogeny. *Trends Neurosci.* **2013**, *36*, 275–284. [CrossRef]
22. Sasabayashi, D.; Takayanagi, Y.; Nishiyama, S.; Takahashi, T.; Furuichi, A.; Kido, M.; Nishikawa, Y.; Nakamura, M.; Noguchi, K.; Suzuki, M. Increased frontal gyrification negatively correlates with executive function in patients with first-episode schizophrenia. *Cereb. Cortex* **2017**, *27*, 2686–2694. [CrossRef]
23. Sasabayashi, D.; Takayanagi, Y.; Takahashi, T.; Nemoto, K.; Furuichi, A.; Kido, M.; Nishikawa, Y.; Nakamura, M.; Noguchi, K.; Suzuki, M. Increased brain gyrification in the schizophrenia spectrum. *Psychiatry Clin. Neurosci.* **2020**, *74*, 70–76. [CrossRef] [PubMed]
24. Oertel-Knöchel, V.; Knöchel, C.; Matura, S.; Stäblein, M.; Prvulovic, D.; Maurer, K.; Linden, D.E.; van de Ven, V. Association between symptoms of psychosis and reduced functional connectivity of auditory cortex. *Schizophr. Res.* **2014**, *160*, 35–42. [CrossRef] [PubMed]
25. Shinn, A.K.; Baker, J.T.; Cohen, B.M.; Öngür, D. Functional connectivity of left Heschl's gyrus in vulnerability to auditory hallucinations in schizophrenia. *Schizophr. Res.* **2013**, *143*, 260–268. [CrossRef] [PubMed]
26. Li, S.; Hu, N.; Zhang, W.; Tao, B.; Dai, J.; Gong, Y.; Tan, Y.; Cai, D.; Lui, S. Dysconnectivity of multiple brain networks in schizophrenia: A meta-analysis of resting-state functional connectivity. *Front. Psychiatry* **2019**, *10*, 482. [CrossRef] [PubMed]
27. Zhang, Q.; Shen, J.; Wu, J.; Yu, X.; Lou, W.; Fan, H.; Shi, L.; Wang, D. Altered default mode network functional connectivity in schizotypal personality disorder. *Schizophr. Res.* **2014**, *160*, 51–56. [CrossRef]
28. World Health Organization. *The ICD-10 Classification of Mental and Behavioural Disorders: Diagnostic Criteria for Research*; World Health Organization: Geneva, Switzerland, 1993.
29. Andreasen, N.C.; Okazaki, Y.; Kitamura, T.; Anzai, N.; Shima, S.; Ohta, T. *The Comprehensive Assessment of Symptoms and History (CASH): An Instrument for Assessing Diagnosis and Psychopathology*; Seiwa Shoten Publishers: Tokyo, Japan, 1995. (In Japanese)
30. Andreasen, N.C.; Okazaki, Y.; Anzai, N.; Ohta, T.; Shima, S.; Kitamura, T. The Japanese version of Scale for the Assessment of Negative Symptoms (SANS). *Jpn. J. Clin. Psychiatry* **1984**, *13*, 999–1010. (In Japanese)
31. Andreasen, N.C.; Okazaki, Y.; Kitamura, T.; Anzai, N.; Ohta, T.; Shima, S.; McDonald-Scott, P. Scale for the Assessment of Positive Symptoms (SAPS). *Arch. Psychiatr. Diag. Clin. Eval.* **1992**, *3*, 365–377. (In Japanese)
32. Kawasaki, Y.; Suzuki, M.; Nohara, S.; Hagino, H.; Matsui, M.; Yamashita, I.; Takahashi, T.; Chitnis, X.; McGuire, P.K.; Seto, H.; et al. Structural brain differences in patients with schizotypal disorder and schizophrenia demonstrated by voxel-based morphometry. *Eur. Arch. Psychiatry Clin. Neurosci.* **2004**, *254*, 406–414. [CrossRef]
33. Suzuki, M.; Zhou, S.-Y.; Takahashi, T.; Hagino, H.; Kawasaki, Y.; Niu, L.; Matsui, M.; Seto, H.; Kurachi, M. Differential contributions of prefrontal and temporolimbic pathology to mechanisms of psychosis. *Brain* **2005**, *128*, 2109–2122. [CrossRef]
34. Nordentoft, M.; Thorup, A.; Petersen, L.; Øhlenschlæger, J.; Melau, M.; Christensen, T.Ø.; Krarup, G. Transition rates from schizotypal disorder to psychotic disorder for first-contact patients included in the OPUS trial. A randomized clinical trial of integrated treatment and standard treatment. *Schizophr. Res.* **2006**, *83*, 29–40. [CrossRef]
35. Takahashi, T.; Suzuki, M.; Tsunoda, M.; Kawamura, Y.; Takahashi, N.; Maeno, N.; Kawasaki, Y.; Zhou, S.Y.; Hagino, H.; Niu, L.; et al. The association of genotypic combination of the DRD3 and BDNF polymorphisms on the adhesio interthalamica and medial temporal lobe structures. *Prog. Neuropsychopharmacol. Biol. Psychiatry* **2008**, *32*, 1236–1342. [CrossRef] [PubMed]
36. Takahashi, T.; Wood, S.J.; Yung, A.R.; Soulsby, B.; McGorry, P.D.; Suzuki, M.; Kawasaki, Y.; Phillips, L.J.; Velakoulis, D.; Pantelis, C. Progressive gray matter reduction of the superior temporal gyrus during transition to psychosis. *Arch. Gen. Psychiatry* **2009**, *66*, 366–376. [CrossRef] [PubMed]

37. Takahashi, T.; Suzuki, M.; Zhou, S.Y.; Tanino, R.; Nakamura, K.; Kawasaki, Y.; Seto, H.; Kurachi, M. A follow-up MRI study of the superior temporal subregions in schizotypal disorder and first-episode schizophrenia. *Schizophr. Res.* **2010**, *119*, 65–74. [CrossRef] [PubMed]
38. Nakamura, M.; Takahashi, T.; Takayanagi, Y.; Sasabayashi, D.; Katagiri, N.; Sakuma, A.; Obara, C.; Koike, S.; Yamasue, H.; Furuichi, A.; et al. Surface morphology of the orbitofrontal cortex in individuals at risk of psychosis. *Eur. Arch. Psychiatry Clin. Neurosci.* **2019**, *269*, 397–406. [CrossRef] [PubMed]
39. Sasabayashi, D.; Takayanagi, Y.; Takahashi, T.; Koike, S.; Yamasue, H.; Katagiri, N.; Sakuma, A.; Obara, C.; Nakamura, M.; Furuichi, A.; et al. Increased occipital gyrification and development of psychotic disorders in individuals with an at-risk mental state: A multicenter study. *Biol. Psychiatry* **2017**, *82*, 737–745. [CrossRef] [PubMed]
40. Takahashi, T.; Suzuki, M.; Zhou, S.Y.; Nakamura, K.; Tanino, R.; Kawasaki, Y.; Seal, M.L.; Seto, H.; Kurachi, M. Prevalence and length of the adhesio interthalamica in schizophrenia spectrum disorders. *Psychiatry Res.* **2008**, *164*, 90–94. [CrossRef] [PubMed]
41. Trzesniak, C.; Kempton, M.J.; Busatto, G.F.; de Oliveira, I.R.; Galvão-de Almeida, A.; Kambeitz, J.; Ferrari, M.C.; Filho, A.S.; Chagas, M.H.; Zuardi, A.W.; et al. Adhesio interthalamica alterations in schizophrenia spectrum disorders: A systematic review and meta-analysis. *Prog. Neuropsychopharmacol. Biol. Psychiatry* **2011**, *35*, 877–886. [CrossRef]
42. Nishikawa, Y.; Takahashi, T.; Takayanagi, Y.; Furuichi, A.; Kido, M.; Nakamura, M.; Sasabayashi, D.; Noguchi, K.; Suzuki, M. Orbitofrontal sulcogyral pattern and olfactory sulcus depth in the schizophrenia spectrum. *Eur. Arch. Psychiatry Clin. Neurosci.* **2016**, *266*, 15–23. [CrossRef]
43. Fervaha, G.; Remington, G. Neuroimaging findings in schizotypal personality disorder: A systematic review. *Prog. Neuropsychopharmacol. Biol. Psychiatry* **2013**, *43*, 96–107. [CrossRef]
44. Lener, M.S.; Wong, E.; Tang, C.Y.; Byne, W.; Goldstein, K.E.; Blair, N.J.; Haznedar, M.M.; New, A.S.; Chemerinski, E.; Chu, K.W.; et al. White matter abnormalities in schizophrenia and schizotypal personality disorder. *Schizophr. Bull.* **2015**, *41*, 300–310. [CrossRef]
45. Kurachi, M. Pathogenesis of schizophrenia: Part II. Temporo-frontal two-step hypothesis. *Psychiatry Clin. Neurosci.* **2003**, *57*, 9–15. [CrossRef] [PubMed]
46. Gavrilescu, M.; Rossell, S.; Stuart, G.W.; Shea, T.L.; Innes-Brown, H.; Henshall, K.; McKay, C.; Sergejew, A.A.; Copolov, D.; Egan, G.F. Reduced connectivity of the auditory cortex in patients with auditory hallucinations: A resting state functional magnetic resonance imaging study. *Psychol. Med.* **2010**, *40*, 1149–1158. [CrossRef] [PubMed]
47. Leonard, C.M.; Eckert, M.A.; Lombardino, L.J.; Oakland, T.; Kranzler, J.; Mohr, C.M.; King, W.M.; Freeman, A. Anatomical risk factors for phonological dyslexia. *Cereb. Cortex* **2001**, *11*, 148–157. [CrossRef] [PubMed]
48. Benner, J.; Wengenroth, M.; Reinhardt, J.; Stippich, C.; Schneider, P.; Blatow, M. Prevalence and function of Heschl's gyrus morphotypes in musicians. *Brain Struct. Funct.* **2017**, *222*, 3587–3603. [CrossRef] [PubMed]
49. Golestani, N.; Price, C.J.; Scott, S.K. Born with an ear for dialects? Structural plasticity in the expert phonetician brain. *J. Neurosci.* **2011**, *31*, 4213–4220. [CrossRef] [PubMed]
50. Concina, G.; Renna, A.; Grosso, A.; Sacchetti, B. The auditory cortex and the emotional valence of sounds. *Neurosci. Biobehav. Rev.* **2019**, *98*, 256–264. [CrossRef] [PubMed]
51. Weinberger, N.M. New perspectives on the auditory cortex: Learning and memory. *Handb. Clin. Neurol.* **2015**, *129*, 117–147. [CrossRef]
52. Patti, M.A.; Troiani, V. Orbitofrontal sulcogyral morphology is a transdiagnostic indicator of brain dysfunction. *Neuroimage Clin.* **2018**, *17*, 910–917. [CrossRef]
53. Watanabe, H.; Nakamura, M.; Ohno, T.; Itahashi, T.; Tanaka, E.; Ohta, H.; Yamada, T.; Kanai, C.; Iwanami, A.; Kato, N.; et al. Altered orbitofrontal sulcogyral patterns in adult males with high-functioning autism spectrum disorders. *Soc. Cogn. Affect. Neurosci.* **2014**, *9*, 520–528. [CrossRef]
54. Sasabayashi, D.; Takahashi, T.; Takayanagi, Y.; Suzuki, M. Anomalous brain gyrification patterns in major psychiatric disorders: A systematic review and trans-diagnostic integration. *Trans. Psychiatry* **2021**. under review.
55. McGorry, P.D.; Hickie, I.B.; Yung, A.R.; Pantelis, C.; Jackson, H.J. Clinical staging of psychiatric disorders: A heuristic framework for choosing earlier, safer and more effective interventions. *Aust. N. Z. J. Psychiatry* **2006**, *40*, 616–622. [CrossRef] [PubMed]

Article

Prolonged P300 Latency in Antipsychotic-Free Subjects with At-Risk Mental States Who Later Developed Schizophrenia

Yuko Higuchi [1,2,3,*], Tomiki Sumiyoshi [3], Takahiro Tateno [1,2], Suguru Nakajima [1,2], Daiki Sasabayashi [1,2], Shimako Nishiyama [1,4], Yuko Mizukami [1], Tsutomu Takahashi [1,2,3] and Michio Suzuki [1,2,3]

[1] Department of Neuropsychiatry, Graduate School of Medicine and Pharmaceutical Sciences, University of Toyama, Toyama 930-0194, Japan; tdtpodim@med.u-toyama.ac.jp (T.T.); snaka@med.u-toyama.ac.jp (S.N.); ds179@med.u-toyama.ac.jp (D.S.); nishiyas@ctg.u-toyama.ac.jp (S.N.); yk1022@med.u-toyama.ac.jp (Y.M.); tsutomu@med.u-toyama.ac.jp (T.T.); suzukim@med.u-toyama.ac.jp (M.S.)
[2] Research Center for Idling Brain Science, University of Toyama, Toyama 930-0194, Japan
[3] National Center of Neurology and Psychiatry, Department of Preventive Intervention for Psychiatric Disorders, National Institute of Mental Health, Tokyo 187-8551, Japan; sumiyot@ncnp.go.jp
[4] Center for Health Care and Human Sciences, University of Toyama, Toyama 930-8555, Japan
* Correspondence: yhiguchi@med.u-toyama.ac.jp; Tel.: +81-76-434-7323

Abstract: We measured P300, an event-related potential, in subjects with at-risk mental states (ARMS) and aimed to determine whether P300 parameter can predict progression to overt schizophrenia. Thirty-three subjects with ARMS, 39 with schizophrenia, and 28 healthy controls participated in the study. All subjects were antipsychotic-free. Subjects with ARMS were followed-up for more than two years. Cognitive function was measured by the Brief assessment of Cognition in Schizophrenia (BACS) and Schizophrenia Cognition Rating Scale (SCoRS), while the modified Global Assessment of Functioning (mGAF) was used to assess global function. Patients with schizophrenia showed smaller P300 amplitudes and prolonged latency at Pz compared to those of healthy controls and subjects with ARMS. During the follow-up period, eight out of 33 subjects with ARMS developed overt psychosis (ARMS-P) while 25 did not (ARMS-NP). P300 latency of ARMS-P was significantly longer than that of ARMS-NP. At baseline, ARMS-P elicited worse cognitive functions, as measured by the BACS and SCoRS compared to ARMS-NP. We also detected a significant relationship between P300 amplitudes and mGAF scores in ARMS subjects. Our results suggest the usefulness of prolonged P300 latency and cognitive impairment as a predictive marker of later development of schizophrenia in vulnerable individuals.

Keywords: P300; event-related potentials; clinical high-risk; psychosis; at risk mental state; schizophrenia; cognition; latency

1. Introduction

Patients with schizophrenia suffer from impairments of several types of cognitive functions which are considered to affect quality of life (QOL) and social functions [1]. Therefore, early detection and intervention into cognitive disturbances of schizophrenia are needed to achieve a satisfactory outcome for patients. For the same reason, the importance of intervention into the prodromal stage of schizophrenia and other psychotic disorders has also been recognized [2–4]. For this purpose, operational criteria to detect putative prodromal symptoms of psychosis have been used worldwide [5], and are designated as ultra-high risk, clinical high risk, or at-risk mental state (ARMS). These criteria allow for the identification of subjects with ~30% risk of developing psychosis over a two-year period [6], mostly schizophrenia-spectrum disorders [7]. For better prediction, the use of objective biomarkers, such as those based on brain morphology, neurophysiology, and neuropsychology, has been proposed [8–12]. For example, event-related potentials (ERPs), such as duration mismatch negativity (MMN) and P300, have been reported to provide sensitive and feasible electrophysiological tools [13,14]. These measures of ERPs have also been suggested to provide biological substrates for some aspects of cognitive disturbances in patients with schizophrenia and ARMS subjects [9,15,16].

P300 was discovered in 1960s and has been shown to reflect a putative electrophysiological basis of cognitive functions, such as attention-dependent information processing and immediate memory [17–19], which are impaired in schizophrenia [20,21]. Specifically, patients with schizophrenia have been reported to elicit smaller amplitudes and pro-longed latencies of P300 compared to those in healthy control subjects [22–24]. In fact, a recent meta-analysis reported that the effect sizes of amplitude reduction and latency prolongation are as large as 0.83 and 0.48, respectively [25]. As in the case for schizophrenia, abnormalities in P300 have been reported in other neuropsychiatric disorders, such as mood disorders (e.g., bipolar disorder and major depression), developmental disorders (e.g., attention deficit hyperactivity disorder), and Parkinson's disease [26–31]. Therefore, P300 may be considered to provide a biomarker of schizophrenia, especially in patients in whom these diseases are excluded.

Potential P300 abnormalities have also been examined in subjects with ARMS [32–38]. To our knowledge, five studies to date have attempted to determine whether P300 parameters (e.g., amplitude and latency) at baseline can predict later onset of overt psychosis [33–37]. Two studies [34,36], but not others [33,35,37] reported differences in amplitude between ARMS subjects who later developed psychosis (ARMS-P) and those who did not (ARMS-NP). On the other hand, these previous ARMS studies did not find associations between baseline P300 latency and later psychosis onset [33,35,37]. These negative results may contradict the concept that prolonged P300 latency would reflect trait abnormality of schizophrenia irrespective of illness stages, including the prodromal stage [25]. The reasons for these inconsistent findings in ARMS remain unclear but may include the difference in clinical profiles of participants, e.g., medication status that has been reported to alter P300 parameters [9,39,40]. Thus, further investigations to examine the potential ability of P300 latency to predict later onset of psychosis in high-risk subjects would be desired.

In this study, we reported P300 amplitudes and latencies in subjects with antipsychotics-free ARMS or schizophrenia in comparison with healthy control subjects. On the basis of P300 abnormalities as a trait marker of schizophrenia [25], we hypothesized that baseline P300 latency in ARMS subjects would predict onset of psychosis. We also explored whether abnormal P300 parameters would be associated with cognitive and functional deficits in these subjects.

2. Materials and Methods

2.1. Participants

Thirty-three ARMS subjects (male/female, 23/10; mean age 19.2 ± 4.6 years), recruited from University of Toyama Hospital or Toyama Prefectural Mental Health Centre [41], as well as 39 schizophrenia patients (male/female, 16/23; mean age 24.4 ± 7.2 years) participated in this study. Diagnosis was made by experienced psychiatrists based on ICD-10 for schizophrenia and the Comprehensive Assessment of At-Risk Mental State (CAARMS) for ARMS [42]. We also recruited 28 healthy volunteers (male/female, 16/12; mean age 21.7 ± 5.0 years) from our community. All subjects were physically healthy and had well hearing ability. A psychiatric and treatment history was collected from the subjects themselves, their families, and medical records. Exclusion criteria included the following: subjects with a history of substance abuse or dependence, seizure, and head injury. Eligible patients were confirmed to be physically healthy by physical examinations and standard laboratory tests. Healthy volunteers and their first-degree relatives did not have any psychiatric disorders. Subjects with an estimated premorbid IQ less than 70 were also excluded.

For the clinical assessments, experienced psychiatrists administered the Positive and Negative Syndrome Scale (PANSS) [43]. The Japanese adult reading test (JART) [44] was performed to estimate premorbid IQ. The Brief Assessment of Cognition in Schizophrenia

(BACS) [45,46], Schizophrenia Cognition Rating Scale (SCoRS) [47–49] and modified Global Assessment of Functioning (mGAF) [50] were used to evaluate cognitive and social functions. BACS was standardized by z-scores, with the mean score of Japanese healthy controls set to zero and the standard deviation set to one [51]. Furthermore, the BACS composite score was calculated by averaging the z-scores of the six primary BACS measurements [45]. The demographic data at baseline evaluation for healthy control, ARMS and schizophrenia is shown in Table 1.

Table 1. Demographic data, cognitive functions and P300 parameters

	H	ARMS	Sch	Effect Size	Group Comparison
	(n = 28)	(n = 33)	(n = 39)		
Male/female	16/12	23/10	16/23	-	$\chi^2 = 6.00, p = 0.05$, n.s.
Age (years)	21.7 (5.0)	19.2 (4.6)	24.4 (7.2)	-	$F(2,97) = 7.93, p = 0.001$ **, ARMS < Sch
Age of onset (years)	-	-	24.4 (6.6)	-	-
Duration of illness (years)	-	-	2.7 (3.0)	-	-
JART [a]	102.5 (7.4)	96.9 (10.0)	99.3 (11.1)	-	$F(2,85) = 1.91, p = 0.15$, n.s.
PANSS: positive symptom	-	13.1 (3.7)	16.7 (5.8)	-	$p = 0.003$ **, ARMS < Sch
negative symptom	-	19.5 (7.2)	19.1 (7.4)	-	$p = 0.81$, n.s.
general psychopathology	-	34.9 (8.9)	36.5 (9.1)	-	$p = 0.45$, n.s.
mGAF	-	46.5 (9.1)	34.1 (8.6)	-	$p < 0.001$ **, ARMS > Sch
SCoRS	-	4.7 (2.2)	5.8 (2.3)	-	$p = 0.069$, n.s.
BACS [a,b]: verbal memory	−0.16 (1.1)	−0.54 (1.4)	−1.46 (1.6)	0.12	$F(2,86) = 5.81, p = 0.004$ **, H, ARMS > Sch
working memory	0.10 (0.8)	−0.9 (1.3)	−1.32 (1.3)	0.15	$F(2,86) = 7.99, p = 0.001$ **, H > ARMS, Sch
motor function	−0.15 (1.0)	−1.31 (1.7)	−2.04 (1.5)	0.18	$F(2,86) = 9.45, p < 0.001$ **, H > ARMS, Sch
verbal fluency	0.096 (1.0)	−0.96 (1.2)	−1.44 (1.3)	0.19	$F(2,86) = 9.84, p < 0.001$ **, H > ARMS, Sch
attention	0.70 (0.8)	−0.22 (1.5)	−1.60 (1.3)	0.32	$F(2,86) = 20.97, p < 0.001$ **, H > ARMS > Sch
executive function	0.29 (1.1)	−0.36 (1.3)	−1.47 (1.9)	0.16	$F(2,86) = 8.64, p < 0.001$ **, H, ARMS > Sch
composite score [c]	0.14 (0.5)	−0.72 (1.0)	−1.55 (1.2)	0.28	$F(2,86) = 17.52, p < 0.001$ **, H > ARMS > Sch
P300 Amplitude (μV):T3	9.26 (4.5)	6.12 (3.1)	5.14 (2.6)	0.20	$F(2,97) = 11.76, p < 0.001$ **, H > ARMS, Sch
T4	9.30 (5.5)	6.50 (4.1)	4.04 (3.0)	0.20	$F(2,97) = 12.19, p < 0.001$ **, H > ARMS, Sch
Fz	13.59 (7.2)	8.46 (6.3)	4.80 (4.2)	0.27	$F(2,97) = 17.89, p < 0.001$ **, H > ARMS > Sch
Cz	19.51 (8.6)	13.08 (6.3)	7.07 (3.6)	0.40	$F(2,97) = 32.33, p < 0.001$ **, H > ARMS > Sch
Pz	20.57 (8.9)	15.66 (4.9)	9.4 (3.9)	0.37	$F(2,97) = 28.39 p < 0.001$ **, H > ARMS > Sch
P300 Latency (msec):T3	327.8 (35.9)	325.5 (32.5)	347.1 (52.9)	0.07	$F(2,97) = 2.78, p = 0.067$, n.s.
T4	326.3 (29.5)	320.1 (39.0)	343.4 (52.6)	0.06	$F(2,97) = 2.88, 0.061$, n.s.
Fz	323.6 (30.9)	322.9 (38.6)	343.9 (52.7)	0.05	$F(2,97) = 2.76, p = 0.068$, n.s.
Cz	314.8 (29.1)	315.3 (36.1)	340.5 (52.2)	0.08	$F(2,97) = 4.43, p = 0.014$ *, H, ARMS < Sch
Pz	313.5 (29.5)	314.9 (32.5)	339.0 (45.7)	0.10	$F(2,97) = 5.17, p = 0.007$ **, H, ARMS < Sch

Values represent mean (SD). ARMS; at-risk mental state, H; healthy controls, Sch; schizophrenia. JART; Japanese Adult Reading Test, PANSS; Positive and Negative Syndrome Scale, mGAF; modified Global Assessment Functioning. P300 data represent peak amplitudes (μV) and latencies (msec) for each group [mean (SD)]. All participants were antipsychotic-free at the time of measurement P300. Demographic differences between groups were examined with one-way analysis of variance (ANOVA), Student's t-test or the chi-square test (* $p < 0.05$, ** $p < 0.01$). Effect sizes are represented in η^2. [a] BACS and JART data were missing for some healthy control patients. [b] BACS was standardized by creating z-scores, with the mean score of Japanese healthy controls set to zero and the standard deviation set to one [45]. [c] BACS composite score was calculated by averaging all z-scores of the six primary measures from the BACS [46].

Subjects with ARMS were clinically followed-up at our hospital. When the severity of psychotic symptoms exceeded the criteria of CAARMS, the subject was regarded as ARMS-P. In this study, eight out of the 33 (24.2%) subjects with ARMS developed schizophrenia during the observation period (1.0 ± 1.1 years). Twenty-five subjects who did not develop psychosis were defined as ARMS-NP. The observation period for ARMS-NP was more than two years, with average 3.5 ± 2.3 years. The demographic data at baseline evaluation for ARMS-NP and ARMS-P is shown in Table 2.

No subject was on antipsychotic medications. All ARMS-NP patients (twenty-five), five of eight ARMS-P patients and thirty one out of thirty-nine schizophrenia patients were antipsychotic naïve. Other subjects were antipsychotic free at least 2 weeks.

This protocol was approved by the Committee on Medical Ethics of the University of Toyama. After complete and detail description of the study was provided, written informed consent was obtained from the participants in agreement with the Declaration of Helsinki. If a subject was under 20 years old, written consent was also obtained from a parent or legal guardian.

Table 2. Demographic data, cognitive functions and P300 parameters in clinical high-risk subjects.

	ARMS-NP (n = 25)	ARMS-P (n = 8)	Group Comparison
Male/female	17/8	6/2	$\chi^2 = 0.14, p = 0.70$, n.s.
Age (years)	18.7 (3.8)	20.5 (6.6)	$p = 0.33$, n.s.
JART	98.1 (9.6)	93.3 (11.1)	$p = 0.25$, n.s.
PANSS: positive symptom	12.9 (4.1)	13.8 (2.1)	$p = 0.53$, n.s.
negative symptom	19.6 (8.0)	19.2 (4.3)	$p = 0.85$, n.s.
general psychopathology	34.1 (9.1)	37.2 (8.4)	$p = 0.40$, n.s.
mGAF	48.6 (9.0)	41.7 (7.9)	$p = 0.096$, n.s.
SCoRS	4.1 (1.9)	6.6 (2.0)	$p = 0.004$ **
BACS: verbal memory	−0.36 (1.4)	−1.1 (1.3)	$p = 0.21$, n.s.
working memory	−0.65 (1.1)	−1.70 (1.8)	$p = 0.060$, n.s.
motor function	−1.09 (1.8)	−2.02 (1.4)	$p = 0.20$, n.s.
verbal fluency	−0.78 (1.1)	−1.50 (1.4)	$p = 0.16$, n.s.
attention	0.06 (1.5)	−1.12 (1.4)	$p = 0.063$, n.s.
executive function	−0.17 (0.96)	−0.94 (2.2)	$p = 0.17$, n.s.
composite score	−0.50 (0.94)	−1.40 (1.25)	$p = 0.038$ *
Amplitude (μV):T3	6.06 (3.0)	6.30 (3.8)	$p = 0.85$, n.s.
T4	7.18 (3.9)	4.37 (4.4)	$p = 0.099$, n.s.
Fz	8.94 (6.6)	6.96 (5.7)	$p = 0.45$, n.s.
Cz	14.14 (6.0)	9.79 (6.7)	$p = 0.094$, n.s.
Pz	16.27 (5.2)	13.76 (3.3)	$p = 0.21$, n.s.
Latency (msec):T3	318.9 (30.5)	346.5 (31.8)	$p = 0.039$ *
T4	317.2 (40.0)	329.0 (36.6)	$p = 0.49$, n.s.
Fz	315.9 (35.7)	344.7 (41.3)	$p = 0.65$, n.s.
Cz	306.5 (34.5)	342.7 (27.3)	$p = 0.011$ *
Pz	307.7 (29.3)	337.5 (33.3)	$p = 0.022$ *

Values represent mean (SD). ARMS; at-risk mental state, ARMS-p; ARMS patients later transitioned to overt psychosis, ARMS-NP; ARMS patients who did not transition to overt psychosis, JART; Japanese Adult Reading Test, PANSS; Positive and Negative Syndrome Scale, mGAF; modified Global Assessment Functioning, SCoRS; Schizophrenia Cognitive Rating Scale, BACS; Brief Assessment of Cognition in Schizophrenia. P300 data represent peak amplitudes (μV) and latencies (msec) for each group [mean (SD)]. Demographic differences between groups were examined with Student's t-test or the chi-square test (* $p < 0.05$, ** $p < 0.01$).

2.2. Electroencephalogram (EEG) Recording

ERPs were recorded at the time of clinical assessments using an auditory odd-ball paradigm, based on an established method [9,22,39]. Subjects were directed to lay awake on a bed, open their eyes, and watch a red circle shown on a display monitor. The patients were observed carefully, and if the patients were in poor conditions (asleep, too many eye blinks or eye movements, frequent body movement, unwilling to participate in the examination), we gave instructions again or stopped the recording.

EEGs were recorded with a 32-channel DC-amplifier (EEG-2100 version 2.22J, Nihon Kohden Corp., Tokyo, Japan). Recordings were performed using 19 or 32 channel Electrocap (Electrocap Inc., Eaton, OH) or in a wave-shielded and sound-attenuated room. Auditory stimuli were delivered binaurally through headphones with variable inter-stimulus intervals ranging from 1.5 to 2.5 s. Target tones of 2000 Hz were randomly presented in a series of standard tones of 1000 Hz, with the presentation probability of 0.2 for target tones. Numbers of the standard and target (deviant) tones were 200 and 50, respectively. All tones were 50 ms in duration with a rise–fall time of 10 ms. Subjects were requested to press a button as promptly and accurately as possible in response to infrequent target tones. EEGs were recorded at 19 (located at FP1, FP2, F3, F4, F7, F8, C3, C4, P3, P4, O1, O2, T3, T4, T5, T6, Fz, Cz, and Pz) or 29 (Fp1, Fp2, F3, F4, F7, F8, FC3, FC4, C3, C4, T3, T4, CP3, CP4, TP7, TP8, P3, P4, T5, T6, O1, O2, FPz, Fz, FCz, Cz, CPz, Pz, and Oz) electrodes with average reference. In this paper, only midline (Fz, Cz, and Pz) and temporal lobe (T3, and T4) electrodes were presented according to a previous study [9]. The bandwidth was 0.16–120 Hz with a 60 Hz notch filter. Electrode impedance was less than 10 kΩ. Data were collected with a sampling rate of 500 Hz. Averaging of ERP waves and related procedures were performed using EPLYZER II software (Kissei Comtec, Co. Ltd. Nagano, Japan). The epoch was 700 ms, including a 100 ms pre-stimulus baseline. EEG responses with target tones were averaged off-line. We averaged all pre-stimulus amplitudes (from -100 to 0 ms) and defined it as zero-point. The peak of P300 was observed 250–400 ms after the target sound started. We defined it as time-window, and a positive maximum peak was detected within this time window by EPLYZAR II software. P300 amplitude was defined as the difference between the zero-point and peak, and its latency was defined as the interval from 0 ms to the timing of the peak. Before averaging ERPs, we manually checked the raw waveforms with care and removed all epochs without a typical P300 shape due to eye movement or blinking, facial muscle movement, sweating, or basic rhythms.

2.3. Statistical Methods

We used Statistical Package for Social Sciences (SPSS) version 25 (SPSS Japan Inc., Tokyo, Japan) for statistical analyses. Groups were compared for demographic and clinical data using a one-way analysis of variance (ANOVA) or Chi-square test. We used analysis of covariance (ANCOVA) with group as a between-subject variable and age as a covariate to evaluate group differences in P300 amplitude and latency, SCoRS score and GAF score. BACS domains were corrected by age and gender, as reported previously [45]. Bonferroni's tests were employed as post hoc analysis to follow-up results yielded by ANCOVA. Correlation analyses were carried out to study the relationship between the amplitude of P300 vs. performance on clinical and neuropsychological tasks by Spearman's rank correlation test. In these correlational analyses, we used amplitudes at Pz as a representative parameter, according to previous studies [52,53].

For data from the six subtests on the BACS, Bonferroni's tests were performed for multiple comparisons. In subjects with ARMS, P300 amplitude and latency were normally distributed, with no differences between ARMS-P and ARMS-NP demographics; therefore, they were compared by an independent sample t-test.

For all statistical analyses, Shapiro–Wilk analysis and Levene's test were performed to test normality, and significance level was defined as $p < 0.05$.

3. Results

3.1. Profiles of Subjects

Demographic and clinical data of the participants with healthy controls, ARMS and schizophrenia is shown in Table 1. There was a significant group difference in age and PANSS positive symptom between ARMS and schizophrenia, while the male/female ratio and JART scores did not differ. mGAF scores in patients with schizophrenia were worse than those of subjects with ARMS. Scores on the composite score of the BACS was lowest for schizophrenia group, followed by ARMS, compared to healthy control group. As shown in Table 2, compared to ARMS-NP group, ARMS-P group was not different in gender, age, JART, PANSS, and mGAF, but ARMS-P had worse scores on the BACS and SCoRS at baseline.

3.2. Group Comparison of P300 in Healthy Control, ARMS, and Schizophrenia

Grand average waveforms of P300 for healthy control, ARMS, and schizophrenia are shown in Figure 1. Average P300 amplitudes and latencies of these three groups at the T3, T4, Fz, Cz, and Pz leads are shown in Table 1. Statistical analysis revealed that patients with schizophrenia showed smallest P300 amplitudes, followed by ARMS and healthy control, at midline electrodes. P300 latencies at Cz and Pz in schizophrenia were longer than those in healthy controls and ARMS. P300 latency in subjects with ARMS do not differ from those in healthy control.

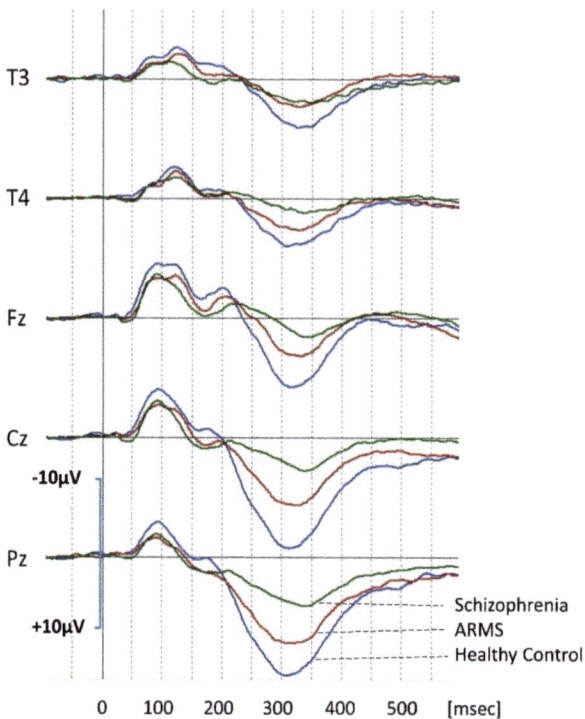

Figure 1. P300 waveforms at the T3, T4, Fz, Cz, and Pz leads. Grand average waveforms in healthy controls (Control, blue lines), subjects with at-risk mental states (ARMS, red lines), and patients with schizophrenia (Schizophrenia, green lines), respectively.

3.3. P300 between ARMS-P and ARMS-NP

Grand average waveforms of P300 in ARMS-P and ARMS-NP are shown in Figure 2. For comparison, waveforms of schizophrenia and controls are also drawn. P300 amplitudes appeared to be most profoundly reduced in patient with schizophrenia, followed by ARMS-P and ARMS-NP, in comparison with healthy controls. However, the difference in amplitude between ARMS-P and ARMS-NP was not significant.

P300 latencies of patients with schizophrenia and ARMS-P appeared to be longer than those of ARMS-NP and healthy controls. Statistical analysis revealed that ARMS-P subjects elicited significantly more prolonged latencies at the T3, Cz, and Pz leads compared with those of ARMS-NP subjects (Table 2).

3.4. Relationship between P300 and Cognitive Functions

We examined correlations between P300 parameters and cognitive functions. As shown in Table 3, in entire (ARMS, schizophrenia, and healthy controls combined) subjects, P300 amplitudes at Pz were significantly positively correlated with mGAF scores, performance on some BACS domains (motor function, attention, and executive function) and BACS composite score. Furthermore, P300 latencies were negatively correlated with composite and attention scores of the BACS. In subjects with ARMS as a whole, scores on the mGAF were positively correlated with P300 amplitudes. Such relationship was found in ARMS-NP ($r_s = 0.57$, $p = 0.019$) but not in ARMS-P subgroups (data not shown). No significant relationships were observed between performance on the BACS and P300 latency in ARMS subjects. In subjects with schizophrenia, BACS composite scores and PANSS general psychopathology mildly correlated with P300 amplitude, but no relationships were observed between latency and other clinical/cognitive measurements.

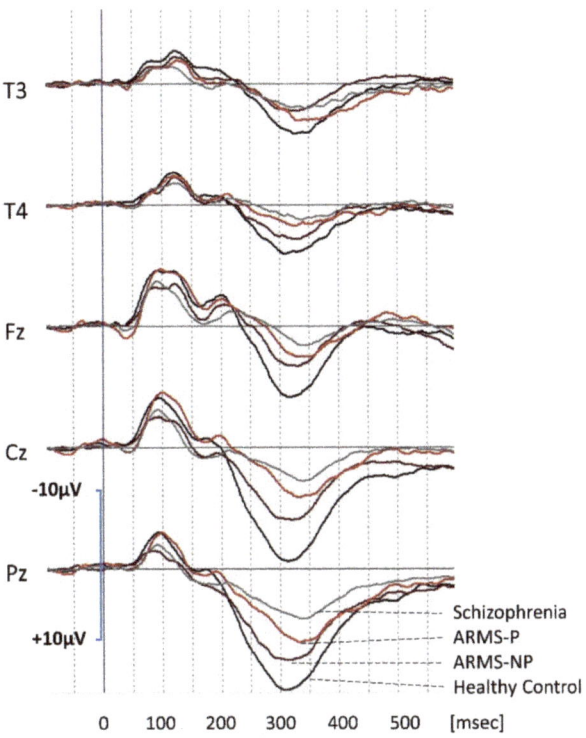

Figure 2. P300 waveforms at the T3, T4, Fz, Cz, and Pz leads. Grand average waveforms for subjects with ARMS who later developed psychosis (ARMS-P; red lines) and those who did not (ARMS non-converters) (ARMS-NP; brown lines). For comparison, waveforms of healthy controls (black lines) and those of patients with schizophrenia (gray lines) are also shown.

Table 3. Correlations between P300 parameters and clinical symptoms.

	Entire Subject [a]				ARMS (n = 33)				Schizophrenia (n = 39)			
	Amplitude (µV)		Latency (msec)		Amplitude (µV)		Latency (msec)		Amplitude (µV)		Latency (msec)	
	r_s	p	r_s	p	r_s	p	r_s	p	r_s	p	r_s	p
JART	−0.03	0.77	0.08	0.44	−0.08	0.65	0.07	0.71	0.10	0.56	0.01	0.95
PANSS: positive symptom	−0.15	0.20	0.02	0.86	−0.08	0.68	0.05	0.78	0.12	0.47	−0.11	0.50
negative symptom	−0.19	0.12	0.21	0.09	−0.30	0.09	0.15	0.41	−0.28	0.10	0.31	0.06
general psychopathology	−0.22	0.07	0.08	0.51	−0.08	0.68	0.17	0.34	−0.34	0.04 *	−0.022	0.90
mGAF	0.46	0.003 **	−0.14	0.29	0.48	0.02 *	0.09	0.67	0.14	0.46	−0.095	0.61
SCoRS	−0.22	0.07	0.17	0.16	−0.11	0.54	0.16	0.36	−0.17	0.33	0.11	0.52
BACS: verbal memory	0.25	0.01	−0.10	0.35	0.02	0.65	−0.02	0.92	0.31	0.06	−0.04	0.80
working memory	0.21	0.04	−0.19	0.06	−0.21	0.23	−0.15	0.40	0.28	0.10	−0.12	0.48
motor function	0.41	<0.001 [b]	−0.22	0.04	0.03	0.86	−0.28	0.10	0.27	0.10	−0.14	0.54
verbal fluency	0.28	0.007	−0.24	0.02	−0.03	0.87	−0.17	0.34	0.17	0.31	−0.85	0.62
attention	0.50	<0.001 [b]	−0.33	0.001 [b]	0.06	0.74	−0.16	0.36	0.43	0.01	−0.24	0.14
executive function	0.36	0.003 [b]	−0.15	0.14	0.06	0.74	−0.002	0.99	0.37	0.03	−0.20	0.22
BACS composite score	0.43	<0.001 **	−0.28	0.006 *	0.01	0.95	−0.22	0.20	0.34	0.04 *	−0.16	0.33

Data were calculated by Spearman's rank correlation (* $p < 0.05$, ** $p < 0.01$). [a] "Entire subject" means schizophrenia, ARMS, and healthy control (n = 100). As shown in Table 1, PANSS, mGAF and SCoRS were measured only in ARMS and schizophrenia patients (n = 72). [b] BACS subdomains survived after Bonferroni's correction for multiple comparison.

4. Discussion

To our knowledge, this is the first report that subjects with ARMS who later developed overt schizophrenia (ARMS-P) elicited prolonged P300 latencies at baseline com-pared to those in subjects who did not develop psychosis. Progression to schizophrenia was also associated with disturbances of cognition and social functioning at baseline, as represented by poorer performances on the BACS in ARMS-P subjects compared to those of ARMS-NP. We further demonstrated a significant correlation between P300 amplitudes and global functioning in ARMS subjects.

As shown on Tables 1 and 2, attention deficits in ARMS-P, but not ARMS-NP subjects, as measured by the BACS, were greater than −1 (z-score), which was comparable to those in overt schizophrenia. Consistent with previous studies [17,19], our results indicated that P300 amplitudes and latencies in the entire patients were significantly associated with performance on the digit symbol substitution test in the BACS (Table 3). These findings accord with the notion that P300 reflects attention-dependent information processing and provides a feasible marker of neurophysiological abnormalities shared by different clinical stages of schizophrenia [17–21,54]. P300 and other EEG parameters have been shown to be influenced by several factors, such as volition and medication status the latter including antipsychotic drugs [9,39,40,55]. Although some previous studies of P300 used subjects with ARMS receiving these drugs [34,35,56], all of the participants studied here were antipsychotic-free, which is one of the strengths of our study.

P300 parameters have been investigated in the context of prediction of people particularly vulnerable to developing psychosis [32–36,38,56,57]. Reduced P300 amplitudes in subjects with ARMS as a whole, studied here, compared to those in healthy controls is consistent with previous findings [32–36,38,56,57]. By contrast, the lack of difference in P300 amplitudes between ARMS-P and ARMS-NP differs from the findings in some previous studies [34,36]. Importantly, no study has reported prolonged latency in ARMS-P subjects compared to ARMS-NP subjects. Part of these discrepant results may be related to the difference in study conditions and/or backgrounds of subjects; one study [34] used longer (100 ms) duration for the target tone, unlike the present study used 50 ms duration of target tone. Further, other studies [34,35,56] used patients who were treated with antipsychotic drugs, while our study concerned only antipsychotic-free patients. The discrepancy in presence/absence of prolonged P300 latency between a previous study [33] that also used antipsychotic-free patients and the current one may be explained by the difference in demographic data, such as age, a factor known to prolong P300 latency [58,59].

The origins of the P300 are considered to involve the temporal-parietal junction, medial temporal cortex, and lateral prefrontal cortex [60,61]. For example, volume reductions of these brain regions have been found to be correlated with decreased P300 amplitudes in ARMS subjects [35,56]. Further, the supramarginal gyrus, a part of temporal-parietal junction whose function is impaired in schizophrenia [62], has been regarded as one of the main generators of P300, because its damage results in deterioration of P300 activity [63]. Thus, the aberrant functions of these brain areas, such as temporal gyrus, may cause prolongation of P300 latency in schizophrenia and ARMS. Further, re-ductions in P300 amplitudes and prolonged latency are also present in unaffected relatives of patients [64–67], suggesting genetic backgrounds for these neurophysiological phenotypes. Specifically, data from a meta-analysis performed by Bramon et al. (2005) indicate a significant prolongation of P300 latency in relatives of schizophrenia patients, while its amplitudes were not affected [64]. Further efforts to characterize these electro-physiological manifestations in the prodromal stage of schizophrenia are likely to broaden the views on trait markers of the illness.

Cognitive and social functioning has been recognized to provide an important target of early intervention for people susceptible to developing psychosis. The SCoRS was developed for measuring daily activity skills in patients with schizophrenia [49]. Further, we found this assessment tool is also useful for evaluation of real-world activities in people with ARMS [47]. Importantly, SCoRS scores in the ARMS-P group were worse than those in ARMS-NP group (Table 2). To our knowledge, our observation is the first to indicate that daily-living skills linked to cognition, evaluated in this way, are more profoundly impaired who later convert to schizophrenia compared to non-converters. These findings overall add to the concept that poor functionality provide a trait marker for psychosis.

There have been attempts to identify neural substrates for neuropsychological disturbances of individuals in early stages of schizophrenia. Accordingly, P300 indices at Pz elicited significant correlations with mGAF and BACS scores in entire subjects (healthy controls, ARMS subjects and patients with schizophrenia combined) (Table 3). These findings are consistent with the concept that changes of cognitive and social functions, measured behaviorally, are reflected by some electrophysiological parameters in individuals with schizophrenia or the clinical high-risk state [9,38,39]. On the other hand, P300 amplitudes were related to mGAF, but not BACS scores in the ARMS subjects. Further study with a larger number of subjects should clarify the contribution of P300 activities to functional outcomes in ARMS.

Finally, it would be worthwhile to discuss the clinical implications of our findings. The present results indicate prolonged P300 latency may provide a potential biomarker for schizophrenia. This is supported by the lack of a significant effect of antipsychotic treatments on P300 latency, unlike the case for its amplitudes, as demonstrated in a meta-analysis [68], suggesting the robustness of P300 latency as a trait-marker of schizophrenia. On the other hand, a number of other candidates for biomarkers of the disease have been reported, and attempts have been made to combine multiple indicators to improve predictive accuracy [69,70]. In this line, P300 latency may help improve diagnostic accuracy when used with other indices.

Several limitations of this study should be considered. First, the small sample size, especially for ARMS-P subjects, might have limited the statistical power and restricted the generalizability of our results. Second, given the evidence of age-related changes of P300 [59,71], the higher age of schizophrenia patients as compared with other groups might have biased our results. However, this may not be relevant to the difference in P300 laten-cy between the ARMS-P and -NP groups (the main find of the current study), as they shared similar ages.

In conclusion, the present study suggests, for the first time, the ability of P300 latency to predict the development of schizophrenia in vulnerable subjects. Our observations also confirm that poor cognitive function and daily-living skills are associated with the risk of development of schizophrenia. When combined with other indices of different modalities, P300 latency may provide a diagnostic marker. Further study is warranted to investigate if P300 latency would be linked to outcomes and other clinical features of individuals at high-risk for schizophrenia and related psychoses.

Author Contributions: Conceptualization, Y.H., T.S., T.T. (Tsutomu Takahashi), and M.S.; methodology, Y.H. and T.S.; investigation for EEG recording and analysis, T.T. (Takahiro Tateno), S.N. (Suguru Nakajima), and Y.H.; investigation for symptom evaluation, D.S., T.T. (Takahiro Tateno), and S.N. (Suguru Nakajima); investigation for neurocognitive evaluation, Y.M. and S.N. (Shimako Nishiyama); writing—original draft preparation, Y.H.; writing—review and editing, T.S., T.T. (Tsutomu Takahashi), and M.S.; project administration, M.S. and Y.H.; funding acquisition, M.S., T.T. (Tsutomu Takahashi), T.S., and Y.H. All authors have read and agreed to the published version of the manuscript.

Funding: This research was funded in part by the Japan Society for the Promotion of Science KAKENHI (grant numbers 18K07550, 16K10205, JP20H03598, JP20H03610 and 26461739), and by the Japan Agency for Medical Research and Development (grant number JP18dk030708, JP19dk0307029 and JP20dk0307099).

Institutional Review Board Statement: The study was conducted in accordance with the Declaration of Helsinki. The Committee on Medical Ethics of Toyama University approved the present study (No. I2013006) on 5 February 2014.

Informed Consent Statement: Informed consent was obtained from all subjects involved in the study. Written informed consent has been obtained from the subjects and their caregivers to publish this paper.

Data Availability Statement: The data presented in this study are available on request from the corresponding author. The data are not publicly available since we do not have permission to share the data.

Acknowledgments: Special thanks to our colleagues, Tomonori Seo, Tomohiro Miyanishi in Department of Neuropsychiatry, University of Toyama Graduate School of Medicine and Pharmaceutical Science to help recording EEG. Further, we would like to thank Kaori Sakata for coordinate subjects' schedule and performing the neuropsychological tests. Kodai Tanaka, Tadasu Matsuoka and Mihoko Nakamura made big effort to evaluate ARMS patients' by CAARMS. Yoichiro Takayanagi and Yasuhiro Kawasaki provided valuable advice about statistical methods and recruitment of patients.

Conflicts of Interest: The authors declare no conflict of interest.

References

1. Green, M.F. What are the functional consequences of neurocognitive deficits in schizophrenia? *Am. J. Psychiatry* **1996**, *153*, 321–330. [CrossRef] [PubMed]
2. McGlashan, T.H.; Zipursky, R.B.; Perkins, D.; Addington, J.; Miller, T.; Woods, S.W.; Hawkins, K.A.; Hoffman, R.E.; Preda, A.; Epstein, I.; et al. Randomized, double-blind trial of olanzapine versus placebo in patients prodromally symptomatic for psychosis. *Am. J. Psychiatry* **2006**, *163*, 790–799. [CrossRef] [PubMed]
3. McGorry, P.D.; Yung, A.R.; Phillips, L.J.; Yuen, H.P.; Francey, S.; Cosgrave, E.M.; Germano, D.; Bravin, J.; McDonald, T.; Blair, A.; et al. Randomized Controlled Trial of Interventions Designed to Reduce the Risk of Progression to First-Episode Psychosis in a Clinical Sample With Subthreshold Symptoms. *Arch. Gen. Psychiatry* **2002**, *59*, 921–928. [CrossRef] [PubMed]
4. Morrison, A.P.; French, P.; Walford, L.; Lewis, S.W.; Kilcommons, A.; Green, J.; Parker, S.; Bentall, R.P. Cognitive therapy for the prevention of psychosis in people at ultra-high risk: Randomised controlled trial. *Br. J. Psychiatry* **2004**, *185*, 291–297. [CrossRef]
5. Fusar-Poli, P.; Borgwardt, S.; Bechdolf, A.; Addington, J.; Riecher-Rossler, A.; Schultze-Lutter, F.; Keshavan, M.; Wood, S.; Ruhrmann, S.; Seidman, L.J.; et al. The psychosis high-risk state: A comprehensive state-of-the-art review. *JAMA Psychiatry* **2013**, *70*, 107–120. [CrossRef] [PubMed]
6. Fusar-Poli, P.; Bonoldi, I.; Yung, A.R.; Borgwardt, S.; Kempton, M.J.; Valmaggia, L.; Barale, F.; Caverzasi, E.; McGuire, P. Predicting psychosis: Meta-analysis of transition outcomes in individuals at high clinical risk. *Arch. Gen. Psychiatry* **2012**, *69*, 220–229. [CrossRef] [PubMed]
7. Fusar-Poli, P.; Bechdolf, A.; Taylor, M.J.; Bonoldi, I.; Carpenter, W.T.; Yung, A.R.; McGuire, P. At Risk for Schizophrenic or Affective Psychoses? A Meta-Analysis of DSM/ICD Diagnostic Outcomes in Individuals at High Clinical Risk. *Schizophr. Bull.* **2013**, *39*, 923–932. [CrossRef]
8. Kawasaki, Y.; Suzuki, M.; Kherif, F.; Takahashi, T.; Zhou, S.-Y.; Nakamura, K.; Matsui, M.; Sumiyoshi, T.; Seto, H.; Kurachi, M. Multivariate voxel-based morphometry successfully differentiates schizophrenia patients from healthy controls. *NeuroImage* **2007**, *34*, 235–242. [CrossRef]
9. Higuchi, Y.; Sumiyoshi, T.; Kawasaki, Y.; Matsui, M.; Arai, H.; Kurachi, M. Electrophysiological basis for the ability of olanzapine to improve verbal memory and functional outcome in patients with schizophrenia: A LORETA analysis of P300. *Schizophr. Res.* **2008**, *101*, 320–330. [CrossRef]
10. Lin, Y.-T.; Liu, C.-M.; Chiu, M.-J.; Liu, C.-C.; Chien, Y.-L.; Hwang, T.-J.; Jaw, F.-S.; Shan, J.-C.; Hsieh, M.H.; Hwu, H.-G. Differentiation of Schizophrenia Patients from Healthy Subjects by Mismatch Negativity and Neuropsychological Tests. *PLOS ONE* **2012**, *7*, e34454. [CrossRef]
11. Takahashi, T.; Zhou, S.-Y.; Nakamura, K.; Tanino, R.; Furuichi, A.; Kido, M.; Kawasaki, Y.; Noguchi, K.; Seto, H.; Kurachi, M.; et al. A follow-up MRI study of the fusiform gyrus and middle and inferior temporal gyri in schizophrenia spectrum. *Prog. Neuro-Psychopharmacol. Biol. Psychiatry* **2011**, *35*, 1957–1964. [CrossRef] [PubMed]
12. Takayanagi, Y.; Takahashi, T.; Orikabe, L.; Mozue, Y.; Kawasaki, Y.; Nakamura, K.; Sato, Y.; Itokawa, M.; Yamasue, H.; Kasai, K.; et al. Classification of First-Episode Schizophrenia Patients and Healthy Subjects by Automated MRI Measures of Regional Brain Volume and Cortical Thickness. *PLoS ONE* **2011**, *6*, e21047. [CrossRef] [PubMed]
13. Niznikiewicz, M.A. Neurobiological approaches to the study of clinical and genetic high risk for developing psychosis. *Psychiatry Res.* **2019**, *277*, 17–22. [CrossRef] [PubMed]
14. Näätänen, R.; Todd, J.; Schall, U. Mismatch negativity (MMN) as biomarker predicting psychosis in clinically at-risk individuals. *Biol. Psychol.* **2016**, *116*, 36–40. [CrossRef] [PubMed]
15. Higuchi, Y.; Sumiyoshi, T.; Ito, T.; Suzuki, M. Perospirone Normalized P300 and Cognitive Function in a Case of Early Psychosis. *J. Clin. Psychopharmacol.* **2013**, *33*, 263–266. [CrossRef]
16. Higuchi, Y.; Sumiyoshi, T.; Seo, T.; Miyanishi, T.; Kawasaki, Y.; Suzuki, M. Mismatch Negativity and Cognitive Performance for the Prediction of Psychosis in Subjects with At-Risk Mental State. *PLoS ONE* **2013**, *8*, e54080. [CrossRef]
17. Polich, J.; Kok, A. Cognitive and biological determinants of P300: An integrative review. *Biol. Psychol.* **1995**, *41*, 103–146. [CrossRef]
18. Johnson, R., Jr. A triarchic model of P300 amplitude. *Psychophysiology* **1986**, *23*, 367–384. [CrossRef]

19. Nieman, D.; Koelman, J.; Linszen, D.; Bour, L.; Dingemans, P.; de Visser, B.O. Clinical and neuropsychological correlates of the P300 in schizophrenia. *Schizophr. Res.* **2002**, *55*, 105–113. [CrossRef]
20. Sutton, S.; Braren, M.; Zubin, J.; John, E.R. Evoked-Potential Correlates of Stimulus Uncertainty. *Science* **1965**, *150*, 1187–1188. [CrossRef]
21. Bashore, T.R.; van der Molen, M.W. Discovery of the P300: A tribute. *Biol. Psychol.* **1991**, *32*, 155–171. [CrossRef]
22. Kawasaki, Y.; Maeda, Y.; Higashima, M.; Nagasawa, T.; Koshino, Y.; Suzuki, M.; Ide, Y. Reduced auditory P300 amplitude, medial temporal volume reduction and psychopathology in schizophrenia. *Schizophr. Res.* **1997**, *26*, 107–115. [CrossRef]
23. Roth, W.T.; Pfefferbaum, A.; Horvath, T.B.; Berger, P.; Kopell, B.S. P3 reduction in auditory evoked potentials of schizophrenics. *Electroencephalogr. Clin. Neurophysiol.* **1980**, *49*, 497–505. [CrossRef]
24. Bruder, G.E.; Tenke, C.E.; Towey, J.P.; Leite, P.; Fong, R.; Stewart, J.E.; McGrath, P.J.; Quitkin, F.M. Brain ERPs of depressed patients to complex tones in an oddball task: Relation of reduced P3 asymmetry to physical anhedonia. *Psychophysiology* **1998**, *35*, 54–63. [CrossRef] [PubMed]
25. Qiu, Y.-Q.; Tang, Y.-X.; Chan, R.C.K.; Sun, X.-Y.; He, J. P300 Aberration in First-Episode Schizophrenia Patients: A Meta-Analysis. *PLoS ONE* **2014**, *9*, e97794. [CrossRef] [PubMed]
26. Hünerli, D.; Emek-Savaş, D.D.; Çavuşoğlu, B.; Çolakoğlu, B.D.; Ada, E.; Yener, G.G. Mild cognitive impairment in Parkinson's disease is associated with decreased P300 amplitude and reduced putamen volume. *Clin. Neurophysiol.* **2019**, *130*, 1208–1217. [CrossRef] [PubMed]
27. Yilmaz, F.T.; Ozkaynak, S.S.; Barcin, E. Contribution of auditory P300 test to the diagnosis of mild cognitive impairment in Parkinson's disease. *Neurol. Sci.* **2017**, *38*, 2103–2109. [CrossRef] [PubMed]
28. Wada, M.; Kurose, S.; Miyazaki, T.; Nakajima, S.; Masuda, F.; Mimura, Y.; Nishida, H.; Ogyu, K.; Tsugawa, S.; Mashima, Y.; et al. The P300 event-related potential in bipolar disorder: A systematic review and meta-analysis. *J. Affect. Disord.* **2019**, *256*, 234–249. [CrossRef]
29. Zhong, B.-L.; Xu, Y.-M.; Xie, W.-X.; Li, Y. Can P300 aid in the differential diagnosis of unipolar disorder versus bipolar disorder depression? A meta-analysis of comparative studies. *J. Affect. Disord.* **2019**, *245*, 219–227. [CrossRef] [PubMed]
30. Peisch, V.; Rutter, T.; Wilkinson, C.L.; Arnett, A.B. Sensory processing and P300 event-related potential correlates of stimulant response in children with attention-deficit/hyperactivity disorder: A critical review. *Clin. Neurophysiol.* **2021**, *132*, 953–966. [CrossRef] [PubMed]
31. Cui, T.; Wang, P.P.; Liu, S.; Zhang, X. P300 amplitude and latency in autism spectrum disorder: A meta-analysis. *Eur. Child Adolesc. Psychiatry* **2016**, *26*, 177–190. [CrossRef]
32. Ozgürdal, S.; Gudlowski, Y.; Witthaus, H.; Kawohl, W.; Uhl, I.; Hauser, M.; Gorynia, I.; Gallinat, J.; Heinze, M.; Heinz, A.; et al. Reduction of auditory event-related P300 amplitude in subjects with at-risk mental state for schizophrenia. *Schizophr. Res.* **2008**, *105*, 272–278. [CrossRef]
33. Bramon, E.; Shaikh, M.; Broome, M.; Lappin, J.; Bergé, D.; Day, F.; Woolley, J.; Tabraham, P.; Madre, M.; Johns, L.; et al. Abnormal P300 in people with high risk of developing psychosis. *NeuroImage* **2008**, *41*, 553–560. [CrossRef] [PubMed]
34. Van Tricht, M.J.; Nieman, D.H.; Koelman, J.H.; van der Meer, J.N.; Bour, L.J.; de Haan, L.; Linszen, D.H. Reduced parietal P300 amplitude is associated with an increased risk for a first psychotic episode. *Biol. Psychiatry* **2010**, *68*, 642–648. [CrossRef] [PubMed]
35. Fusar-Poli, P.; Crossley, N.; Woolley, J.; Carletti, F.; Perez-Iglesias, R.; Broome, M.; Johns, L.; Tabraham, P.; Bramon, E.; McGuire, P. White matter alterations related to P300 abnormalities in individuals at high risk for psychosis: An MRI–EEG study. *J. Psychiatry Neurosci.* **2011**, *36*, 239–248. [CrossRef] [PubMed]
36. Nieman, D.H.; Ruhrmann, S.; Dragt, S.; Soen, F.; Van Tricht, M.J.; Koelman, J.H.T.M.; Bour, L.J.; Velthorst, E.; Becker, H.E.; Weiser, M.; et al. Psychosis Prediction: Stratification of Risk Estimation With Information-Processing and Premorbid Functioning Variables. *Schizophr. Bull.* **2014**, *40*, 1482–1490. [CrossRef]
37. Tang, Y.; Wang, J.; Zhang, T.; Xu, L.; Qian, Z.; Cui, H.; Tang, X.; Li, H.; Whitfield-Gabrieli, S.; Shenton, M.E.; et al. P300 as an index of transition to psychosis and of remission: Data from a clinical high risk for psychosis study and review of literature. *Schizophr. Res.* **2020**, *226*, 74–83. [CrossRef] [PubMed]
38. Kim, M.; Lee, T.H.; Kim, J.-H.; Hong, H.; Lee, T.Y.; Lee, Y.; Salisbury, D.F.; Kwon, J.S. Decomposing P300 into correlates of genetic risk and current symptoms in schizophrenia: An inter-trial variability analysis. *Schizophr. Res.* **2018**, *192*, 232–239. [CrossRef] [PubMed]
39. Sumiyoshi, T.; Higuchi, Y.; Itoh, T.; Matsui, M.; Arai, H.; Suzuki, M.; Kurachi, M.; Sumiyoshi, C.; Kawasaki, Y. Effect of perospirone on P300 electrophysiological activity and social cognition in schizophrenia: A three-dimensional analysis with sLORETA. *Psychiatry Res. Neuroimaging* **2009**, *172*, 180–183. [CrossRef] [PubMed]
40. Umbricht, D.; Javitt, D.; Novak, G.; Bates, J.; Pollack, S.; Lieberman, J.; Kane, J. Effects of clozapine on auditory event-related potentials in schizophrenia. *Biol. Psychiatry* **1998**, *44*, 716–725. [CrossRef]
41. Mizuno, M.; Suzuki, M.; Matsumoto, K.; Murakami, M.; Takeshi, K.; Miyakoshi, T.; Ito, F.; Yamazawa, R.; Kobayashi, H.; Nemoto, T.; et al. Clinical practice and research activities for early psychiatric intervention at Japanese leading centres. *Early Interv. Psychiatry* **2009**, *3*, 5–9. [CrossRef] [PubMed]
42. Yung, A.R.; Yuen, H.P.; McGorry, P.D.; Phillips, L.J.; Kelly, D.; Dell'Olio, M.; Francey, S.M.; Cosgrave, E.M.; Killackey, E.; Stanford, C.; et al. Mapping the Onset of Psychosis: The Comprehensive Assessment of At-Risk Mental States. *Aust. N. Z. J. Psychiatry* **2005**, *39*, 964–971. [CrossRef]

43. Kay, S.R.; Fiszbein, A.; Opler, L.A. The positive and negative syndrome scale (PANSS) for schizophrenia. *Schizophr. Bull.* **1987**, *13*, 261–276. [CrossRef]
44. Matsuoka, K.; Uno, M.; Kasai, K.; Koyama, K.; Kim, Y. Estimation of premorbid IQ in individuals with Alzheimer's disease using Japanese ideographic script (Kanji) compound words: Japanese version of National Adult Reading Test. *Psychiatry Clin. Neurosci.* **2006**, *60*, 332–339. [CrossRef]
45. Kaneda, Y.; Sumiyoshi, T.; Keefe, R.; Ishimoto, Y.; Numata, S.; Ohmori, T. Brief Assessment of Cognition in Schizophrenia: Validation of the Japanese version. *Psychiatry Clin. Neurosci.* **2007**, *61*, 602–609. [CrossRef] [PubMed]
46. Keefe, R.S.; Goldberg, T.; Harvey, P.D.; Gold, J.M.; Poe, M.P.; Coughenour, L. The Brief Assessment of Cognition in Schizophrenia: Reliability, sensitivity, and comparison with a standard neurocognitive battery. *Schizophr. Res.* **2004**, *68*, 283–297. [CrossRef] [PubMed]
47. Higuchi, Y.; Sumiyoshi, T.; Seo, T.; Suga, M.; Takahashi, T.; Nishiyama, S.; Komori, Y.; Kasai, K.; Suzuki, M. Associations between daily living skills, cognition, and real-world functioning across stages of schizophrenia; a study with the Schizophrenia Cognition Rating Scale Japanese version. *Schizophr. Res. Cogn.* **2017**, *7*, 13–18. [CrossRef] [PubMed]
48. Kaneda, Y.; Ueoka, Y.; Sumiyoshi, T.; Yasui-Furukori, N.; Ito, T.; Higuchi, Y.; Suzuki, M.; Ohmori, T. Schizophrenia Cognition Rating Scale Japanese version (SCoRS-J) as a co-primary measure assessing cognitive function in schizophrenia. *Nihon Shinkei Seishin Yakurigaku Zasshi* **2011**, *31*, 259–262.
49. Keefe, R.S.; Poe, M.; Walker, T.M.; Kang, J.W.; Harvey, P.D. The Schizophrenia Cognition Rating Scale: An Interview-Based Assessment and Its Relationship to Cognition, Real-World Functioning, and Functional Capacity. *Am. J. Psychiatry* **2006**, *163*, 426–432. [CrossRef] [PubMed]
50. Hall, R.C. Global Assessment of Functioning. *J. Psychosom. Res.* **1995**, *36*, 267–275. [CrossRef]
51. Kaneda, Y.; Ohmori, T.; Okahisa, Y.; Sumiyoshi, T.; Pu, S.; Ueoka, Y.; Takaki, M.; Nakagome, K.; Sora, I. Measurement and Treatment Research toImprove Cognition in Schizophrenia Consensus Cognitive Battery: Validation of the Japanese version. *Psychiatry Clin. Neurosci.* **2013**, *67*, 182–188. [CrossRef] [PubMed]
52. Takahashi, S.; Tanabe, E.; Yara, K.; Matsuura, M.; Matsushima, E.; Kojima, T. Impairment of exploratory eye movement in schizophrenia patients and their siblings. *Psychiatry Clin. Neurosci.* **2008**, *62*, 487–493. [CrossRef] [PubMed]
53. Hall, M.-H.; Jensen, J.E.; Du, F.; Smoller, J.W.; O'Connor, L.; Spencer, K.M.; Öngür, D. Frontal P3 event-related potential is related to brain glutamine/glutamate ratio measured in vivo. *Neuroimage* **2015**, *111*, 186–191. [CrossRef] [PubMed]
54. Michie, P.T.; Kent, A.; Stienstra, R.; Castine, R.; Johnston, J.; Dedman, K.; Wichmann, H.; Box, J.; Rock, D.; Rutherford, E.; et al. Phenotypic markers as risk factors in schizophrenia: Neurocognitive functions. *Aust. N. Z. J. Psychiatry* **2000**, *34*, 74–85. [CrossRef]
55. Jackson, A.; Seneviratne, U. EEG changes in patients on antipsychotic therapy: A systematic review. *Epilepsy Behav.* **2019**, *95*, 1–9. [CrossRef] [PubMed]
56. Fusar-Poli, P.; Crossley, N.; Woolley, J.; Carletti, F.; Perez-Iglesias, R.; Broome, M.; Johns, L.; Tabraham, P.; Bramon, E.; McGuire, P. Gray matter alterations related to P300 abnormalities in subjects at high risk for psychosis: Longitudinal MRI-EEG study. *Neuroimage* **2011**, *55*, 320–328. [CrossRef] [PubMed]
57. Van der Stelt, O.; Lieberman, J.A.; Belger, A. Auditory P300 in high-risk, recent-onset and chronic schizophrenia. *Schizophr. Res.* **2005**, *77*, 309–320. [CrossRef]
58. Mori, Y.; Kurosu, S.; Hiroyama, Y.; Niwa, S.-I. Prolongation of P300 latency is associated with the duration of illness in male schizophrenia patients. *Psychiatry Clin. Neurosci.* **2007**, *61*, 471–478. [CrossRef]
59. Van Dinteren, R.; Arns, M.; Jongsma, M.L.; Kessels, R.P. P300 development across the lifespan: A systematic review and meta-analysis. *PLoS ONE* **2014**, *9*, e87347. [CrossRef] [PubMed]
60. Soltani, M.; Knight, R.T. Neural origins of the P300. *Crit. Rev. Neurobiol.* **2000**, *14*, 199–224. [CrossRef] [PubMed]
61. Linden, D.E.J. The P300: Where in the Brain Is It Produced and What Does It Tell Us? *Neuroscience* **2005**, *11*, 563–576. [CrossRef] [PubMed]
62. Shenton, M.E.; Dickey, C.C.; Frumin, M.; McCarley, R.W. A review of MRI findings in schizophrenia. *Schizophr. Res.* **2001**, *49*, 1–52. [CrossRef]
63. Yamaguchi, S.; Knight, R.T. Anterior and posterior association cortex contributions to the somatosensory P300. *J. Neurosci.* **1991**, *11*, 2039–2054. [CrossRef] [PubMed]
64. Bramon, E.; McDonald, C.; Croft, R.J.; Landau, S.; Filbey, F.; Gruzelier, J.H.; Sham, P.C.; Frangou, S.; Murray, R.M. Is the P300 wave an endophenotype for schizophrenia? A meta-analysis and a family study. *NeuroImage* **2005**, *27*, 960–968. [CrossRef]
65. Blackwood, D.H.R.; Clair, D.M.S.; Muir, W.J.; Duffy, J.C. Auditory P300 and Eye Tracking Dysfunction in Schizophrenic Pedigrees. *Arch. Gen. Psychiatry* **1991**, *48*, 899–909. [CrossRef]
66. Turetsky, B.I.; Cannon, T.D.; Gur, R.E. P300 subcomponent abnormalities in schizophrenia: III. Deficits In unaffected siblings of schizophrenic probands. *Biol. Psychiatry* **2000**, *47*, 380–390. [CrossRef]
67. Winterer, G.; Egan, M.F.; Raedler, T.; Sanchez, C.; Jones, D.W.; Coppola, R.; Weinberger, D.R. P300 and Genetic Risk for Schizophrenia. *Arch. Gen. Psychiatry* **2003**, *60*, 1158–1167. [CrossRef]
68. Bramon, E.; Rabe-Hesketh, S.; Sham, P.; Murray, R.M.; Frangou, S. Meta-analysis of the P300 and P50 waveforms in schizophrenia. *Schizophr. Res.* **2004**, *70*, 315–329. [CrossRef] [PubMed]
69. Lieberman, J.A.; Small, S.A.; Girgis, R.R. Early Detection and Preventive Intervention in Schizophrenia: From Fantasy to Reality. *Am. J. Psychiatry* **2019**, *176*, 794–810. [CrossRef]

70. Schmidt, A.; Cappucciati, M.; Radua, J.; Rutigliano, G.; Rocchetti, M.; Dell'Osso, L.; Politi, P.; Borgwardt, S.; Reilly, T.; Valmaggia, L.; et al. Improving Prognostic Accuracy in Subjects at Clinical High Risk for Psychosis: Systematic Review of Predictive Models and Meta-analytical Sequential Testing Simulation. *Schizophr. Bull.* **2016**, *43*, 375–388. [CrossRef] [PubMed]
71. Bourisly, A.K. Effects of aging on P300 between late young-age and early middle-age adulthood: An electroencephalogram event-related potential study. *Neuroreport* **2016**, *27*, 999–1003. [CrossRef] [PubMed]

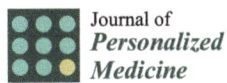

Article

Cannabis Use Induces Distinctive Proteomic Alterations in Olfactory Neuroepithelial Cells of Schizophrenia Patients

Marta Barrera-Conde [1,2], Karina Ausin [3], Mercedes Lachén-Montes [3], Joaquín Fernández-Irigoyen [3], Liliana Galindo [4,5], Aida Cuenca-Royo [1], Cristina Fernández-Avilés [2], Víctor Pérez [5,6], Rafael de la Torre [1,2,7], Enrique Santamaría [3] and Patricia Robledo [1,2,*]

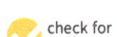

1. Integrative Pharmacology and Systems Neuroscience, Neuroscience Research Program, IMIM-Hospital del Mar Research Institute, 08003 Barcelona, Spain; mbarrera1@imim.es (M.B.-C.); acuenca@imim.es (A.C.-R.); RTorre@imim.es (R.d.l.T.)
2. Department of Experimental and Health Sciences, University Pompeu Fabra, 08003 Barcelona, Spain; cristina.fernandeza@upf.edu
3. Clinical Neuroproteomics Unit, Proteomics Platform, Navarrabiomed, Complejo Hospitalario de Navarra (CHN), Universidad Pública de Navarra (UPNA), IdisNA, Proteored-ISCIII, 31006 Pamplona, Spain; karina.ausin.perez@navarra.es (K.A.); mercedes.lachen.montes@navarra.es (M.L.-M.); jokfer@gmail.com (J.F.-I.); enrique.santamaria.martinez@navarra.es (E.S.)
4. Department of Psychiatry, University of Cambridge, Cambridgeshire and Peterborough NHS Foundation Trust, Cambridge CB2 1TN, UK; lg532@cam.ac.uk
5. Neuropsychiatry and Addictions Institute (INAD) of Parc de Salut Mar, 08003 Barcelona and CIBER de Salud Mental, Spain; 61155@parcdesalutmar.cat
6. Department of Psychiatry and Legal Medicine, Autonomous University of Barcelona, 08193 Barcelona, Spain
7. Centro de Investigación Biomédica en Red de Fisiopatología de la Obesidad y Nutrición, Instituto de Salud Carlos III, 28029 Madrid, Spain
* Correspondence: probledo@imim.es; Tel.: +34-93-316-0455

Abstract: A close epidemiological link has been reported between cannabis use and schizophrenia (SCZ). However, biochemical markers in living humans related to the impact of cannabis in this disease are still missing. Olfactory neuroepithelium (ON) cells express neural features and offer a unique advantage to study biomarkers of psychiatric diseases. The aim of our study was to find exclusively deregulated proteins in ON cells of SCZ patients with and without a history of cannabis use. Thus, we compared the proteomic profiles of SCZ non-cannabis users (SCZ/nc) and SCZ cannabis users (SCZ/c) with control subjects non-cannabis users (C/nc) and control cannabis users (C/c). The results revealed that the main cascades affected in SCZ/nc were cell cycle, DNA replication, signal transduction and protein localization. Conversely, cannabis use in SCZ patients induced specific alterations in metabolism of RNA and metabolism of proteins. The levels of targeted proteins in each population were then correlated with cognitive performance and clinical scores. In SCZ/c, the expression levels of 2 proteins involved in the metabolism of RNA (MTREX and ZNF326) correlated with several cognitive markers and clinical signs. Moreover, use duration of cannabis negatively correlated with ZNF326 expression. These findings indicate that RNA-related proteins might be relevant to understand the influence of cannabis use on SCZ.

Keywords: cannabis; schizophrenia; proteomics; olfactory neuroepithelium; metabolism; RNA; ZNF326; MTREX

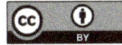

1. Introduction

The complexity of schizophrenia (SCZ), involving intricate interactions between environmental factors and genetics, hinders the identification of the molecular mechanisms underlying its development [1]. State of the art techniques are being used to find biomarkers and ease clinical practice. In this sense, proteomic tools, allowing the study of a large number of proteins at a time, can provide an integrated picture of the biological dysfunctions associated with SCZ [2]. Serum, plasma and cerebrospinal fluid studies reveal an effect on proteins related to the innate immune system and a highly reported downregulation of Apolipoprotein A-I1 (APOA1) [3–5], which might mediate the impact of SCZ on the peripheral immune response [6,7]. On the other hand, postmortem brain studies have shown deregulations in metabolic pathways, calcium signalling and cytoskeleton assembly in several brain areas in SCZ [8–10]. However, other neuropsychiatric conditions present similar affectations [11]. In fact, the two most referenced biomarkers of SCZ, namely Fructose-bisphosphate aldolase C (ALDOC) and Glial fibrillary acidic protein (GFAP), are also altered in major depression and bipolar disorder [12]. Thus, postmortem brains from individuals diagnosed with different mental conditions appear to have great similarities that hamper the identification of exclusive biomarkers for SCZ. Additionally, the impossibility of correlating these biochemical findings with cognitive dysfunctions and environmental cues specific for each condition highlights the necessity to use other substrates. In this context, the olfactory neuroepithelium (ON) has emerged as a useful tool. This specialized epithelial tissue can be easily obtained from living subjects and it contains multipotent progenitors that express neural markers [13–16]. Therefore, the main advantage of ON cells is that ongoing environmental factors and molecular alterations can be evaluated during the progression of the disease.

Years of epidemiological research in psychotic disorders suggest that cannabis use is a specific environmental factor for SCZ. The incidence of cannabis use is two to four times higher among SCZ patients, and its consumption doubles the risk of psychosis in a dose- and time-dependent manner [17,18]. Moreover, an endocannabinoid system imbalance, including alterations in the expression of the cannabinoid receptor 1 (CB_1) in postmortem brains and a diminished production of the enzymes involved in the synthesis of endocannabinoids, has been observed in postmortem and peripheral samples of SCZ patients [19,20]. Additionally, cannabis and SCZ have a shared effect on some cellular functions. Indeed, protein metabolism via AKT/mTOR, cytoskeleton organization, and calcium signalling are affected in human samples from SCZ patients [2], and after cannabinoid exposure in cultured cells [21,22] and mice models [23,24]. Moreover, plasmatic samples from heavy cannabis users and SCZ patients share an effect on oxidative stress response [7,25]. However, whether the coexistence of both factors has equal or distinct consequences is less clear. In fact, in a synchrotron-based infrared spectroscopy study, significant differences in the protein spectra were reported in ON cells from SCZ cannabis users compared to non-users [26]. Additionally, we recently demonstrated that the functional signature of the CB_1 and serotonin 2A receptor (CB_1-$5HT_{2A}R$) heteromer in ON cells is differentially regulated in SCZ patients depending on cannabis use [27].

Therefore, the aim of this study was to find exclusively deregulated proteins in ON cells of SCZ patients with and without a history of chronic cannabis use. We applied mass spectrometry-based quantitative proteomics followed by a functional analysis to characterize the proteomic changes specifically induced by cannabis use in ON cells from SCZ patients, as compared to controls that use cannabis or not. The primary outcome of the study, i.e., the expression levels of the target proteins, were correlated with cannabis consumption, and with secondary cognitive and clinical outcomes associated with SCZ.

2. Materials and Methods

2.1. Study Design

SCZ patients without a history of chronic cannabis use (SCZ/nc, n = 5), SCZ patients with a reported history of chronic cannabis use (SCZ/c, n = 5), chronic cannabis users without any psychiatric diagnosis (C/c, n = 5), and control subjects non-cannabis users (C/nc, n = 5) between 18 and 45 years old (both males and females), were recruited to conduct a cross-sectional study. Every subject gave written informed consent after a complete description of the study and the procedures involved. Cannabis users had to consume more than 5 cannabis cigarettes per week during at least 6 months. On the day of testing, subjects were told to refrain from cannabis use for at least 12 h before testing to avoid the potential confounding of acute cannabis intoxication in both neuropsychological and proteomic studies. The exclusion criteria were: (i) meeting criteria for any severe mental disorder according to the Diagnostic and Statistical Manual of Mental Disorders, Fifth Edition (DSM-5); (ii) history of severe mental illness among first degree relatives; (iii) history of severe congenital, medical or neurological illness; (iv) show medical conditions with nasal repercussions (rhinitis or bleeding); and (v) use of other drugs of abuse. SCZ-diagnosed participants were receiving antipsychotic medication at the time of the study. All subjects underwent a physical, psychiatric and neuropsychological evaluation, as previously described [16]. This study was approved by the local Institutional ethics committee (CEIC-PSMAR).

2.2. Clinical and Neuropsychological Evaluation

Neuropsychological assessments were carried out in all subjects. Executive functions were tested with the semantic verbal fluency test. Attention performance was evaluated using the direct spatial span (SSP) and digit direct series. Working memory was addressed using the inverse spatial span and digit inverse series using the Cambridge neuropsychological test automated battery (CANTAB 2017), and the digit span of the Wechsler Adult Intelligence Scale (WAIS-III). Emotional recognition was evaluated with the CANTAB test. Clinical outcomes included the global assessment of functioning (GAF), and the neurological soft signs (NSS) scores.

2.3. Quantification of Cannabis Metabolites

To estimate the amount of cannabis consumed by cannabis users, the plasma concentrations of its main non-psychoactive metabolite, namely, 11-nor-9-carboxy-Δ-9-THC (THC-COOH), were calculated. Briefly, 1 mL of plasma was transferred into a glass tube and spiked with d3-Δ-9-THC as the internal standard. A protein precipitation with 2 mL of 0.1% formic acid in acetonitrile was performed prior to a solid phase extraction with Oasis Prime HLB 3 cm^3, 60 mg column (Waters Co., Milford, MA, USA). The supernatant was diluted with MilliQ water and loaded. Subsequently, 2 mL of 25% of methanol was added twice. Elution was carried out twice with 2 mL of 90:10 acetonitrile:methanol (ACN:MeOH). The organic phase was evaporated to dryness under a nitrogen stream at < 39 °C and <15 psi pressure. Analytes were reconstituted in 50 µL of 90:10 ACN:MeOH and 50 µL of MilliQ water. Quantification of THC-COOH in plasma was performed using an Agilent 1200 series HPLC system (Agilent Technologies) coupled to a 6410 Triple Quadrupole LC-MS (Agilent Technologies) mass spectrometer with an electrospray interface.

2.4. Nasal Exfoliation and Cell Culture

ON samples were obtained by nasal brushing. Samples from the middle and upper turbinates were maintained in 250 µL of cold Dulbecco's Modified Eagle Medium/Ham F-12 (DMEM/F12) enriched with 10% FBS, 2% glutamine and 1% streptomycin–penicillin (GibcoBRL), as previously described [27]. At 80% confluence, cells were expanded using 0.25% trypsin (GibcoBRL) and replated in 75 cm^2 flasks. Then, cells were expanded until passage four was reached and stored in liquid nitrogen with 20% FBS and 10% dimethyl sulfoxide (Sigma-Aldrich, Madrid, Spain). The aliquots from all subjects (n = 20) were unfrozen at the same time and harvested in 75 cm^2 flasks under standard conditions using enriched DMEM/F12 medium.

2.5. Quantitative Proteomics in ON Cells

Physical protein extraction was performed using sterile scrappers and PBS 1X. After centrifugation, the pellet was kept frozen at −80 °C until homogenization using lysis buffer (7 M urea, 2 M thiourea, and 50 mM DTT). The homogenates were then subjected to in-solution digestion, peptide purification and reconstitution prior to mass spectrometric analysis (MS/MS). Data acquisition was performed as previously described [28] using ProteinPilot v5.0 (Sciex) as a search engine, ParagonTM Algorithm (v.4.0.0.0) [29] for database searching and a non-lineal fitting method to calculate the false discovery rate (FDR) (1% Global FDR or better). Data analysis was performed by sequential window acquisition of all theoretical mass spectra–mass spectrometry (SWATH-MS), and the TripleTOF 5600+ mass-spectrometer was configured as previously described [30]. The library generation-associated ProteinPilot group file was loaded into PeakView® 2.1 (Sciex), and peaks from SWATH runs were extracted with a peptide confidence threshold of 99% confidence (Unused Score ≥ 1.3) and FDR lower than 1%. ProteinPilot was used to extract the MS/MS spectra of the assigned peptides, and only proteins quantified with at least two unique peptides were considered. For more detailed information about the SWATH-MS library generation, please refer to the extended experimental procedures in the Supplementary Information.

2.6. Pathway Analysis, Statistics and Bioinformatics

The peer-reviewed pathway database REACTOME [31] was used to functionally characterize the proteomic alterations detected in every comparison. This database hierarchically classifies cellular functions in 27 cascades. We established a 0.01 *p*-value threshold, and the functional proteome results obtained were ordered based on their FDR. All calculations were performed using SPSS (SPSS Inc., Chicago, IL, USA). Normality and homoscedasticity for continuous variables were tested using Shapiro–Wilk W and Levene tests. Demographic categorical variables were evaluated using Chi-squared tests and continuous normally distributed variables were evaluated using one-way ANOVAs followed by the least significance difference (LSD) post-hoc test. Neuropsychological calculations were corrected for tobacco use duration. Not normally distributed variables were compared using Kruskal–Wallis and Dunn's post-hoc test. Vulcano plot representations and Spearman correlation plots were depicted using GraphPad prism 8.0 Software (La Jolla California, CA, USA). Venn diagrams for proteomic comparisons were designed using BioVenn platform [32].

3. Results

3.1. Demographics and Neuropsychological Outcomes

The demographic data are shown in Table 1. The groups did not differ in age, sex or dosage of tobacco use. However, SCZ/c showed a significantly higher duration of tobacco use (years) when compared to all other groups ($p < 0.05$). The analysis of cannabis use patterns between C/c and SCZ/c revealed no significant differences. The neuropsychological evaluation (Table 2) revealed significantly lower verbal fluency scores for SCZ/nc and SCZ/c as compared to C/nc ($p < 0.05$), but not when compared to C/c. GAF scores were significantly lower in SCZ/nc and SCZ/c when compared to C/nc and C/c ($p < 0.001$). Finally, significantly more NSS were present in SCZ patients regardless of cannabis use when compared to C/nc ($p < 0.01$) and C/c ($p < 0.05$).

3.2. Plasmatic Concentrations of THC-COOH

The plasmatic concentrations of THC-COOH were not significantly different between the groups (C/c: 34.92 ± 17.55 ng/mL; SCZ/c: 11.22 ± 15.91 ng/mL).

3.3. Proteomic Analyses

Our proteomic workflow was fundamentally based on a triangular approach [33], whereby a relatively small number of cases and controls are analyzed by hypothesis-free discovery proteomics in great depth, leading to the quantification of thousands of proteins. Using this workflow, we observed specific changes in protein abundance in C/nc vs. SCZ patients and in SCZ/nc vs. SCZ/c, underpinning the importance of analyzing independent factors (disease/cannabis), instead of merely contrasting SCZ versus control cases. Firstly, C/c, SCZ/nc and SCZ/c were compared to C/nc subtracting exclusively deregulated proteins for each population. Then, each group of SCZ patients was compared to C/c to subtract the effect of cannabis use on control subjects. In the end, each group of SCZ (SCZ/nc and SCZ/c) was compared to obtain proteomic biomarkers that were only affected by SCZ or by SCZ plus cannabis use. For the summary followed in the proteomic data analysis, see Supplementary Figure S1.

Table 1. Demographic characteristics of the different groups included in the study.

	Control Subjects (C/nc)	Cannabis Users (C/c)	Schizophrenia Non-Cannabis (SCZ/nc)	Schizophrenia Cannabis (SCZ/c)
Age (years)	31.4 ± 5.5	29.2 ± 5.6	37 ± 10.1	41.4 ± 6.2
Gender (M-F)	3/2	4/1	2/3	5/0
Tobacco use				
Users—n (%)	5 (100%)	4 (80%)	4 (80%)	5 (100%)
Units per week $^\mu$	53.8 ± 50.2	36.4 ± 40.6	91.2 ± 91.0	147 ± 62.6
Use duration (years) $^\mu$	11.4 ± 4.9	10.4 ± 10.0	5.8 ± 6.8	24.2 ± 9.6 *,+,#
Cannabis use				
Age first use (years) $^\mu$	-	15.4 ± 2.5	-	17.2 ± 3
Units per week $^\mu$	-	16.2 ± 10.2	-	19.4 ± 14.6
Use duration (years) $^\mu$	-	12.2 ± 7.2	-	17.6 ± 11.5
Antipsychotic treatment				
Clozapine/Olanzapine	-	-	1/5	3/5
Aripiprazole	-	-	2/5	1/5
Paliperidone	-	-	1/5	1/5
Risperidone	-	-	1/5	-

Data are shown as mean ± SD. * $p < 0.05$ vs. C/nc; + $p < 0.05$ vs. C/c; # $p < 0.05$ vs. SCZ/nc. (μ) Indicates continuous non-normally distributed variables.

Table 2. Neuropsychological and clinical data of the different groups.

	Control Subjects (C/nc)	Cannabis Users (C/c)	Schizophrenia Non-Cannabis (SCZ/nc)	Schizophrenia Cannabis (SCZ/c)
Direct series score	8.8 ± 0.4	8.2 ± 1.8	7.4 ± 1.5	8.8 ± 2.2
Inverse series score $^\mu$	6.3 ± 1.3	8.2 ± 5.5	4.4 ± 1.5	8.8 ± 2.1
Verbal fluency score	26 ± 1.2	22.8 ± 4.5	18.8 ± 6.9	17.2 ± 5.3 *,+
Direct spatial span	7.4 ± 0.6	5.6 ± 1.9	5.2 ± 1.5	5.6 ± 1.7
Inverse spatial span	7.6 ± 2.9	5.8 ± 1.5	5.6 ± 3	5.6 ± 1.7
Emotional recognition	65.9 ± 8.6	73.8 ± 7.4	58.2 ± 22.5	58.9 ± 10.2
Global assessment of functioning $^\mu$	99 ± 5	96 ± 5.5	67 ± 8.4 ***,+,++	63 ± 2.7 ***,+,++
Neurological soft signs $^\mu$	2.8 ± 1.1	5.2 ± 3.1	14.8 ± 8.6 **,+	13.2 ± 2.3 **,+

Data are shown as mean ± SD of the mean. * $p < 0.05$, ** $p < 0.01$, *** $p < 0.001$ versus C/nc; + $p < 0.05$; ++ $p < 0.01$ versus C/c. (μ) Indicates continuous non-normally distributed variables.

3.3.1. Quantitative and Functional Proteomic Profile of ON Cells from SCZ Patients as Compared to C/nc

The proteomic analysis of ON cells from C/c, SCZ/nc and SCZ/c as compared to C/nc showed 1185, 1209 and 1584 deregulated proteins, respectively. The Venn diagrams (Figure 1a) showed that in C/c, 550 proteins were upregulated (554 in SCZ/nc and 758 in SCZ/c). On the other hand, 635 proteins were downregulated in C/c (655 in SCZ/nc and 826 in SCZ/c); 371 proteins were commonly upregulated in C/c, SCZ/nc and SCZ/c; 211 were exclusively upregulated in SCZ/c and 44 in SCZ/nc. In addition, 474 proteins were commonly downregulated in C/c, SCZ/nc and SCZ/c; 169 were exclusively downregulated in SCZ/c and 37 in SCZ/nc. In total, 845 proteins were commonly deregulated in C/c, SCZ/nc and SCZ/c as compared to C/nc. The pathway analysis of the 845 commonly deregulated proteins (Figure 1b) revealed programmed cell death (37 proteins; $\log_{(10)}$FDR = 4.5), metabolism of proteins (225 proteins; $\log_{(10)}$FDR = 4.2), extracellular matrix organization (47 proteins; $\log_{(10)}$FDR = 3.5), vesicle-mediated transport (87 proteins;

log$_{(10)}$FDR = 2.7), immune system (241 proteins; log$_{(10)}$FDR = 2.0), protein localization (22 proteins; log$_{(10)}$FDR = 1.4) and cellular responses to external stimuli (67 proteins; log$_{(10)}$FDR = 1.2).

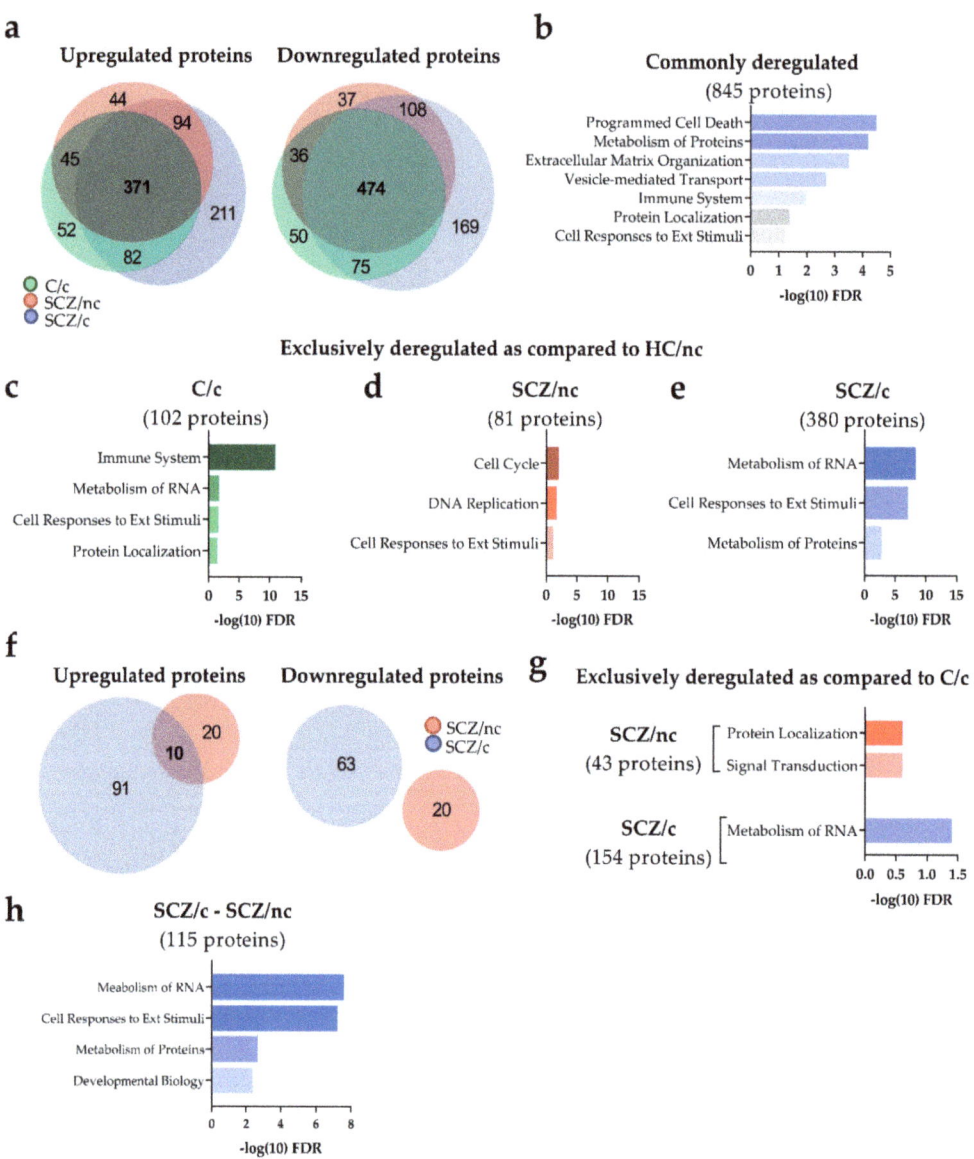

Figure 1. Characterization of the proteome of ON cells from control subjects non-cannabis users (C/nc), control cannabis users (C/c), schizophrenia patients non-cannabis users (SCZ/nc) and schizophrenia patients cannabis users (SCZ/c). (**a**) Proteomic alterations in C/c, SCZ/nc and SCZ/c as compared to C/nc. The upregulated and downregulated proteins in C/c-C/nc, SCZ/nc-C/nc and SCZ/c-C/nc are represented in two different Venn diagrams. (**b**) Enrichment pathway analysis of the 845 proteins commonly deregulated in C/c, SCZ/nc and SCZ/c as compared to C/nc. (**c**) Enrichment pathway analysis of the exclusively deregulated proteins in C/c, (**d**) SCZ/nc (**e**) and SCZ/c versus C/nc. (**f**) Proteomic alterations in SCZ/nc and SCZ/c as compared to C/c. The upregulated and downregulated proteins when SCZ/nc-C/c and SCZ/c-C/c are compared are represented in two Venn diagrams. (**g**) Functional characterization of the 43 proteins deregulated in SCZ/nc

and the 154 proteins deregulated in SCZ/c as compared to C/c. (h) Functional characterization of the 115 proteins deregulated in SCZ/c as compared to SCZ/nc. Data from the pathway analysis are represented as minus the logarithm (10) of the FDR.

The exclusive impact of cannabis on C/c was represented by 102 proteins (Figure 1c), wherein the main pathways affected included the immune system (79 proteins; $\log_{(10)}$FDR = 10.9), metabolism of RNA (21 proteins; $\log_{(10)}$FDR = 1.7), cellular responses to external stimuli (19 proteins; $\log_{(10)}$FDR = 1.6) and protein localization (7 proteins; $\log_{(10)}$FDR = 1.4). When comparing the two groups of SCZ vs. C/nc, we detected a substantial difference (Figure 1d). SCZ/nc only showed 81 exclusively deregulated proteins, whereas 380 were deregulated in SCZ/c. The functional characterization of the 81 proteins deregulated in SCZ/nc indicated that most of them were involved in cell cycle (16 proteins; $\log_{(10)}$FDR = 2.0), DNA replication (6 proteins; $\log_{(10)}$FDR = 1.7) and cellular responses to external stimuli (11 proteins; $\log_{(10)}$FDR = 1.2). On the other hand, the 380 proteins deregulated in SCZ/c (Figure 1e) were associated with metabolism of RNA (61 proteins; $\log_{(10)}$FDR = 8.3), cellular responses to external stimuli (54 proteins; $\log_{(10)}$FDR = 7.1) and metabolism of proteins (104 proteins; $\log_{(10)}$FDR = 2.8).

3.3.2. Quantitative and Functional Proteomic Profile of ON Cells from SCZ Patients as Compared to C/nc

To identify disease-exclusive protein markers, and tease out the effect of cannabis use, the exclusively deregulated proteins in SCZ/nc and SCZ/c were compared to C/c (Figure 1f). In total, 53 proteins were deregulated in SCZ/nc, whereas 164 proteins were differentially expressed in SCZ/c. In SCZ/nc, 30 proteins were upregulated and 101 in SCZ/c.

On the other hand, 23 proteins were downregulated in SCZ/nc and 63 in SCZ/c. The Venn diagram revealed that only 10 proteins were commonly upregulated in SCZ/nc and SCZ/c as compared to C/c, wherein none were commonly downregulated. The functional characterization of the 43 exclusively deregulated proteins in SCZ/nc (Figure 1g) indicated that signal transduction (2 proteins; $\log_{(10)}$FDR = 0.6) and protein localization (2 proteins; $\log_{(10)}$FDR = 0.6) were the mainly enriched functions. The 154 exclusively deregulated proteins in SCZ/c unveiled metabolism of RNA (21 proteins; $\log_{(10)}$FDR = 1.4) as the only deregulated cascade. Thus, the profile of deregulated protein pathways in SCZ/c patients as compared to C/c is quantitatively larger and functionally different to the profile observed in SCZ/nc. To further evaluate the specific proteins involved SCZ/nc vs. SCZ/c, we assessed their functional differences. The results showed that 115 proteins were differentially expressed (Figure 1h). These proteins were associated with metabolism of RNA (28 proteins; $\log_{(10)}$FDR = 7.6), cellular responses to external stimuli (27 proteins; $\log_{(10)}$FDR = 7.2), metabolism of proteins (40 proteins; $\log_{(10)}$FDR = 2.7) and developmental biology (25 proteins; $\log_{(10)}$FDR = 2.4). A detailed list of the proteins involved in each comparison can be found in the Supplement Material.

3.3.3. Specific Proteins Markers of SCZ Depending on Cannabis Use

To identify specific protein markers in ON cells of SCZ/nc, we designed a Venn diagram including the 81 proteins exclusively deregulated in SCZ/nc as compared to C/nc; the 115 proteins differently expressed in SCZ/nc as compared to SCZ/c; and the 43 proteins exclusively different between SCZ/nc and C/c (Figure 2a). In total, 3 proteins were commonly deregulated in these comparisons: (i) Cyclin-dependent-like kinase 5 (CDK5), (ii) LSM2 Homolog, U6 Small Nuclear RNA and mRNA Degradation-Associated (LSM2), and (iii) Tyrosine-tRNA ligase, mitochondrial (YARS2). The expression of CDK5 was significantly reduced in SCZ/nc ($p < 0.01$) as compared to C/nc. In addition, a significant increase in the expression of this protein was observed in SCZ/c when compared to SCZ/nc ($p < 0.01$) (Figure 2b). LSM2 was downregulated in SCZ/nc as compared to C/nc ($p < 0.01$) and vs. C/c ($p < 0.01$), and presented a different expression in SCZ/c vs. SCZ/nc

($p < 0.01$) (Figure 2c). YARS2 was significantly downregulated in SCZ/nc as compared to C/c ($p < 0.01$), and vs. SCZ/c ($p < 0.01$) (Figure 2d).

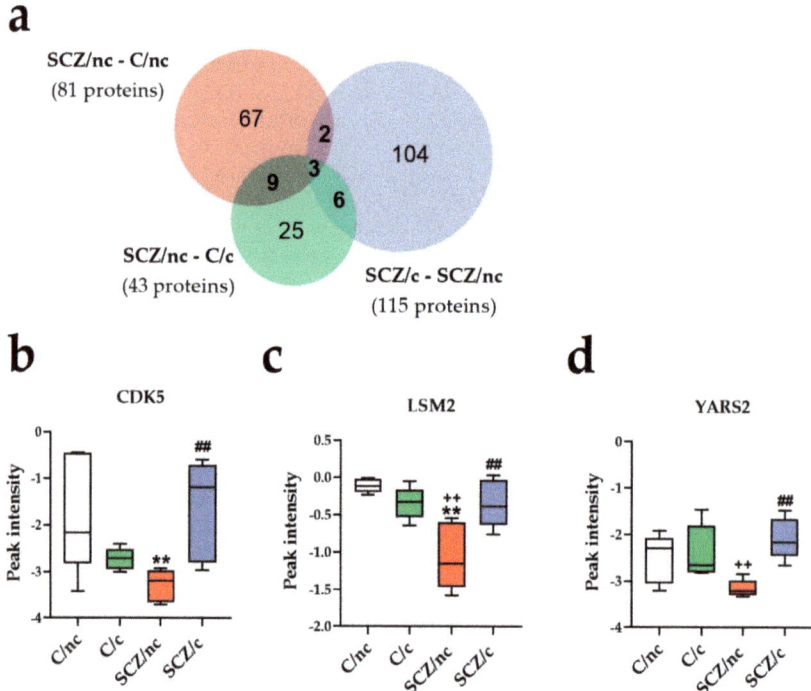

Figure 2. Specific proteomic markers of schizophrenia patients non-cannabis users (SCZ/nc). (**a**) Venn diagram comparing SCZ/nc to control subjects non-cannabis users (C/nc), control cannabis users (C/c) and schizophrenia patients cannabis users (SCZ/c). Graphical representation of CDK5 (**b**), LSM2 (**c**) and YARS2 (**d**), which were commonly deregulated in SCZ/c as compared to C/nc, C/c and SCZ/nc. ** $p < 0.01$; versus C/nc; ++ $p < 0.01$ versus C/c; ## $p < 0.01$ versus SCZ/nc.

To identify specific protein markers in the ON cells of SCZ/c, the 380 proteins exclusively deregulated in SCZ/c as compared to C/nc, the 115 proteins differently expressed in SCZ/c as compared to SCZ/nc, and the 154 proteins exclusively differing between SCZ/c and C/c, were compared (Figure 3a). Seven proteins were commonly deregulated in these three comparisons; (i) CDK5 regulatory subunit-associated protein 3 (CDKRAP3); (ii) Haloacid dehalogenase-like hydrolase domain-containing 5 (HDHD5); (iii) Exosome RNA helicase MTR4 (MTREX); (iv) Unconventional myosin-Ib (MYO1B); (v) 40S ribosomal protein S20 (RPS20); (vi) Nucleoporin SEH1 (SEH1L), and (vii) DBIRD complex subunit ZNF326 (ZNF326). CDK5RAP3 was significantly upregulated in SCZ/c as compared to C/nc, C/c and SCZ/nc ($p < 0.001$, $p < 0.05$, $p < 0.05$, respectively) (Figure 3b). HDHD5 was not significantly altered when the four groups were compared together. MTREX was downregulated in SCZ/c ($p < 0.001$) and SCZ/nc ($p < 0.05$) as compared to C/nc. SCZ/c showed a significant downregulation in its expression as compared to C/c ($p < 0.05$) (Figure 3c). MYO1B was significantly upregulated in SCZ/c as compared to C/nc ($p < 0.01$) and C/c and SCZ/nc ($p < 0.05$) (Figure 3d). RPS20 was downregulated in SCZ/c only, as compared to non-cannabis users ($p < 0.001$ vs. C/nc and $p < 0.05$ vs. SCZ/nc) (Figure 3e). SEH1L was significantly upregulated in SCZ/c as compared to C/nc ($p < 0.01$), C/c and SCZ/nc ($p < 0.05$) (Figure 3f). Finally, ZNF326 was significantly upregulated in SCZ/c as compared to C/nc ($p < 0.001$) and C/c and SCZ/nc ($p < 0.05$) (Figure 3g).

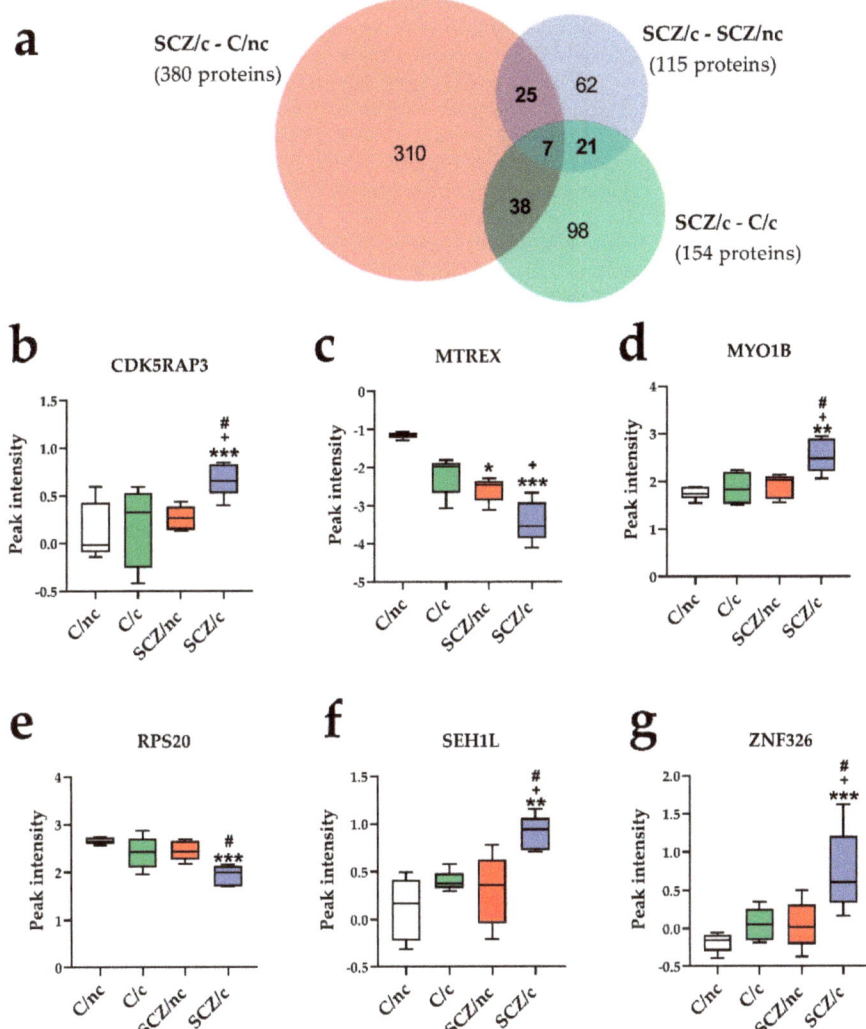

Figure 3. Specific proteome markers of schizophrenia patients cannabis users (SCZ/c). (**a**) Venn diagram comparing SCZ/c to control subjects non-cannabis users (C/nc), schizophrenia patients non-cannabis users (SCZ/nc), and control cannabis users (C/c). Graphical representation of CDK5RAP3 (**b**), MTREX (**c**), MYO1B (**d**), RPS20 (**e**), SEH1L (**f**), and ZNF326 (**g**), which were commonly deregulated in SCZ/c as compared to C/nc, C/c and SCZ/c. Data are represented as the mean ± minimum to maximum peak intensity. * $p < 0.05$; ** $p < 0.01$; *** $p < 0001$ versus C/nc; + $p < 0.05$ versus C/c; # $p < 0.05$; versus SCZ/nc.

3.4. Correlations between Specific Protein Markers, Cannabis Use and Cognitive Performance

A Spearman correlation plot was designed to evaluate the association between the expression levels of target proteins identified in SCZ/nc and in SCZ/c with cognitive performance, cannabis use patterns, and clinical signs in the entire population. For proteins related to SCZ/nc, the results showed that higher LSM2 expression was correlated with better GAF ($r = 0.50$, $p < 0.05$) and less NSS ($r = -0.54$, $p < 0.05$), whereas higher YARS2 levels were associated with better attentional performance in the direct series score test ($r = 0.53$, $p < 0.05$) (Data not shown). For proteins related to SCZ/c, MYO1B negatively correlated with plasmatic THC-COOH concentration (r = −0.80, $p < 0.05$) (Figure 4a), and ZNF326 positively correlated with cannabis use duration (r = 0.81, $p < 0.01$) (Figure 4b). MTREX showed a positive correlation with attentional performance in the direct spatial span test (r = 0.52, $p < 0.05$) (Figure 4c), and with better verbal fluency scores (r = 0.50, $p < 0.05$) (Figure 4d). Moreover, MTREX positively correlated with GAF (r = 0.73, $p < 0.001$) (Figure 4e), and correlated negatively with NSS (r = −0.65, $p < 0.01$) (Figure 4f). In addition, ZNF326 negatively correlated with attention in the direct spatial span test (r = −0.57, $p < 0.01$) (Figure 4j); with working memory in the inverse spatial span test (r = −0.51, $p < 0.05$) (Figure 4g); and with emotional recognition scores (r = −0.55, $p < 0.05$) (Figure 4h). Finally, higher ZNF326 correlated with lower GAF (r = −0.49, $p < 0.05$) (Figure 4i) and higher NSS (r = 0.52, $p < 0.05$) (Figure 4j). CDK5RAP3 correlated with GAF (r = −0.5, $p < 0.05$) and NSS (r = 0.47, $p < 0.05$) (Supplement Figure S2a,b). MYO1B levels were negatively correlated with GAF scores (r = −0.56, $p < 0.05$) and positively with NSS (r = 0.48, $p < 0.05$) (Supplementary Figure S2c,d). Finally, RPS20 was positively associated with GAF (r = −0.50, $p < 0.05$) (Supplementary Figure S2e), while SEH1L showed a significant negative correlation with this parameter (r = 0.48, $p < 0.05$) (Supplementary Figure S2f).

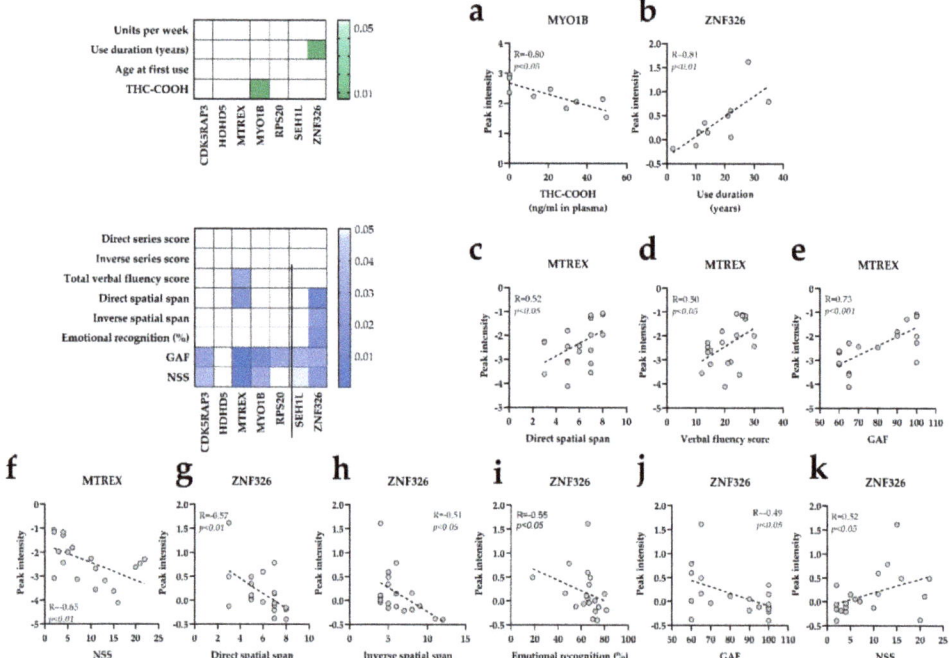

Figure 4. Association studies of protein markers, cannabis use and neurocognitive performance. (**a**) THC-COOH (ng/mL plasma) and MYO1B correlation. (**b**) Use duration and ZNF326 spearman correlation. (**c**) MTREX and direct spatial span correlation. (**d**) MTREX and verbal fluency score correlation. (**e**) MTREX and GAF correlation. (**f**) MTREX and NSS correlation. (**g**) ZNF326 and direct spatial span correlation. (**h**) ZNF326 and inverse spatial span correlation. (**i**) ZNF326 and emotional recognition correlation. (**j**) ZNF326 and GAF correlation. (**k**) ZNF326 and NSS correlation. In the correlation matrixes, only the significant correlations are colored. Darker squares indicate lower p-values.

4. Discussion

In this study we revealed a quantitative shared impact of cannabis use and SCZ. These results are consistent with recent GWAS studies showing a significant common genetic risk of SCZ and cannabis use [29]. Interestingly, when assessing the exclusively deregulated proteins, we observed a functional selectivity among the different groups. Thus, the most significantly deregulated pathway in C/c was the immune system cascade, while in SCZ/c metabolism of RNA, cell responses to external stimuli and metabolism of proteins showed strong and significant alterations. In SCZ/nc, smaller but significant deregulations were observed in cell cycle, DNA replication and cell responses to external stimuli cascades. These findings indicate that despite the common proteomic changes induced by cannabis use and SCZ, there might be specific changes prompted in the proteome depending on whether these two factors are present together or separately. In fact, when we subtracted the effect of cannabis comparing both groups of SCZ patients with C/c, we found a more similar profile between SCZ/nc and C/c, with small deregulations in protein localization and signal transduction, than in SCZ/c and C/c, which showed larger changes only in metabolism of RNA. Moreover, when the exclusively deregulated proteins were compared in both groups of SCZ patients, differences were obtained for metabolism of RNA and cellular responses to external stimuli. Again, these comparisons revealed functional differences in the proteomic alterations induced by the presence of SCZ depending on whether patients use cannabis or not.

Therefore, to identify specific proteins that could be proteomic markers of SCZ with or without the concomitant use of cannabis, we assessed separately the commonly deregulated proteins in SCZ/nc and in SCZ/c with respect to all the other groups. In SCZ/nc, we found three protein markers: CDK5, LSM2 and YARS2. These proteins were significantly downregulated in SCZ/nc, but not in SCZ/c. CDK5 is a cyclin-dependent kinase that controls the development of the central nervous system [34]. In the mature brain, it is associated with cognitive processes [35], and in vitro, it modulates oxidative stress responses [36]. According to the REACTOME database, it participates in developmental biology, which functionally differentiates SCZ/nc from SCZ/c. The observed reduction in CDK5 expression is consistent with previous studies showing a significant decline in CDK5 expression in postmortem brain samples of antipsychotic-treated SCZ patients, but not in drug-naïve individuals [37]. Markedly, our data indicate that cannabis use may counteract the effects of SCZ on CDK5. Further studies may shed light on whether cannabis use also opposes antipsychotic efficiency through this mechanism. Secondly, the downregulation of LSM2, which encodes for a key protein of the spliceosome [38], is in agreement with previously reported global changes in alternative splicing in SCZ patients [39]. LSM2 participates in metabolism of RNA, which differentiated SCZ/nc from SCZ/c, and presented a positive correlation with GAF and a negative correlation with NSS, indicating that it may be relevant for the clinical alterations observed in SCZ. Thirdly, we show a decrease in YARS2, a tyrosyl-tRNA synthetase located in the mitochondria, involved in metabolism of proteins, which differentiated SCZ/nc from SCZ/c. Its downregulation may lead to respiratory chain dysfunctions causing mitochondrial oxidative stress [40], which has been observed in postmortem brain samples from SCZ patients [41,42]. Moreover, lower levels of YARS2 could be correlated with worse attention performance, consistent with previous studies reporting that an oxidative imbalance increases negative symptoms' severity in SCZ patients [43]. Once more, cannabis use seems to counteract the molecular changes in YARS2 in ON cells of SCZ/c, hypothetically via CB_1 receptors expressed in the mitochondrial membranes [44], which have been proven to modulate respiration in this organelle [45].

In SCZ/c, we identified expression level changes in seven proteins: CDK5RAP3, HDHD5, MYO1B, MTREX, RPS20, SEH1L, and ZNF326. CDK5RAP3, a regulator of CDK5, was significantly upregulated in SCZ/c with respect to all other groups. It is genetically associated with SCZ [46], and participates in cell cycle. It modulates hippocampal aging because its transcriptional upregulation lowers neurogenesis [47]. Higher levels of this protein were associated with less GAF and more NSS in the entire population. MYO1B, SEH1L and RPS20 were also deregulated, specifically in SCZ/c, and were associated with clinical outcomes (GAF and NSS). They are involved in the metabolism of proteins cascade, which includes the AKT-mTOR pathway that is thought to play a role in the interaction between

SCZ and cannabinoids exposure in humans [48] and in mice models [24]. In fact, MYO1B, SEH1L and RPS20 directly or indirectly interact with AKT-mTOR [49–51]. Interestingly, we found a negative correlation between MYO1B and plasmatic concentrations of THC-COOH in SCZ/c and C/c. THC-COOH is the last molecule arising from Δ^9-tetrahidrocannabinol degradation [52], which might point to the role of this unconventional myosin in cannabis metabolism. Finally, MTREX and ZNF326, which are involved in the metabolism of RNA cascade, were found to be deregulated in SCZ/c as compared to the rest of the groups. In fact, metabolism of RNA was consistently deregulated in SCZ/c in every functional comparison. Although prior studies have found deregulations in ribosomal and RNA-related proteins in human samples from SCZ patients [53,54], our data revealed functional differences in metabolism of RNA exclusively linked to the coexistence of cannabis consumption and SCZ. According to REACTOME, MTREX and ZNF326 are involved in the same step of pre-mRNA processing prior to protein translation. However, we found that MTREX was significantly downregulated in SCZ/nc and SCZ/c, while ZNF326 was upregulated in SCZ/c, but both of these alterations correlated with worse cognitive performance and more clinical signs of SCZ. Thus, a lower peak intensity of MTREX was associated with worse spatial attention, verbal fluency, and GAF scores, but with more NSS. On the other hand, higher peak intensity levels of ZNF326 were related with worse attention, working memory, emotional recognition, and clinical signs. Moreover, cannabis use duration positively correlated with ZNF326 expression. These data indicate that either a decrease in MTREX or an increase in ZNF326 expression may have a negative effect on RNA metabolism, which could impact neurocognitive functioning.

The results of our study need to be interpreted considering its strengths and limitations. The main strength of our data relies on the translational power of ON cell models to investigate biomarkers of neuropsychiatric disorders, such as SCZ. In addition, the evaluation of cannabis' effects on separate cohorts of SCZ patients is unique, since there is an absence of studies comparing these populations. The main limitation of our study was the small number of subjects per group, thus, additional follow-up studies on a larger scale, including longitudinal and epidemiological studies, will be needed to further corroborate these findings.

In summary, we revealed a quantitative shared effect of SCZ and cannabis use in the proteomic profile of ON cells, consistent with the genetic similarities previously described [29]. We found that cannabis use in controls has a significant impact on the immune system, while it alters metabolism of RNA and metabolism of proteins in SCZ patients. Additionally, SCZ/nc show small but significant differences in cell cycle, DNA replication, proteins localization and signal transduction. In this group, we identified significant changes in two functionally relevant proteins (YARS2 and LSM2) associated to attentional processes, GAF and NSS scores. On the other hand, in ON cells from SCZ/c we found significant changes in six proteins relevant to clinical scores (MYO1B, MTREX, ZNF326, RPS20, CDK5RAP3, SEH1L) and two for cannabis use (MYO1B, ZNF326). Moreover, in SCZ/c, we identified consistent deregulation in metabolism of RNA in every comparison, and expression levels of MTREX and ZNF326, which take part in this pathway, correlated with several aspects of cognitive performance.

Supplementary Materials: The following are available online at https://www.mdpi.com/2075-4426/11/3/160/s1, Supplementary Figure S1, Supplementary Figure S2, Supplementary Material.

Author Contributions: Experimental design, M.B.-C., P.R.; methodology, M.B.-C., K.A., M.L.-M., J.F.-I., E.S., P.R.; software, M.B.-C., K.A., M.L.-M., J.F.-I., E.S., P.R.; investigation, M.B.-C., C.F.-A., L.G., A.C.-R., P.R.; writing—original draft preparation, M.B.-C., P.R.; writing—review and editing, M.B.-C. and P.R.; supervision, R.d.l.T., V.P., E.S., P.R.; project administration, R.d.l.T., V.P., P.R.; funding acquisition, E.S., J.F.-I., P.R. All authors have read and agreed to the published version of the manuscript.

Funding: This work was supported by grants from DIUE de la Generalitat de Catalunya (2017-SGR-1497), Instituto de Salud Carlos III, (PI18/00053 to P.R.) FIS-FEDER FUNDS, the Spanish Ministry of Science Innovation and Universities (PID2019-110356RB-I00 to ES and JFI), and Department of Economic and Business Development from Government of Navarra (ref. 0011-1411-2020-000028) to ES. The Proteomics Platform of Navarrabiomed is a member of Proteored (PRB3-ISCIII) and is supported by grant PT17/0019/009 to J.F.-I., of the PE I + D + I 2013-2016 funded by ISCIII and FEDER. We would like to acknowledge the Clinical Research Unit at the IMIM-Hospital del Mar Research Institute for their expertise in nasal brushing, especially Marta Pérez Otero and Dr. Ana M. Aldea Perona. The authors thank all the PRIDE Team for helping with the mass spectrometric data deposit in ProteomeXChange/PRIDE. The Clinical Neuroproteomics Unit of Navarrabiomed is a member of the Spanish Olfactory Network (ROE) (supported by grant RED2018-102662-T funded by Spanish Ministry of Science and Innovation).

Institutional Review Board Statement: The study was conducted according to the guidelines of the Declaration of Helsinki, and approved by the Ethics Committee of the Parc de Salut Mar Clinical Research (CEIC; protocol code IMIMFTCL/SC/1, 13-3-2015).

Informed Consent Statement: Informed consent was obtained from all subjects involved in the study.

Data Availability Statement: In All MS raw data and search results files have been deposited into the ProteomeXchange Consortium (http://proteomecentral.proteomexchange.org) via the PRIDE partner repository with the dataset identifiers PXD020739 (Reviewer account details: Username: reviewer15955@ebi.ac.uk; Password: UDhwtjVV).

Conflicts of Interest: The authors declare no conflict of interest.

References

1. Van Os, J.; Rutten, B.P.F.; Poulton, R. Gene-environment interactions in schizophrenia: Review of epidemiological findings and future directions. *Schizophr. Bull.* **2008**, *34*, 1066–1082. [CrossRef]
2. Nascimento, J.M.; Martins-De-Souza, D. The proteome of schizophrenia. *NPJ Schizophr.* **2015**, *1*, 14003. [CrossRef]
3. Jaros, J.A.J.; Martins-de-Souza, D.; Rahmoune, H.; Rothermundt, M.; Leweke, F.M.; Guest, P.C.; Bahn, S. Protein phosphorylation patterns in serum from schizophrenia patients and healthy controls. *J. Proteom.* **2012**, *76*, 43–55. [CrossRef] [PubMed]
4. Yang, Y.; Wan, C.; Li, H.; Zhu, H.; La, Y.; Xi, Z.; Chen, Y.; Jiang, L.; Feng, G.; He, L. Altered levels of acute phase proteins in the plasma of patients with schizophrenia. *Anal. Chem.* **2006**, *78*, 3571–3576. [CrossRef] [PubMed]
5. Huang, J.T.J.; Wang, L.; Prabakaran, S.; Wengenroth, M.; Lockstone, H.E.; Koethe, D.; Gerth, C.W.; Gross, S.; Schreiber, D.; Lilley, K.; et al. Independent protein-profiling studies show a decrease in apolipoprotein A1 levels in schizophrenia CSF, brain and peripheral tissues. *Mol. Psychiatry* **2008**, *13*, 1118–1128. [CrossRef] [PubMed]
6. Khandaker, G.M.; Dantzer, R. Is there a role for immune-to-brain communication in schizophrenia? *Psychopharmacology* **2016**, *233*, 1559–1573. [CrossRef]
7. Boiko, A.S.; Mednova, I.A.; Kornetova, E.G.; Semke, A.V.; Bokhan, N.A.; Loonen, A.J.M.; Ivanova, S.A. Apolipoprotein serum levels related to metabolic syndrome in patients with schizophrenia. *Heliyon* **2019**, *5*, e02033. [CrossRef]
8. Föcking, M.; Dicker, P.; English, J.A.; Schubert, K.O.; Dunn, M.J.; Cotter, D.R. Common proteomic changes in the hippocampus in schizophrenia and bipolar disorder and particular evidence for involvement of cornu ammonis regions 2 and 3. *Arch. Gen. Psychiatry* **2011**, *68*, 477–488. [CrossRef] [PubMed]
9. Martins-de-Souza, D.; Maccarrone, G.; Wobrock, T.; Zerr, I.; Gormanns, P.; Reckow, S.; Falkai, P.; Schmitt, A.; Turck, C.W. Proteome analysis of the thalamus and cerebrospinal fluid reveals glycolysis dysfunction and potential biomarkers candidates for schizophrenia. *J. Psychiatr. Res.* **2010**, *44*, 1176–1189. [CrossRef]
10. Wesseling, H.; Chan, M.K.; Tsang, T.M.; Ernst, A.; Peters, F.; Guest, P.C.; Holmes, E.; Bahn, S. A combined metabonomic and proteomic approach identifies frontal cortex changes in a chronic phencyclidine rat model in relation to human schizophrenia brain pathology. *Neuropsychopharmacology* **2013**, *38*, 2532–2544. [CrossRef]
11. Beasley, C.L.; Pennington, K.; Behan, A.; Wait, R.; Dunn, M.J.; Cotter, D. Proteomic analysis of the anterior cingulate cortex in the major psychiatric disorders: Evidence for disease-associated changes. *Proteomics* **2006**, *6*, 3414–3425. [CrossRef]
12. Saia-Cereda, V.M.; Cassoli, J.S.; Martins-de-Souza, D.; Nascimento, J.M. Psychiatric disorders biochemical pathways unraveled by human brain proteomics. *Eur. Arch. Psychiatry Clin. Neurosci.* **2017**, *267*, 3–17. [CrossRef] [PubMed]
13. Willard, S.L.; Sinclair, D.; Mirza, N.; Turetsky, B.; Berretta, S.; Hahn, C. Translational potential of olfactory mucosa for the study of neuropsychiatric illness. *Transl. Psychiatry* **2015**, *5*, e527-12. [CrossRef]
14. Mackay-Sim, A. Concise review: Patient-derived olfactory stem cells: New models for brain diseases. *Stem Cells* **2012**, *30*, 2361–2365. [CrossRef]
15. Benítez-King, G.; Riquelme, A.; Ortíz-López, L.; Berlanga, C.; Rodríguez-Verdugo, M.S.; Romo, F.; Calixto, E.; Solís-Chagoyán, H.; Jímenez, M.; Montaño, L.M.; et al. A non-invasive method to isolate the neuronal linage from the nasal epithelium from schizophrenic and bipolar diseases. *J. Neurosci. Methods* **2011**, *201*, 35–45. [CrossRef]

16. Galindo, L.; Moreno, E.; Lopez-Armenta, F.; Guinart, D.; Cuenca-Royo, A.; Izquierdo-Serra, M.; Xicota, L.; Fernandez, C.; Menoyo, E.; Fernandez-Fernandez, J.M.; et al. Cannabis Users Show Enhanced Expression of CB1-5HT2A Receptor Heteromers in Olfactory Neuroepithelium Cells. *Mol. Neurobiol.* **2018**, *55*, 6347–6361. [CrossRef]
17. Ortiz-Medina, M.B.; Perea, M.; Torales, J.; Ventriglio, A.; Vitrani, G.; Aguilar, L.; Roncero, C. Cannabis consumption and psychosis or schizophrenia development. *Int. J. Soc. Psychiatry* **2018**, *64*, 690–704. [CrossRef]
18. Di Forti, M.; Quattrone, D.; Freeman, T.P.; Tripoli, G.; Gayer-Anderson, C.; Quigley, H.; Rodriguez, V.; Jongsma, H.E.; Ferraro, L.; La Cascia, C.; et al. The contribution of cannabis use to variation in the incidence of psychotic disorder across Europe (EU-GEI): A multicentre case-control study. *Lancet Psychiatry* **2019**, *6*, 427–436. [CrossRef]
19. Muguruza, C.; Morentin, B.; Meana, J.J.; Alexander, S.P.H.; Callado, L.F. Endocannabinoid system imbalance in the postmortem prefrontal cortex of subjects with schizophrenia. *J. Psychopharmacol.* **2019**, *33*, 1132–1140. [CrossRef]
20. Bioque, M.; García-Bueno, B.; MacDowell, K.S.; Meseguer, A.; Saiz, P.A.; Parellada, M.; Gonzalez-Pinto, A.; Rodriguez-Jimenez, R.; Lobo, A.; Leza, J.C.; et al. Peripheral endocannabinoid system dysregulation in first-episode psychosis. *Neuropsychopharmacology* **2013**, *38*, 2568–2577. [CrossRef] [PubMed]
21. Twitchell, W.; Brown, S.; Mackie, K. Cannabinoids inhibit n- and p/q-type calcium channels in cultured rat hippocampal neurons. *J. Neurophysiol.* **1997**, *78*, 43–50. [CrossRef]
22. Fisyunov, A.; Tsintsadze, V.; Min, R.; Burnashev, N.; Lozovaya, N. Cannabinoids modulate the P-type high-voltage-activated calcium currents in Purkinje neurons. *J. Neurophysiol.* **2006**, *96*, 1267–1277. [CrossRef]
23. Miller, M.L.; Chadwick, B.; Dickstein, D.L.; Purushothaman, I.; Egervari, G.; Rahman, T.; Tessereau, C.; Hof, P.R.; Roussos, P.; Shen, L.; et al. Adolescent exposure to Δ 9 -tetrahydrocannabinol alters the transcriptional trajectory and dendritic architecture of prefrontal pyramidal neurons. *Mol. Psychiatry* **2019**, *24*, 588–600. [CrossRef] [PubMed]
24. Ibarra-Lecue, I.; Mollinedo-Gajate, I.; Meana, J.J.; Callado, L.F.; Diez-Alarcia, R.; Urigüen, L. Chronic cannabis promotes pro-hallucinogenic signaling of 5-HT2A receptors through Akt/mTOR pathway. *Neuropsychopharmacology* **2018**, *43*, 2028–2035. [CrossRef] [PubMed]
25. Jayanthi, S.; Buie, S.; Moore, S.; Herning, R.I.; Better, W.; Wilson, N.M.; Contoreggi, C.; Cadet, J.L. Heavy marijuana users show increased serum apolipoprotein C-III levels: Evidence from proteomic analyses. *Mol. Psychiatry* **2010**, *15*, 101–112. [CrossRef]
26. Saladrigas-Manjón, S.; Dučić, T.; Galindo, L.; Fernández-Avilés, C.; Pérez, V.; de la Torre, R.; Robledo, P. Effects of cannabis use on the protein and lipid profile of olfactory neuroepithelium cells from schizophrenia patients studied by synchrotron-based FTIR spectroscopy. *Biomolecules* **2020**, *10*, 329. [CrossRef]
27. Guinart, D.; Moreno, E.; Galindo, L.; Cuenca-Royo, A.; Barrera-Conde, M.; Pérez, E.J.; Fernández-Avilés, C.; Correll, C.U.; Canela, E.I.; Casadó, V.; et al. Altered Signaling in CB1R-5-HT2AR Heteromers in Olfactory Neuroepithelium Cells of Schizophrenia Patients is Modulated by Cannabis Use. *Schizophr. Bull.* **2020**, *46*, 1547–1557. [CrossRef]
28. Lachén-Montes, M.; Mendizuri, N.; Ausín, K.; Pérez-Mediavilla, A.; Azkargorta, M.; Iloro, I.; Elortza, F.; Kondo, H.; Ohigashi, I.; Ferrer, I.; et al. Smelling the Dark Proteome: Functional Characterization of PITH Domain-Containing Protein 1 (C1orf128) in Olfactory Metabolism. *J. Proteome Res.* **2020**, *19*, 4826–4843. [CrossRef]
29. Pasman, J.A.; Verweij, K.J.H.; Gerring, Z.; Stringer, S.; Sanchez-roige, S.; Treur, J.L.; Abdellaoui, A.; Nivard, M.G.; Baselmans, B.M.L.; Ong, J.; et al. A Causal Influence of Schizophrenia. *Nat. Neurosci.* **2018**, *21*, 1161–1170. [CrossRef]
30. Gillet, L.C.; Navarro, P.; Tate, S.; Röst, H.; Selevsek, N.; Reiter, L.; Bonner, R.; Aebersold, R. Targeted data extraction of the MS/MS spectra generated by data-independent acquisition: A new concept for consistent and accurate proteome analysis. *Mol. Cell. Proteom.* **2012**, *11*, 1–17. [CrossRef]
31. Jassal, B.; Matthews, L.; Viteri, G.; Gong, C.; Lorente, P.; Fabregat, A.; Sidiropoulos, K.; Cook, J.; Gillespie, M.; Haw, R.; et al. The reactome pathway knowledgebase. *Nucleic Acids Res.* **2020**, *48*, D498–D503. [CrossRef]
32. Hulsen, T.; de Vlieg, J.; Alkema, W. BioVenn—A web application for the comparison and visualization of biological lists using area-proportional Venn diagrams. *BMC Genom.* **2008**, *9*, 488. [CrossRef]
33. Geyer, P.E.; Holdt, L.M.; Teupser, D.; Mann, M. Revisiting biomarker discovery by plasma proteomics. *Mol. Syst. Biol.* **2017**, *13*, 942. [CrossRef]
34. Cruz, J.C.; Tseng, H.C.; Goldman, J.A.; Shih, H.; Tsai, L.H. Aberrant Cdk5 activation by p25 triggers pathological events leading to neurodegeneration and neurofibrillary tangles. *Neuron* **2003**, *40*, 471–483. [CrossRef]
35. Nishi, A.; Bibb, J.A.; Matsuyama, S.; Hamada, M.; Higashi, H.; Nairn, A.C.; Greengard, P. Regulation of DARPP-32 dephosphorylation at PKA- and Cdk5-sites by NMDA and AMPA receptors: Distinct roles of calcineurin and protein phosphatase-2A. *J. Neurochem.* **2002**, 832–841. [CrossRef] [PubMed]
36. Jimenez-Blasco, D.; Santofimia-Castaño, P.; Gonzalez, A.; Almeida, A.; Bolaños, J.P. Astrocyte NMDA receptors' activity sustains neuronal survival through a Cdk5-Nrf2 pathway. *Cell Death Differ.* **2015**, *22*, 1877–1889. [CrossRef] [PubMed]
37. Ramos-Miguel, A.; Javier Meana, J.; García-Sevilla, J.A. Cyclin-dependent kinase-5 and p35/p25 activators in schizophrenia and major depression prefrontal cortex: Basal contents and effects of psychotropic medications. *Int. J. Neuropsychopharmacol.* **2013**, *16*, 683–689. [CrossRef]
38. Bertram, K.; Agafonov, D.E.; Dybkov, O.; Haselbach, D.; Leelaram, M.N.; Will, C.L.; Urlaub, H.; Kastner, B.; Lührmann, R.; Stark, H. Cryo-EM Structure of a Pre-catalytic Human Spliceosome Primed for Activation. *Cell* **2017**, *170*, 701–713.e11. [CrossRef]
39. Reble, E.; Dineen, A.; Barr, C.L. The contribution of alternative splicing to genetic risk for psychiatric disorders. *Genes Brain Behav.* **2018**, *17*, 1–12. [CrossRef] [PubMed]

40. Riley, L.G.; Cooper, S.; Hickey, P.; Rudinger-Thirion, J.; McKenzie, M.; Compton, A.; Lim, S.C.; Thorburn, D.; Ryan, M.T.; Giegé, R.; et al. Mutation of the mitochondrial tyrosyl-tRNA synthetase gene, YARS2, causes myopathy, lactic acidosis, and sideroblastic anemia—MLASA syndrome. *Am. J. Hum. Genet.* **2010**, *87*, 52–59. [CrossRef] [PubMed]
41. Rezin, G.T.; Amboni, G.; Zugno, A.I.; Quevedo, J.; Streck, E.L. Mitochondrial dysfunction and psychiatric disorders. *Neurochem. Res.* **2009**, *34*, 1021–1029. [CrossRef] [PubMed]
42. Maurer, I.; Zierz, S.; Möller, H.J. Evidence for a mitochondrial oxidative phosphorylation defect in brains from patients with schizophrenia. *Schizophr. Res.* **2001**, *48*, 125–136. [CrossRef]
43. Gunes, M.; Altindag, A.; Bulut, M.; Demir, S.; Ibiloglu, A.O.; Kaya, M.C.; Atli, A.; Aksoy, N. Oxidative metabolism may be associated with negative symptoms in schizophrenia. *Psychiatry Clin. Psychopharmacol.* **2017**, *27*, 54–61. [CrossRef]
44. Melser, S.; Zottola, A.C.P.; Serrat, R.; Puente, N.; Grandes, P.; Marsicano, G.; Hebert-Chatelain, E. *Functional Analysis of Mitochondrial CB1 Cannabinoid Receptors (mtCB1) in the Brain*, 1st ed.; Elsevier Inc.: Amsterdam, The Netherlands, 2017; Volume 593.
45. Bénard, G.; Massa, F.; Puente, N.; Lourenço, J.; Bellocchio, L.; Soria-Gómez, E.; Matias, I.; Delamarre, A.; Metna-Laurent, M.; Cannich, A.; et al. Mitochondrial CB 1 receptors regulate neuronal energy metabolism. *Nat. Neurosci.* **2012**, *15*, 558–564. [CrossRef] [PubMed]
46. Camargo, L.M.; Collura, V.; Rain, J.C.; Mizuguchi, K.; Hermjakob, H.; Kerrien, S.; Bonnert, T.P.; Whiting, P.J.; Brandon, N.J. Disrupted in Schizophrenia 1 interactome: Evidence for the close connectivity of risk genes and a potential synaptic basis for schizophrenia. *Mol. Psychiatry* **2007**, *12*, 74–86. [CrossRef]
47. Shetty, G.A.; Hattiangady, B.; Shetty, A.K. Neural stem cell- and neurogenesis-related gene expression profiles in the young and aged dentate gyrus. *Age* **2013**, *35*, 2165–2176. [CrossRef] [PubMed]
48. Di Forti, M.; Iyegbe, C.; Sallis, H.; Kolliakou, A.; Falcone, M.A.; Paparelli, A.; Sirianni, M.; La Cascia, C.; Stilo, S.A.; Marques, T.R.; et al. Confirmation that the AKT1 (rs2494732) genotype influences the risk of psychosis in cannabis users. *Biol. Psychiatry* **2012**, *72*, 811–816. [CrossRef]
49. Platani, M.; Samejima, I.; Samejima, K.; Kanemaki, M.T.; Earnshaw, W.C. Seh1 targets GATOR2 and Nup153 to mitotic chromosomes. *J. Cell Sci.* **2018**, *131*, jcs213140. [CrossRef]
50. Salas-Cortes, L.; Ye, F.; Tenza, D.; Wilhelm, C.; Theos, A.; Louvard, D.; Raposo, G.; Coudrier, E. Myosin Ib modulates the morphology and the protein transport within multi-vesicular sorting endosomes. *J. Cell Sci.* **2005**, *118*, 4823–4832. [CrossRef]
51. Yu, Y.; Xiong, Y.; Montani, J.P.; Yang, Z.; Ming, X.F. Arginase-II activates mTORC1 through myosin-1b in vascular cell senescence and apoptosis. *Cell Death Dis.* **2018**, *9*, 313. [CrossRef]
52. Sharma, P.; Murthy, P.; Bharath, M.M.S. Chemistry, metabolism, and toxicology of cannabis: Clinical implications. *Iran. J. Psychiatry* **2012**, *7*, 149–156. [PubMed]
53. English, J.A.; Fan, Y.; Föcking, M.; Lopez, L.M.; Hryniewiecka, M.; Wynne, K.; Dicker, P.; Matigian, N.; Cagney, G. Reduced protein synthesis in schizophrenia patient-derived olfactory cells. *Transl. Psychiatry* **2015**, *5*, e663. [CrossRef] [PubMed]
54. Ibarra-Lecue, I.; Diez-Alarcia, R.; Morentin, B.; Meana, J.J.; Callado, L.F.; Urigüen, L. Ribosomal Protein S6 Hypofunction in Postmortem Human Brain Links mTORC1-Dependent Signaling and Schizophrenia. *Front. Pharmacol.* **2020**, *11*, 344. [CrossRef] [PubMed]

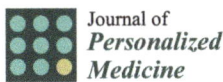

Communication

Genetic Polymorphisms of *5-HT* Receptors and Antipsychotic-Induced Metabolic Dysfunction in Patients with Schizophrenia

Diana Z. Paderina [1], Anastasiia S. Boiko [1], Ivan V. Pozhidaev [1], Anna V. Bocharova [2], Irina A. Mednova [1], Olga Yu. Fedorenko [1], Elena G. Kornetova [1,3], Anton J.M. Loonen [4,*], Arkadiy V. Semke [1], Nikolay A. Bokhan [1,3] and Svetlana A. Ivanova [1,3]

1. Mental Health Research Institute, Tomsk National Research Medical Center of the Russian Academy of Sciences, 634014 Tomsk, Russia; osmanovadiana@mail.ru (D.Z.P.); anastasya-iv@yandex.ru (A.S.B.); craig1408@yandex.ru (I.V.P.); irinka145@yandex.ru (I.A.M.); f_o_y@mail.ru (O.Y.F.); kornetova@sibmail.com (E.G.K.); asemke@tnimc.ru (A.V.S.); bna909@gmail.com (N.A.B.); ivanovaniipz@gmail.com (S.A.I.)
2. Research Institute of Medical Genetics, Tomsk National Research Medical Center of the Russian Academy of Sciences, 634050 Tomsk, Russia; anna.bocharova@medgenetics.ru
3. Siberian State Medical University, 634050 Tomsk, Russia
4. Unit of PharmacoTherapy, -Epidemiology & -Economics, Groningen Research Institute of Pharmacy, University of Groningen, 9713AV Groningen, The Netherlands
* Correspondence: a.j.m.loonen@rug.nl

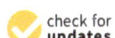

Abstract: Background: Antipsychotic-induced metabolic syndrome (MetS) is a multifactorial disease with a genetic predisposition. Serotonin and its receptors are involved in antipsychotic-drug-induced metabolic disorders. The present study investigated the association of nine polymorphisms in the four 5-hydroxytryptamine receptor (*HTR*) genes *HTR1A*, *HTR2A*, *HTR3A*, and *HTR2C* and the gene encoding for the serotonin transporter *SLC6A4* with MetS in patients with schizophrenia. Methods: A set of nine single-nucleotide polymorphisms of genes of the serotonergic system was investigated in a population of 475 patients from several Siberian regions (Russia) with a clinical diagnosis of schizophrenia. Genotyping was performed and the results were analyzed using chi-square tests. Results: Polymorphic variant rs521018 (*HTR2C*) was associated with higher body mass index in patients receiving long-term antipsychotic therapy, but not with drug-induced metabolic syndrome. Rs1150226 (*HTR3A*) was also associated but did not meet Hardy–Weinberg equilibrium. Conclusions: Our results indicate that allelic variants of *HTR2C* genes may have consequences on metabolic parameters. MetS may have too complex a mechanistic background to be studied without dissecting the syndrome into its individual (causal) components.

Keywords: schizophrenia; antipsychotics; body mass index; weight gain; metabolic syndrome; serotonin; genes; pharmacogenetics

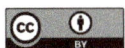

1. Introduction

Antipsychotics are important therapeutic agents for patients with schizophrenia, but long-term use of these drugs increases the risk of developing type 2 diabetes mellitus, hyperlipidemia, and hypertension [1–6]. These drugs are known to increase the prevalence of metabolic syndrome (MetS), which is a clustering of well-known cardiovascular risk factors and is known to be augmented in a variety of psychiatric disorders [6]. Apart from increasing the likelihood of serious cardiovascular and malignant pathologies, significant weight gain can also affect compliance and cause a decrease in the quality of life of patients with schizophrenia, since, in addition to the stigma of schizophrenia, there is the stigma of obesity [7].

Several G protein-coupled receptors, mainly dopamine, serotonin, and noradrenaline receptors, are traditional molecular targets for antipsychotics [8]. The efficacy of classical antipsychotics was mainly associated with the antagonism of dopamine type 2 (D2) receptors. Atypical antipsychotics are far more complex D2 receptor antagonists and act beyond D2 antagonism, involving other receptor targets that regulate dopamine and other neurotransmitters. Therefore, atypical antipsychotics have fewer adverse effects like parkinsonism, hyperprolactinemia, apathy, etc., which are all linked to the strong blockade of D2 receptors [9]. A variety of mechanisms contribute to how treatment with antipsychotic drugs results in metabolic syndrome [3,10,11]. Roughly three components can be distinguished, related to behavioral (reward-seeking, neuropsychoimmunological), hypothalamic endocrine (appetite/satiety), and peripheral (adipocytes, immune system, abdominal organs) regulation [10]. Serotonergic (serotonin, 5-Hydroxytryptamine, 5-HT) neurotransmission appears to be involved in all three of them as well as in the pathophysiology of schizophrenia [12]. Circuits regulating the intensity of reward-seeking and distress-avoiding behaviors are controlled by the habenuloid complex via ascending monoaminergic terminals originating in the upper brainstem [13–15]. Mesencephalic 5-HT neurons projecting to the striatum, prefrontal cortex, and amygdaloid complex increase the intensity of distress-avoiding behavior directly and also indirectly by inhibiting dopaminergic and adrenergic neurons [16–18]. Serotonergic neurotransmission also has a key role concerning obesity through both cerebral and peripheral mechanisms [11,19,20]. Moreover, most atypical antipsychotic drugs have a considerable affinity to certain 5-HT receptors [18,21,22].

Seven types of 5-HT receptors have been identified, all but one (5-HT3) being G-protein coupled receptors (GPCRs) [18,23]. When also considering subtypes, at least 13 of these GPCRs can be distinguished [23]. 5-HT1A is a post-synaptic receptor in limbic forebrain structures and a somatodendritic autoreceptor of 5-HT neurons of the raphe nuclei. 5-HT1A is also expressed by cholinergic neurons within both the brain and the gastrointestinal system. 5-HT1A inhibits neuronal firing and neurotransmitter release via Gi/o-protein-coupled K$^+$ channels (GIRK channels) [23]. Receptors of type 5-HT2 are widely distributed within the brain [24] but also have an important role in vascular contractility (5-HT2A, 5-HT2B), colonic motor function (5-HT2B), and voiding (5-HT2C) [18,23,25–27]. 5-HT2 subtypes are coupled to Gq/11, which increases inositol 1,4,5-triphosphate levels and facilitates neuronal depolarization but, due to the activation of GABAergic interneurons, frequently inhibit their targets [18]. A characteristic of 5-HT2C (and, to a lesser extent, 5-HT2A) is constitutive activity, which enables clozapine to have inverse agonistic effects [28]. 5-HT3 subtypes are expressed by central and peripheral neurons where they induce rapid depolarization/repolarization by the opening of non-selective cation channels [23]. 5-HT3 within the lower brainstem is involved in vomiting and consists of 5-HT3A subunits, while 5-HT3 subtypes on the peripheral (autonomic and somatosensory) neurons have profound effects on the cardiovascular system and regulate motility and secretion throughout the whole gastrointestinal system [23]. This peripheral 5-HT3 consists of a heteromeric combination of 5-HT3A and 5-HT3B subunits.

Several HTR genes are involved in the regulation of metabolic homeostasis, including HTR1B, HTR1F, HTR2A/2C, HTR3, and HTR6 [11,19,20]. As MetS has a significant genetic component [29,30], genes encoding for these 5-HT receptors can be considered good candidates for genetic association studies particularly aimed at studying the molecular mechanism responsible for drug-induced weight gain. Most often studied are single-nucleotide polymorphisms (SNPs) of the HTR2A and HTR2C genes, since the effect of atypical antipsychotics on hypothalamic 5-HT2A/2C, in particular, is believed to contribute to drug-induced weight gain [7,10,11,31]. Moreover, polymorphic variants of the HTR2A gene are associated with higher body mass index (BMI) [32], greater waist circumference, and other components of metabolic syndrome [33]. Single-nucleotide polymorphisms of the HTR2C gene are also associated with obesity, weight gain, and BMI [34–38]. In a study by Yuan et al. [38], several haplotypes of the promoter region of HTR2C were identified and associated with obesity and diabetes. A pharmacogenetic study of other genes of the serotonergic system (*HTR3A, HTR3B*) did not reveal associations with weight gain induced by antipsychotics [39].

Studying the association of functional genetic variants with specific clinical phenomena can be applied to elucidate their mechanistic background [40]. We applied this investigational method several times in attempts to clarify a possible role of *5-HT* neurotransmission in the mechanism of two side effects of (atypical) antipsychotic drugs: dyskinesia [41–44] and hyperprolactinemia [45]. Therefore, studying the contribution of *5-HT* neurotransmission in the mechanisms of MetS can be considered a logical next step. However, due to the complex involvement of genuine metabolic as well as endocrine, immunological, and behavioral mechanisms [46–50], body weight is also considered in this study.

2. Materials and Methods

2.1. Patients

This study was conducted according to the protocol approved by the Bioethical Committee of the Mental Health Research Institute of the Tomsk National Research Medical Center of the Russian Academy of Sciences (Protocol 187, approval on 24.04.2018). After obtaining informed consent we recruited 475 patients with schizophrenia being treated at the clinics of the Research Institute of Mental Health of the Tomsk National Research Medical Center, the Tomsk Clinical Psychiatric Hospital, the Hospital of the Siberian State Medical University, the Kemerovo Regional Clinical Psychiatric Hospital, and the N.N. Solodnikova Clinical Psychiatric Hospital of Omsk in the Russian Federation.

The main criteria for the inclusion of patients in the study were a verified diagnosis of schizophrenia according to ICD-10 (International Classification of Diseases, 10th revision) criteria as assessed by applying a structured clinical interview (Structured Clinical Interview for the DSM [SCID]), age 18–65 years, the patient's informed consent, Caucasian appearance, and the absence of severe organic pathology or somatic disorders in the stage of decompensation.

The antipsychotic and concomitant therapy received at the time of the examination (drugs, dosages used, duration of current drug use) were assessed, as well as previous antipsychotic and concomitant somatic therapy during the preceding six months. We used the chlorpromazine equivalent (CPZeq) daily dosage to standardize the dose, efficacy, and side effects of antipsychotics [51].

MetS was diagnosed according to the criteria of the International Diabetes Federation (IDF, 2005) [52], including the definition of abdominal obesity (waist circumference more than 94 cm in men, or more than 80 cm in women) and the presence of any two of the following four signs:

1. Concentration of triglycerides (TG) above 1.7 mmol/L, or lipid-lowering therapy;
2. Concentration of high-density lipoproteins (HDL) of less than 1.03 mmol/L in men, or less than 1.29 mmol/L in women;
3. Blood pressure (BP) greater than or equal to 130/85 mm Hg, or the usage of antihypertensive therapy;
4. Concentration of glucose in blood serum greater than or equal to 5.6 mmol/L, or previously diagnosed type 2 diabetes mellitus.

2.2. Genetic Analysis

Blood samples for biochemical and pharmacogenetic studies were taken by antecubital venipuncture in vacutainer tubes with SiO_2 as a clot activator (to obtain serum) or with EDTA (to isolate genomic DNA by the standard phenol–chloroform method).

Genotyping of nine single-nucleotide polymorphisms (SNPs) of genes of the serotonergic system *HTR1A* (rs1423691, rs878567), *HTR2A* (rs6314), *HTR3A* (rs2276302, rs1150226), *HTR2C* (rs1414334, rs521018, rs498177), and *SLC6A4* (rs16965628) was carried out using a MassARRAY® Analyzer 4 mass spectrometer (Agena Bioscience ™) and a QuantStudio ™

3D Digital PCR System Life Technologies amplifier (Applied Biosystems) using TaqMan Validated SNP Genotyping Assay kits (Applied Biosystems) based at The Core Facility "Medical Genomics", Tomsk National Research Medical Center of the Russian Academy of Sciences.

2.3. Statistical Analysis

Statistical analysis was carried out using SPSS software, release 23.0. The Hardy–Weinberg equilibrium (HWE) of genotypic frequencies was tested by the chi-square test. Pearson's chi-squared test was used for between-group comparisons of genotypic and allelic frequencies at a significance level of $p < 0.05$. Assessment of the association of genotypes and alleles of the studied polymorphic variants of genes with a pathological phenotype was carried out using the odds ratio (OR) with a 95% confidence interval for the odds ratio (95% CI).

3. Results

A total of 475 patients receiving long-term antipsychotic therapy were examined. Metabolic syndrome was diagnosed in 126 patients (26.5%). Table 1 presents the main demographic and clinical parameters of the studied patient groups.

Table 1. Demographic and clinical parameters of the studied patient groups.

Parameter		Patients without MetS, $n = 349$ (73.5%)	Patients with MetS, $n = 126$ (26.5%)	p-Value
Gender	Women	142 (40.7%)	72 (57.1%)	0.001
	Men	207 (59.3%)	54 (42.9%)	
Age, years M ± SD		38.72 ± 11.43	43.75 ± 11.72	<0.0001
duration of illness, years Me [Q1; Q3]		12.0 [6.0; 20.0]	17.0 [9.0; 22.0]	0.001
CPZeq, dose Me [Q1; Q3]		400.0 [225.0; 750.0]	400.0 [203.0; 741.0]	0.919
Body mass index (BMI) M ± SD		24.45 ± 4.83	30.45 ± 6.36	<0.0001

Note. Me [Q1; Q3]—median and quartiles (first and third); MetS: metabolic syndrome; CPZeq: chlorpromazine equivalent; M ± SD—mean and standard deviation.

In our sample, MetS was more often diagnosed in women with schizophrenia. The patients with MetS were significantly older ($p < 0.0001$), and the duration of illness in these patients was significantly longer than that in patients without MetS ($p = 0.001$). The study groups also showed significant differences in body mass index ($p < 0.0001$).

Deviation from the HWE was found for the rs1150226 polymorphic variant of the *HTR3A* gene; hence, this polymorphism was excluded from further consideration. As the *HTR2C* gene is located on the X chromosome, its polymorphic variants should not meet HWE. Taking this localization into account, the distributions of the genotype and allele frequencies of the studied *HTR2C* genes (rs1414334, rs521018, and rs498177) were analyzed separately in the groups of women ($n = 214$) and men ($n = 261$).

There were no statistically significant differences in any of the eight studied SNPs of genes of the serotonergic system and metabolic syndrome in patients with schizophrenia receiving antipsychotic therapy for a long time. Statistically significant associations were, however, revealed in groups of patients with BMI of <25 and BMI of >25 (Table 2).

Statistically significant differences in the distribution of genotype frequencies were found for the polymorphic variant rs521018 of the *HTR2C* gene in the group of women with schizophrenia ($p = 0.033$). Carriage of the heterozygous genotype GT causes a predisposition to increased weight gain in women receiving antipsychotic treatment (OR 1.97; 95% CI: 1.09–3.55).

Table 2. Distributions of alleles and genotypes of HTR2C single-nucleotide polymorphism (SNPs) in groups of patients with body mass index (BMI) values of <25 and >25.

SNP	Genotypes, Alleles	BMI < 25	BMI > 25	OR	95% CI	χ^2	p Value
HTR2C rs521018	GG	12 (13.8)	5 (5.2)	0.34	0.12–1.02	6.85	0.033
	GT	38 (43.7)	58 (60.4)	1.97	1.09–3.55		
	TT	37 (42.5)	33 (34.4)	0.71	0.39–1.29		
	G	62 (35.6)	68 (35.4)	0.99	0.65–1.52	0.00	0.965
	T	112 (64.4)	124 (64.6)	1.01	0.66–1.55		

4. Discussion

The complexity of 5-HT signaling lies in the large number of receptor genes encoding for seven main 5-HT receptor types with several further subtypes, dimerization with other receptor proteins, and RNA editing and alternative splicing of receptor transcripts [20,23,53,54]. Several serotonin receptors are involved in the regulation of metabolic homeostasis, such as 5-HT1A, 5-HT2A, 5-HT2C, 5-HT3, and 5-HT6 [7,11,20]. Agonists of 5-HT1A and 5-HT2C have opposite effects on food intake: 5-HT1A receptors increase food intake, while 5-HT2C receptors decrease appetite [55,56]. The selective 5-HT2C agonist lorcaserin has been approved in the USA for supportive treatment in weight management [57]. Among all 5-HT receptors, the 5-HT2C are most strongly involved in the pharmacological action of serotonin [54]. Particularly, 5-HT2C expressed by a subset of pro-opiomelanocortin neurons in the hypothalamic arcuate nucleus and the brainstem nucleus of the solitary tract have a crucial role in mediating anti-orexigenic activity [56,58]. In humans, antagonization of the 5-HT2C receptor by atypical antipsychotics such as clozapine and olanzapine leads to weight gain [59–61].

In our study, we failed to establish an association between eight HTR genotypes and MetS. This may be due to the limited number of patients with MetS, but it is more likely due to the complex involvement of serotonergic transmission as well as other neurotransmitters in the mechanisms of the separate components of MetS. When studying one of these (indirect) components, we could find a relationship between rs521018 of HTR2C and increased body weight.

Many allelic variants of the HTR2C gene have been studied in the context of weight gain induced by antipsychotic therapy. These include rs6318*G, rs3813928*A, rs1414334*C, rs498207*A, rs518147*C, rs498177*C, and rs521018*T. A study by Mulder and colleagues showed that the rs1414334*C allele is associated with MetS in patients taking clozapine (OR 9.20; 95% CI 1.95–43.45) or risperidone (OR 5.35; 95% CI 1.26–22.83) [62]. In a study by Bai et al., the polymorphic variant rs498177 showed a significant association with MetS in female patients, and allele C was associated with an increased risk of MetS ($p = 0.0007$) [63]. However, the haplotype of the polymorphic variants rs521018*A and rs498177*C in the HTR2C gene significantly reduces the risk of MetS (adjusted $p = 0.0108$) in women [63].

Unfortunately, rs1150226 of HTR3A did not meet the HWE criterion as the A allele was significantly associated with higher BMI (data not shown). Antipsychotic drugs can also interfere with the expression of various receptors and the release of neurotransmitters. Polymorphic variants of the HTR3A gene (rs2276302, rs1062613, and rs1150226) have been shown to be associated with the response to clozapine therapy [64], which may contribute to weight gain [37,60]. Antipsychotics such as clozapine and olanzapine cause significant metabolic overload but are considered effective treatments for patients who do not respond to other therapies. Therefore, rs1150226 should be studied again in an independent patient population.

Further study of the molecular genetic factors of MetS and the mechanisms by which antipsychotics affect metabolic parameters is necessary to assess the risk of metabolic disorders and the implementation and individual approach to therapeutic tactics. It is possibly useful to expand the studied sample and to include in the analysis other risk factors for the development of MetS, such as the antipsychotic therapy used, smoking, and lifestyle, as well as to study individual components of MetS in patients.

5. Conclusions

Our study did not show an association of serotonin receptor genes with MetS in patients with schizophrenia. However, associations of one of the studied polymorphic variants with an increased BMI were revealed. Metabolic syndrome is a complicated symptoms complex that consists of separate components, including obesity, dyslipidemia, impaired glucose metabolism, and arterial hypertension. Serotonin is involved in these pathophysiological processes to varying degrees. We suggest that the involvement of serotonergic neurotransmission in MetS should be better studied after dissecting the syndrome into its individual (causal) components.

Author Contributions: Conceptualization, A.S.B., E.G.K., A.J.M.L. and S.A.I.; methodology, A.S.B., E.G.K., A.J.M.L. and S.A.I.; software, A.V.B.; validation, D.Z.P., A.S.B. and O.Y.F.; formal analysis, D.Z.P.; investigation, D.Z.P., A.S.B., I.V.P., A.V.B. and I.A.M.; resources, N.A.B. and S.A.I.; data curation, A.S.B. and E.G.K.; writing—original draft preparation, D.Z.P. and A.J.M.L.; writing—review and editing, A.J.M.L., O.Y.F. and S.A.I.; visualization, D.Z.P. and A.J.M.L.; supervision, A.V.S., N.A.B., and S.A.I.; project administration, S.A.I.; funding acquisition, A.S.B. All authors have read and agreed to the published version of the manuscript.

Funding: This research was funded by the Russian Science Foundation (project no. 19-75-10012).

Institutional Review Board Statement: This study was conducted according to the guidelines of the Declaration of Helsinki and approved by the Ethics Committee of the Mental Health Research Institute of the Tomsk National Research Medical Center of the Russian Academy of Sciences (protocol 187 approved on 24 April 2018).

Informed Consent Statement: Informed consent was obtained from all subjects involved in the study.

Data Availability Statement: The datasets generated for this study will not be made publicly available, but they are available on reasonable request to Svetlana A. Ivanova (ivanovaiipz@gmail.com), following approval of the Board of Directors of the MHRI, in line with local guidelines and regulations.

Acknowledgments: The authors are grateful to the Tomsk Clinical Psychiatric Hospital (Sergey M. Andreev), the Kemerovo Regional Clinical Psychiatric Hospital (Veronika A. Sorokina), and the N.N. Solodnikova Clinical Psychiatric Hospital of Omsk (Andrey I. Cheperin) for their help in recruiting patients for this investigation.

Conflicts of Interest: The authors declare no conflict of interest. The funders had no role in the design of the study; in the collection, analyses, or interpretation of data; in the writing of the manuscript; or in the decision to publish the results.

References

1. De Hert, M.; Detraux, J.; van Winkel, R.; Yu, W.; Correll, C.U. Metabolic and cardiovascular adverse effects associated with antipsychotic drugs. *Nat. Rev. Endocrinol.* **2011**, *8*, 114–126. [CrossRef]
2. O'Neill, S.; O'Driscoll, L. Metabolic syndrome: A closer look at the growing epidemic and its associated pathologies. *Obes. Rev.* **2015**, *16*, 1–12. [CrossRef]
3. Rojo, L.E.; Gaspar, P.A.; Silva, H.; Risco, L.; Arena, P.; Cubillos-Robles, K.; Jara, B. Metabolic syndrome and obesity among users of second generation antipsychotics: A global challenge for modern psychopharmacology. *Pharmacol. Res.* **2015**, *101*, 74–85. [CrossRef]
4. Freyberg, Z.; Aslanoglou, D.; Shah, R.; Ballon, J.S. Intrinsic and Antipsychotic Drug-Induced Metabolic Dysfunction in Schizophrenia. *Front. Neurosci.* **2017**, *11*, 432. [CrossRef]
5. Ijaz, S.; Bolea, B.; Davies, S.; Savović, J.; Richards, A.; Sullivan, S.; Moran, P. Antipsychotic polypharmacy and metabolic syndrome in schizophrenia: A review of systematic reviews. *BMC Psychiatry* **2018**, *18*, 275. [CrossRef] [PubMed]
6. Penninx, B.W.J.H.; Lange, S.M.M. Metabolic syndrome in psychiatric patients: Overview, mechanisms, and implications. *Dialogues Clin. Neurosci.* **2018**, *20*, 63–73. [CrossRef] [PubMed]
7. Panariello, F.; De Luca, V.; de Bartolomeis, A. Weight gain, schizophrenia and antipsychotics: New findings from animal model and pharmacogenomic studies. *Schizophr. Res. Treatment* **2011**, *2011*, 459284. [CrossRef]

8. Stępnicki, P.; Kondej, M.; Kaczor, A.A. Current Concepts and Treatments of Schizophrenia. *Molecules* **2018**, *23*, 2087. [CrossRef] [PubMed]
9. Aringhieri, S.; Carli, M.; Kolachalam, S.; Verdesca, V.; Cini, E.; Rossi, M.; McCormick, P.J.; Corsini, G.U.; Maggio, R.; Scarselli, M. Molecular targets of atypical antipsychotics: From mechanism of action to clinical differences. *Pharmacol. Ther.* **2018**, *192*, 20–41. [CrossRef] [PubMed]
10. Ballon, J.S.; Pajvani, U.; Freyberg, Z.; Leibel, R.L.; Lieberman, J.A. Molecular pathophysiology of metabolic effects of antipsychotic medications. *Trends Endocrinol. Metab.* **2014**, *25*, 593–600. [CrossRef] [PubMed]
11. Namkung, J.; Kim, H.; Park, S. Peripheral Serotonin: A New Player in Systemic Energy Homeostasis. *Mol. Cells* **2015**, *38*, 1023–1028. [CrossRef]
12. Selvaraj, S.; Arnone, D.; Cappai, A.; Howes, O. Alterations in the serotonin system in schizophrenia: A systematic review and meta-analysis of postmortem and molecular imaging studies. *Neurosci. Biobehav. Rev.* **2014**, *45*, 233–245. [CrossRef] [PubMed]
13. Loonen, A.J.M.; Ivanova, S.A. Circuits regulating pleasure and happiness: Evolution and role in mental disorders. *Acta Neuropsychiatr.* **2018**, *30*, 29–42. [CrossRef] [PubMed]
14. Loonen, A.J.M.; Ivanova, S.A. The evolutionary old forebrain as site of action to develop new psychotropic drugs. *J. Psychopharmacol.* **2018**, *32*, 1277–1285. [CrossRef] [PubMed]
15. Loonen, A.J.M.; Ivanova, S.A. Evolution of circuits regulating pleasure and happiness with the habenula in control. *CNS Spectr.* **2019**, *24*, 233–238. [CrossRef] [PubMed]
16. Loonen, A.J.M.; Ivanova, S.A. Circuits regulating pleasure and happiness in major depression. *Med. Hypotheses* **2016**, *87*, 14–21. [CrossRef]
17. Loonen, A.J.M.; Ivanova, S.A. Circuits Regulating Pleasure and Happiness-Mechanisms of Depression. *Front. Hum. Neurosci.* **2016**, *10*, 571. [CrossRef]
18. Loonen, A.J.M.; Ivanova, S.A. Role of 5-HT2C receptors in dyskinesia. *Int. J. Pharm. Pharm. Sci.* **2016**, *8*, 5–10. Available online: https://innovareacademics.in/journals/index.php/ijpps/article/view/8736 (accessed on 4 March 2021).
19. Voigt, J.P.; Fink, H. Serotonin controlling feeding and satiety. *Behav. Brain Res.* **2015**, *277*, 14–31. [CrossRef]
20. Wyler, S.C.; Lord, C.C.; Lee, S.; Elmquist, J.K.; Liu, C. Serotonergic Control of Metabolic Homeostasis. *Front. Cell Neurosci.* **2017**, *11*, 277. [CrossRef]
21. Reynolds, G.P. Receptor mechanisms in the treatment of schizophrenia. *J. Psychopharmacol.* **2004**, *18*, 340–345. [CrossRef]
22. Meltzer, H.Y. Serotonergic mechanisms as targets for existing and novel antipsychotics. *Handb. Exp. Pharmacol.* **2012**, *212*, 87–124. [CrossRef]
23. Hannon, J.; Hoyer, D. Molecular biology of 5-HT receptors. *Behav. Brain Res.* **2008**, *195*, 198–213. [CrossRef]
24. Leysen, J.E. 5-HT2 receptors. *Curr. Drug Targets CNS Neurol. Disord.* **2004**, *3*, 11–26. [CrossRef]
25. Lychkova, A.É. Serotoninergic regulation of colonic motor function. *Ter. Arkh.* **2013**, *85*, 89–92. Available online: https://ter-arkhiv.ru/0040-3660/article/view/31237 (accessed on 4 March 2021).
26. Matsumoto-Miyai, K.; Yoshizumi, M.; Kawatani, M. Regulatory Effects of 5-Hydroxytryptamine Receptors on Voiding Function. *Adv. Ther.* **2015**, *32* (Suppl. S1), 3–15. [CrossRef] [PubMed]
27. Padhariya, K.; Bhandare, R.; Canney, D.; Velingkar, V. Cardiovascular Concern of 5-HT2B Receptor and Recent Vistas in the Development of Its Antagonists. *Cardiovasc. Hematol. Disord. Drug Targets* **2017**, *17*, 86–104. [CrossRef] [PubMed]
28. Aloyo, V.J.; Berg, K.A.; Spampinato, U.; Clarke, W.P.; Harvey, J.A. Current status of inverse agonism at serotonin2A (5-HT2A) and 5-HT2C receptors. *Pharmacol. Ther.* **2009**, *121*, 160–173. [CrossRef] [PubMed]
29. Karunakaran, S.; Clee, S.M. Genetics of metabolic syndrome: Potential clues from wild-derived inbred mouse strains. *Physiol. Genom.* **2018**, *50*, 35–51. [CrossRef]
30. Stančáková, A.; Laakso, M. Genetics of metabolic syndrome. *Rev. Endocr. Metab. Disord.* **2014**, *15*, 243–252. [CrossRef] [PubMed]
31. Kroeze, W.K.; Hufeisen, S.J.; Popadak, B.A.; Renock, S.M.; Steinberg, S.; Ernsberger, P.; Jayathilake, K.; Meltzer, H.Y.; Roth, B.L. H1-histamine receptor affinity predicts short-term weight gain for typical and atypical antipsychotic drugs. *Neuropsychopharmacology* **2003**, *28*, 519–526. [CrossRef]
32. Li, P.; Tiwari, H.K.; Lin, W.Y.; Allison, D.B.; Chung, W.K.; Leibel, R.L.; Yi, N.; Liu, N. Genetic association analysis of 30 genes related to obesity in a European American population. *Int. J. Obes.* **2014**, *38*, 724–729. [CrossRef]
33. Halder, I.; Muldoon, M.F.; Ferrell, R.E.; Manuck, S.B. Serotonin Receptor 2A (*HTR2A*) Gene Polymorphisms Are Associated with Blood Pressure, Central Adiposity, and the Metabolic Syndrome. *Metab. Syndr. Relat. Disord.* **2007**, *5*, 323–330. [CrossRef] [PubMed]
34. Chen, C.; Chen, W.; Chen, C.; Moyzis, R.; He, Q.; Lei, X.; Li, J.; Wang, Y.; Liu, B.; Xiu, D.; et al. Genetic variations in the serotoninergic system contribute to body-mass index in Chinese adolescents. *PLoS ONE* **2013**, *8*, e58717. [CrossRef]
35. Opgen-Rhein, C.; Brandl, E.J.; Müller, D.J.; Neuhaus, A.H.; Tiwari, A.K.; Sander, T.; Dettling, M. Association of *HTR2C*, but not LEP or INSIG2, genes with antipsychotic-induced weight gain in a German sample. *Pharmacogenomics* **2010**, *11*, 773–780. [CrossRef] [PubMed]
36. Reynolds, G.P.; Zhang, Z.J.; Zhang, X.B. Association of antipsychotic drug-induced weight gain with a 5-HT2C receptor gene polymorphism. *Lancet* **2002**, *359*, 2086–2087. [CrossRef]
37. Reynolds, G.P.; Zhang, Z.; Zhang, X. Polymorphism of the promoter region of the serotonin 5-HT(2C) receptor gene and clozapine-induced weight gain. *Am. J. Psychiatry* **2003**, *160*, 677–679. [CrossRef] [PubMed]

38. Yuan, X.; Yamada, K.; Ishiyama-Shigemoto, S.; Koyama, W.; Nonaka, K. Identification of polymorphic loci in the promoter region of the serotonin 5-HT2C receptor gene and their association with obesity and type II diabetes. *Diabetologia* **2000**, *43*, 373–376. [CrossRef] [PubMed]
39. Zai, C.C.; Tiwari, A.K.; Chowdhury, N.I.; Brandl, E.J.; Shaikh, S.A.; Freeman, N.; Lieberman, J.A.; Meltzer, H.Y.; Kennedy, J.L.; Müller, D.J. Association Study of Serotonin 3 Receptor Subunit Gene Variants in Antipsychotic-Induced Weight Gain. *Neuropsychobiology* **2016**, *74*, 169–175. [CrossRef]
40. Loonen, A.J.M.; Wilffert, B.; Ivanova, S.A. Putative role of pharmacogenetics to elucidate the mechanism of tardive dyskinesia in schizophrenia. *Pharmacogenomics* **2019**, *20*, 1199–1223. [CrossRef] [PubMed]
41. Al Hadithy, A.F.Y.; Ivanova, S.A.; Pechlivanoglou, P.; Semke, A.; Fedorenko, O.; Kornetova, E.; Ryadovaya, L.; Brouwers, J.R.B.J.; Wilffert, B.; Bruggeman, R.; et al. Tardive dyskinesia and DRD3, HTR2A and HTR2C gene polymorphisms in Russian psychiatric inpatients from Siberia. *Prog. Neuropsycho. Pharmacol. Biol. Psychiatry* **2009**, *33*, 475–481. [CrossRef] [PubMed]
42. Ivanova, S.A.; Loonen, A.J.M.; Pechlivanoglou, P.; Freidin, M.B.; Al Hadithy, A.F.Y.; Rudikov, E.V.; Zhukova, I.A.; Govorin, N.V.; Sorokina, V.A.; Fedorenko, O.Y.; et al. NMDA receptor genotypes associated with the vulnerability to develop dyskinesia. *Transl. Psychiatry* **2012**, *2*, e67. [CrossRef] [PubMed]
43. Ivanova, S.A.; Loonen, A.J.M.; Bakker, P.R.; Freidin, M.B.; Ter Woerds, N.J.; Al Hadithy, A.F.Y.; Semke, A.V.; Fedorenko, O.Y.; Brouwers, J.R.B.J.; Bokhan, N.A.; et al. Likelihood of mechanistic roles for dopaminergic, serotonergic and glutamatergic receptors in tardive dyskinesia: A comparison of genetic variants in two independent patient populations. *SAGE Open Med.* **2016**, *4*, 2050312116643673. [CrossRef] [PubMed]
44. Pozhidaev, I.V.; Paderina, D.Z.; Fedorenko, O.Y.; Kornetova, E.G.; Semke, A.V.; Loonen, A.J.M.; Bokhan, N.A.; Wilffert, B.; Ivanova, S.A. 5-Hydroxytryptamine Receptors and Tardive Dyskinesia in Schizophrenia. *Front. Mol. Neurosci.* **2020**, *13*, 63. [CrossRef] [PubMed]
45. Ivanova, S.A.; Osmanova, D.Z.; Freidin, M.B.; Fedorenko, O.Y.; Boiko, A.S.; Pozhidaev, I.V.; Semke, A.V.; Bokhan, N.A.; Agarkov, A.A.; Wilffert, B.; et al. Identification of 5-hydroxytryptamine receptor gene polymorphisms modulating hyperprolactinaemia in antipsychotic drug-treated patients with schizophrenia. *World J. Biol. Psychiatry* **2017**, *18*, 239–246. [CrossRef] [PubMed]
46. Boiko, A.S.; Mednova, I.A.; Kornetova, E.G.; Semke, A.V.; Bokhan, N.A.; Loonen, A.J.M.; Ivanova, S.A. Apolipoprotein serum levels related to metabolic syndrome in patients with schizophrenia. *Heliyon* **2019**, *5*, e02033. [CrossRef]
47. Boiko, A.S.; Mednova, I.A.; Kornetova, E.G.; Bokhan, N.A.; Semke, A.V.; Loonen, A.J.M.; Ivanova, S.A. Cortisol and DHEAS Related to Metabolic Syndrome in Patients with Schizophrenia. *Neuropsychiatr. Dis. Treat.* **2020**, *16*, 1051–1058. [CrossRef]
48. Kornetova, E.G.; Kornetov, A.N.; Mednova, I.A.; Dubrovskaya, V.V.; Boiko, A.S.; Bokhan, N.A.; Loonen, A.J.M.; Ivanova, S.A. Changes in Body Fat and Related Biochemical Parameters Associated With Atypical Antipsychotic Drug Treatment in Schizophrenia Patients With or Without Metabolic Syndrome. *Front. Psychiatry* **2019**, *10*, 803. [CrossRef]
49. Kornetova, E.G.; Kornetov, A.N.; Mednova, I.A.; Lobacheva, O.A.; Gerasimova, V.I.; Dubrovskaya, V.V.; Tolmachev, I.V.; Semke, A.V.; Loonen, A.J.M.; Bokhan, N.A.; et al. Body Fat Parameters, Glucose and Lipid Profiles, and Thyroid Hormone Levels in Schizophrenia Patients with or without Metabolic Syndrome. *Diagnostics* **2020**, *10*, 683. [CrossRef]
50. Mednova, I.A.; Boiko, A.S.; Kornetova, E.G.; Parshukova, D.A.; Semke, A.V.; Bokhan, N.A.; Loonen, A.J.M.; Ivanova, S.A. Adipocytokines and Metabolic Syndrome in Patients with Schizophrenia. *Metabolites* **2020**, *10*, 410. [CrossRef]
51. Andreasen, N.C.; Pressler, M.; Nopoulos, P.; Miller, D.; Ho, B.C. Antipsychotic dose equivalents and dose-years: A standardized method for comparing exposure to different drugs. *Biol. Psychiatry* **2010**, *67*, 255–262. [CrossRef] [PubMed]
52. Alberti, K.G.; Zimmet, P.; Shaw, J. Metabolic syndrome—a new world-wide definition. A Consensus Statement from the International Diabetes Federation. *Diabet. Med.* **2006**, *23*, 469–480. [CrossRef]
53. Łukasiewicz, S.; Polit, A.; Kędracka-Krok, S.; Wędzony, K.; Maćkowiak, M.; Dziedzicka-Wasylewska, M. Hetero-dimerization of serotonin 5-HT(2A) and dopamine D(2) receptors. *Biochim. Biophys. Acta* **2010**, *1803*, 1347–1358. [CrossRef] [PubMed]
54. Palacios, J.M.; Pazos, A.; Hoyer, D. A short history of the 5-HT2C receptor: From the choroid plexus to depression, obesity and addiction treatment. *Psychopharmacology* **2017**, *234*, 1395–1418. [CrossRef] [PubMed]
55. Dourish, C.T.; Hutson, P.H.; Curzon, G. Characteristics of feeding induced by the serotonin agonist 8-hydroxy-2-(di-n-propylamino) tetralin (8-OH-DPAT). *Brain Res. Bull.* **1985**, *15*, 377–384. [CrossRef]
56. Xu, Y.; Jones, J.E.; Kohno, D.; Williams, K.W.; Lee, C.E.; Choi, M.J.; Anderson, J.G.; Heisler, L.K.; Zigman, J.M.; Lowell, B.B.; et al. 5-HT2CRs expressed by pro-opiomelanocortin neurons regulate energy homeostasis. *Neuron* **2008**, *60*, 582–589. [CrossRef]
57. Higgins, G.A.; Fletcher, P.J.; Shanahan, W.R. Lorcaserin: A review of its preclinical and clinical pharmacology and therapeutic potential. *Pharmacol. Ther.* **2020**, *205*, 107417. [CrossRef]
58. D'Agostino, G.; Lyons, D.; Cristiano, C.; Lettieri, M.; Olarte-Sanchez, C.; Burke, L.K.; Greenwald-Yarnell, M.; Cansell, C.; Doslikova, B.; Georgescu, T.; et al. Nucleus of the Solitary Tract Serotonin 5-HT2C Receptors Modulate Food Intake. *Cell Metab.* **2018**, *28*, 619–630. [CrossRef]
59. Malhotra, N.; Grover, S.; Chakrabarti, S.; Kulhara, P. Metabolic syndrome in schizophrenia. *Indian J. Psychol. Med.* **2013**, *35*, 227–240. [CrossRef]
60. Papanastasiou, E. The prevalence and mechanisms of metabolic syndrome in schizophrenia: A review. *Ther. Adv. Psychopharmacol.* **2013**, *3*, 33–51. [CrossRef] [PubMed]

61. Pillinger, T.; McCutcheon, R.A.; Vano, L.; Mizuno, Y.; Arumuham, A.; Hindley, G.; Beck, K.; Natesan, S.; Efthimiou, O.; Cipriani, A.; et al. Comparative effects of 18 antipsychotics on metabolic function in patients with schizophrenia, predictors of metabolic dysregulation, and association with psychopathology: A systematic review and network meta-analysis. *Lancet Psychiatry* **2020**, *7*, 64–77. [CrossRef]
62. Mulder, H.; Cohen, D.; Scheffer, H.; Gispen-de Wied, C.; Arends, J.; Wilmink, F.W.; Franke, B.; Egberts, A.C. *HTR2C* gene polymorphisms and the metabolic syndrome in patients with schizophrenia: A replication study. *J. Clin. Psychopharmacol.* **2009**, *29*, 16–20. [CrossRef]
63. Bai, Y.M.; Chen, T.T.; Liou, Y.J.; Hong, C.J.; Tsai, S.J. Association between *HTR2C* polymorphisms and metabolic syndrome in patients with schizophrenia treated with atypical antipsychotics. *Schizophr. Res.* **2011**, *125*, 179–186. [CrossRef] [PubMed]
64. Souza, R.P.; de Luca, V.; Meltzer, H.Y.; Lieberman, J.A.; Kennedy, J.L. Influence of serotonin 3A and 3B receptor genes on clozapine treatment response in schizophrenia. *Pharm. Genom.* **2010**, *20*, 274–276. [CrossRef] [PubMed]

Article

Schizophrenia-Like Behavioral Impairments in Mice with Suppressed Expression of Piccolo in the Medial Prefrontal Cortex

Atsumi Nitta [1,*], Naotaka Izuo [1], Kohei Hamatani [1], Ryo Inagaki [1], Yuka Kusui [1], Kequan Fu [1,2], Takashi Asano [1], Youta Torii [3], Chikako Habuchi [3], Hirotaka Sekiguchi [3], Shuji Iritani [3], Shin-ichi Muramatsu [4,5], Norio Ozaki [3] and Yoshiaki Miyamoto [1]

1. Department of Pharmaceutical Therapy and Neuropharmacology, Faculty of Pharmaceutical Sciences, Graduate School of Pharmaceutical Sciences, University of Toyama, Toyama 930-0194, Japan; ntk3izuo@pha.u-toyama.ac.jp (N.I.); kohei-1572@kem.biglobe.ne.jp (K.H.); ryo.inagaki.a2@tohoku.ac.jp (R.I.); d2062302@ems.u-toyama.ac.jp (Y.K.); fukequan6962@hotmail.com (K.F.); tasano@pha.u-toyama.ac.jp (T.A.); miyamoto@josai.ac.jp (Y.M.)
2. Jiangsu Key Laboratory of New Drug Research and Clinical Pharmacy, Xuzhou Medical University, Xuzhou 221004, China
3. Department of Psychiatry, Graduate School of Medicine, Nagoya University, Nagoya 466-8550, Japan; youtat@med.nagoya-u.ac.jp (Y.T.); akariha1029@yahoo.co.jp (C.H.); sguchi77@gmail.com (H.S.); iritani@med.nagoya-u.ac.jp (S.I.); ozaki-n@med.nagoya-u.ac.jp (N.O.)
4. Open Innovation Center, Division of Neurological Gene Therapy, Jichi Medical University, Shimotsuke 329-0498, Japan; muramats@jichi.ac.jp
5. Center for Gene and Cell Therapy, The Institute of Medical Science, The University of Tokyo, Tokyo 108-8639, Japan
* Correspondence: nitta@pha.u-toyama.ac.jp; Tel.: +81-76-415-8822 (ext. 8923); Fax: +81-76-415-8826

Abstract: Piccolo, a presynaptic cytomatrix protein, plays a role in synaptic vesicle trafficking in the presynaptic active zone. Certain single-nucleotide polymorphisms of the Piccolo-encoding gene *PCLO* are reported to be associated with mental disorders. However, a few studies have evaluated the relationship between Piccolo dysfunction and psychotic symptoms. Therefore, we investigated the neurophysiological and behavioral phenotypes in mice with Piccolo suppression in the medial prefrontal cortex (mPFC). Downregulation of Piccolo in the mPFC reduced regional synaptic proteins, accompanied with electrophysiological impairments. The Piccolo-suppressed mice showed an enhanced locomotor activity, impaired auditory prepulse inhibition, and cognitive dysfunction. These abnormal behaviors were partially ameliorated by the antipsychotic drug risperidone. Piccolo-suppressed mice received mild social defeat stress showed additional behavioral despair. Furthermore, the responses of these mice to extracellular glutamate and dopamine levels induced by the optical activation of mPFC projection in the dorsal striatum (dSTR) were inhibited. Similarly, the Piccolo-suppressed mice showed decreased depolarization-evoked glutamate and -aminobutyric acid elevations and increased depolarization-evoked dopamine elevation in the dSTR. These suggest that Piccolo regulates neurotransmission at the synaptic terminal of the projection site. Reduced neuronal connectivity in the mPFC-dSTR pathway via suppression of Piccolo in the mPFC may induce behavioral impairments observed in schizophrenia.

Keywords: piccolo; presynaptic cytomatrix protein; medial prefrontal cortex; dorsal striatum; schizophrenia; optogenetics

1. Introduction

Psychiatric disorders appear as abnormal behavioral and mental patterns that cause severe distress or disability to the individual. Schizophrenia, one of serious psychiatric disorders, is characterized by three major symptoms, positive and negative symptom and cognitive deficit, as well as an accompanying neurological phenomenon [1–3]. Current clinical treatments for schizophrenia have been proven effective for positive symptoms, with only a few being effective for negative symptoms and cognitive deficit. Therefore, elucidating pathophysiological conditions related to schizophrenia is imperative for the early development of highly effective therapeutic treatments.

Many genetic and environmental risk factors are commonly involved in schizophrenia, and the overlap between such risk factors plays a potential role in its development. In addition, some parts of the brain such as the frontal cortex, amygdala, hippocampus, and thalamus are involved in schizophrenia, and the disconnection between such parts in the brain, rather than impairment in one part of the brain, results in its symptoms. Especially, many patients with schizophrenia exhibit functional, structural, and metabolic abnormalities in the prefrontal cortex (PFC) in neuroimaging studies reporting on the effects of antipsychotic medications and cognitive remediation therapy [4]. The dopaminergic dysfunction in the PFC and high density of the binding of the antipsychotic drug chlorpromazine in the PFC in schizophrenic patients support this notion [5]. D2 receptors are typically distributed in the subcortical regions, such as the striatum; however, functional brain imaging studies have shown that the density of striatal D2 receptors is altered in schizophrenia patients without medication [6]. Therefore, it is thought that altered neuronal activity and connection in the PFC by the genetic and environmental insults is associated with the pathophysiology of schizophrenia [7–9].

Piccolo, a presynaptic protein encoded by the *PCLO* gene, plays a role in synaptic vesicle trafficking by interacting with several proteins in the presynaptic active zone [10–14]. Ultrastructurally, the presynaptic active zone is an electron-dense, largely detergent-resistant cytomatrix comprising multiple scaffolding proteins, including Munc18, SNAP-25, and Piccolo [15,16], hypothesized to function as synaptic vesicle regulators in neurotransmission process due to their interaction [17]. Piccolo has been reported to be involved in cognitive function, synaptic plasticity, and psychostimulant-induced psychosis [18,19]. A genome-wide association study showed that single-nucleotide polymorphisms (SNPs) in the *PCLO* gene were significantly associated with bipolar disorder and major depressive disorder. Indeed, the SNP rs13438494 in intron 24 of *PCLO*, which disturbs the splicing pattern of PCLO mRNA to decrease expression [20], is associated with bipolar disorder [21]. Symptoms of drug dependence-related parameters, such as the age of first exposure to a psychostimulant, tobacco dependence, and fentanyl requirement for pain relief in human, have been associated with Piccolo SNPs [22]. In addition, SNP rs2522833 in exon 19 of *PCLO*, causing amino acid substitution (from serine to alanine) in the Ca^{2+} binding C2A domain of Piccolo, induce the mild increase of synaptic transmission [23]. Its C allele is the top risk variant of major depressive disorder [24] and also associated with the reduced regional brain volume [25,26], lower memory performance [27], and increased activity in the left amygdala during processing of fearful faces [28]. There is no consensus of the clinical association between the functional status of Piccolo and mental disorders. Piccolo physiologically expresses at the terminals of glutamatergic and GABAergic neurons [11]. Since Piccolo alteration in its function or expression could change the balance of circuit activity, the phenotypic effects to the brain circuits and behavior are necessary to be investigated.

Therefore, in the present study, we investigate whether or not the suppressed expression of the *Pclo* gene in the medial PFC (mPFC) of mice using adeno-associated virus (AAV) *Pclo* miRNA vectors affects the neurophysiological function. We also investigated whether or not a causal relationship between Piccolo dysfunction and behavioral impairments in mental disorders could be established.

2. Materials and Methods

2.1. Animals

Seven-week-old C57BL/6J male mice (Nihon SLC, Hamamatsu, Japan) were used for this study to avoid the effects of the estrous cycle. The weights of the mice ranged from 21–26 g. The number of mice used was described in each experiment. The mice were housed in a 12-h light–dark cycle (lights on at 8:00) with food and water available ad libitum.

All procedures were performed in accordance with the National Institutes of Health Guide for the Care and Use of Laboratory Animals and Guidelines for the Care and Use of Laboratory Animals at the University of Toyama (Approval No. A2018PHA-5).

2.2. Drugs

Risperidone (Sigma-Aldrich, St. Luis, MO, USA, R3030, 0.01 mg/kg) dissolved with saline was administered by intraperitoneal (i.p.) injections 30 min before each behavioral test. Especially, administration was performed on each day of the novel object recognition and fear-conditioning test. Saline was injected to the control mice as a vehicle. Bicuculine and NBQX were purchased from Tocris Bioscience (Bristol, UK).

2.3. Production and Microinjection of AAV Vector

This study used an AAV vector production protocol described in earlier studies [29,30]. Viral vectors (AAV1) were designed to express an antisense sequence for *Pclo* (TGCTGATC-CCAAACTGTCACCTCCAAGTTTTGGCCACTGACTGACTTGG AGGTCAGTTTGGGAT) and an enhanced GFP sequence (AAV- *Pclo* miRNA/EGFP vectors) based on murine miR-155 as a backbone (BLOCK-iT; Invitrogen Japan K493500, Thermo Fisher Scientific, Tokyo, Japan) under cytomegalovirus promotor. Viral vectors containing only the enhanced GFP sequence (AAV-EGFP vectors) were used as controls. All procedures were performed in accordance with the Guideline for Recombinant DNA Experiment by the Ministry of Education, Culture, Sports, Science and Technology, Japan and were approved by the Gene Recombination Experiment Safety Committee at the University of Toyama (Approval No. G2015PHA-14).

The microinjection of AAV vectors (0.7 µL/side, 0.1 µL/min) into the mPFC of the mice (+1.6 mm anterior, ±0.3 mm lateral from the bregma, and +1.6 mm ventral from the skull) according to the brain atlas [31] was performed as described in a previous report [32]. The mice were used for experiments four weeks after the AAV-injections. Four weeks after AAV injection, behavioral experiments were conducted in the following order: locomotor activity test, spatial working test, novel object recognition test, and spatial working test. After the serial experiments, samples from these mice were used for immunostaining, Western blotting, or quantitative real-time polymerase chain reaction (PCR). Another group of mice was used for electrophysiological recordings or in vivo microdialysis four weeks after the AAV-injection.

2.4. Quantitative Real-Time PCR

All reactions were performed in duplicate using the following cycling protocol: enzyme heat activation for 10 min at 95 °C, 40 cycles of denaturation at 95 °C for 30 s, annealing at 59 °C for 40 s, and extension at 72 °C for 60 s. Piccolo primers used for real-time PCR were as follows: 5'-TGCCTGGTTTCTTCTCAGATGT-3' (forward: 753–774 base pairs [bp]) and 5'-GAGTCTGATATCAAATCAAAAGGGT-3' (reverse: 816–840 bp), 5'-GTCAAAACAGCCAGCAGTCC-3' (forward: 14,607–14,626 bp) and 5'-GTCCATGAG-ATCGGAGATGG-3' (reverse: 14,752–14,771 bp). A 36B4 transcript quantified using the forward primer 5'-ACCCTGAAGTGCTCGACATC-3' and reverse primer 5'-AGGAAGGCCTT-GACCTTTTC-3' was used as the internal control.

2.5. Western Blotting

Western blotting was performed using standard methods [33] with the following primary antibodies: anti-Piccolo (abcam ab20664, Cambridge, UK; 1:1000), anti-phospho-synapsin I (Phosphosolutions 1560-6267, Aurora, CA, USA; 1:1000), anti-synapsin I (Enzo Life Sciences BML-SA495, Farmingdale, NY, USA; 1:1000), anti-synaptophysin (Sigma-Aldrich S5768; 1:1000), anti-munc18 (BD Biosciences 610336, San Jose, CA, USA; 1:1000), anti-SNAP-25 (BD Biosciences 610366; 1:1000), and anti-α-Tubulin (Santa Cruz Biotechnology sc-5546, Santa Cruz, CA, USA; 1:1000). Proteins were detected using horseradish peroxidase-conjugated secondary antibodies (GE Healthcare, Amersham, UK; NA9310, 1:5000) and the ECL Prime kit (GE Healthcare, RPN2332).

2.6. Electrophysiological Recordings

A 64-channel multi-electrode dish system (Alpha MED Sciences, Tokyo, Japan) was employed, as described in an earlier study [18]. We used MED-P515A probes (Alpha MED Sciences) with a 150-µM interpolar distance as electrodes, a chamber depth of 10 mm, and 64 planar microelectrodes in an 8×8 array. For paired pulse facilitation, two field excitatory postsynaptic potentials (fEPSPs) were evoked with twin pulses at interpulse intervals of 20, 60, and 100 ms. The ratio of the second versus the first potential was determined. Long-term potentiation (LTP) was elicited by theta burst stimulation (TBS; 20 trains, each train of 4 pulses at 100 Hz, intertrain interval of 200 ms, total train duration of 40 ms). After the TBS stimulation, fEPSPs were recorded for 60 min at 1-min intervals per slice.

2.7. In Vivo Microdialysis

In vivo microdialysis was performed as described in a previous study [34,35]. The guide cannula was placed into the mPFC (+1.6 mm anterior, 0.3 mm lateral from the bregma, and +1.6 mm ventral from the skull) or dSTR (1.2 mm anterior, 1.0 mm lateral from the bregma and 2.7 mm ventral from the skull) (26). Dialysate was collected at a flow rate of 0.5 or 1.0 µL/min for dopamine (DA) or glutamate (Glu) in 10- or 15-min fractions, respectively, and injected into the high-performance liquid chromatography (HPLC) system (HTEC-500; Eicom, Kyoto, Japan). To measure GABA, dialysate was collected at a flow rate of 1.0 µL/min in 30-min fractions using a fraction collector and mixed with a cocktail of ortho-phthalaldehyde (4 mmol/L) and carboxylic acid solutions (pH 9.5) containing 0.04% mercaptoethanol for 1.5 min. The mixed dialysate solution was continuously autoinjected into the HPLC system.

2.8. Optogenetic Stimulation

For optogenetic stimulation, AAV- *Pclo* miRNA/EGFP or AAV-EGFP vectors mixed with AAV9 vectors expressing ChIEF under the human synapsin promoter were microinjected into the mPFC (+1.7 mm anterior, 0.3 mm lateral from the bregma, and +1.5 mm ventral from the skull) (Paxinos and Franklin, 2008). ChIEF is a light-sensitive protein that is generated by introducing some mutagenesis to the original channelrhodopsin 2 (ChR2), and its activation in response to the light resembles more natural spiking patterns than ChR2 [36]. Four weeks after the microinjection, guide cannula (AGFL-4, Eicom) for an optical fiber and in vivo microdialysis probe (A-FL-4-01, Eicom) were implanted in the dSTR (+1.2 mm anterior, 1.0 mm lateral from the bregma and 2.7 mm ventral from the skull). For optogenetic stimulation, the mice received blue light pulses (pulse width, 15 ms; frequency, 10 Hz; intensity, 5 mW, laser, 473 nm) for 15 min (ESFI-700, Eicom) under the control of stimulation scheduler (ESST-800, Eicom).

2.9. Behavioral Analyses

- Locomotor activity test

To measure the locomotor activity in a novel environment, a mouse was placed in a transparent acrylic cage ($45 \times 45 \times 40$ cm), and its locomotion was measured every 5 min for a total duration of 60 min using a Scanet MV-40 (Melquest, Toyama, Japan).

- PPI test

An SR-LAB system (San Diego, CA, USA) was used to measure the startle response and prepulse inhibition (PPI). The test session began by placing a mouse in a plastic cylinder and leaving it undisturbed for 10 min. The background noise level in each chamber was 70 dB. The intensity of the startle stimulus was 120 dB. The prepulse sound (74 or 78, 82, and 86 dB) was presented 100 ms before the startle stimulus. Four combinations of prepulse and startle stimuli were used (74 and 120, 78 and 120, 82 and 120, and 86 and 120 dB). The extreme outliers determined by Smirnov–Grubbs test were removed.

- Novel object recognition test

Mice were individually habituated to an open-field box (30 × 30 × 45 cm) for 3 days. During the acquisition phase, two objects were placed symmetrically in the center of the chamber for 10 min, and the mouse's exploratory behavior was analyzed. Twenty-four hours later, one object was replaced by a novel object, and the exploratory behavior of the mouse was analyzed again for 10 min. Discrimination of novel object was assessed by counting the total time and number of contacts.

- Contextual learning test

In the contextual learning test, the mice were trained and tested for two consecutive days. The test was performed in operant chambers. Contextual fear conditioning was measured using the FCC mode system (Melquest, Toyama, Japan). Training involved allowing the subjects to freely explore the operant chamber for 2 min. Thereafter, electrical foot shocks (0.6 mA, five seconds) with an auditory cue were automatically delivered through a grid floor using customized programming four times with 15-second intervals. The mice were returned to their home cages after completing the conditioning procedure. Twenty-four hours after training, the mice were brought back to the same chamber, and freezing behavior was observed and recorded for 4 min.

- Y-maze test (spontaneous alternation behaviors)

The Y-maze test was conducted using an apparatus with three identical arms. In this test, a mouse was placed at the end of one arm of the apparatus and allowed to move freely during an 8-min session. An alternation was defined as entry into all three arms on consecutive choices. The percentage of spontaneous alternation behavior was calculated as follows: [(Alternations)/(Total number of arms entered − 2)] × 100.

- Mild social defeat stress exposure

Before the social interaction and forced swimming tests, the mice were subjected to subthreshold levels of social defeat stress. This consisted of three consecutive 5-min defeat sessions in a single day, with 15 min of rest between each session. During this time, the mice were directly exposed to an aggressive male ICR mouse (>8 weeks old; Nihon SLC). The social interaction test was performed 48 h after the exposure and subsequently followed by the forced swimming test 96 h after the exposure.

- Social interaction test

The social interaction test comprised two 150-s phases, separated by a duration of 30 s. During the first phase, a stress-exposed mouse was placed in the open-field arena (45 × 45 × 40 cm) of an empty wire-mesh enclosure (8 × 10 × 8 cm). During the second phase, the mouse was placed in the open-field arena, with an ICR mouse present in the wire-mesh enclosure. The social interaction time, i.e., the duration in which the subject mouse stayed within the interaction zone (14 × 27 cm around the wire-mesh enclosure) was measured. During the 30-s break between each phase, the subject mouse was transferred back to its home cage. The ICR mouse used for the test had no previous interaction with the subject mouse.

- Forced swimming test

The forced swimming test was performed as previously described in a previous study [32]. In brief, the mice were placed in a transparent polycarbonate cylinder (21 cm in diameter × 22.5 cm high) containing water at 22 °C at a depth of 18 cm. The mice were then forced to swim for 6 min. The duration of immobility was measured in 1-min as a period using a SCANET MV-40AQ (Melquest).

2.10. Statistical Analyses

All data are expressed as the mean ± standard error of the mean. Statistical differences between the two groups were determined using Student's *t*-test. Statistical analyses related to the behavioral test was re-performed by one-way ANOVA and *post-hoc* multiple comparisons using Tukey's test. In the microdialysis analysis, statistical differences were determined by a repeated measures two-way ANOVA followed by Bonferroni's *post-hoc* test when F ratios were significant ($p < 0.05$). All statistical analyses were performed by Prism version 5 (Graph Pad Software, San Diego, CA, USA).

3. Results

3.1. Mice with a Suppressed Piccolo Expression in the mPFC

First, mice with a suppressed Piccolo expression in the mPFC (miPiccolo mice) were produced via AAV- *Pclo* miRNA/EGFP vector microinjection (Figure 1A, upper panel). Immunohistochemical studies showed an obvious EGFP expression in the mPFC of miPiccolo mice (Figure 1A, lower panel). The *Pclo* mRNA expression in the mPFC of miPiccolo mice was downregulated to about half that of control Mock mice (Student's *t*-test, n = 6, *Pclo* (753–840): $p = 0.0001$, *Pclo* (14607–14771): $p = 0.0401$; Figure 1B). The Piccolo protein expression in the miPiccolo mice was also suppressed in the mPFC (Student's *t*-test, n = 6, $p = 0.0122$; Figure 1C). The miPiccolo mice also showed a decreased expression of presynaptic protein SNAP-25 in the mPFC, while the Munc18 and Synaptophysin levels remained unchanged (Student's *t*-test, n = 6, SNAP-25: $p = 0.0007$, Munc18: $p = 0.4016$, Synaptophysin: $p = 0.6339$; Figure 1D). Furthermore, the degree of phosphorylation at the CaMKII regulatory site in Synapsin I (Ser603) was lower in miPiccolo than in Mock mice (Student's *t*-test, n = 6, $p = 0.0038$; Figure 1E).

3.2. Diminished Synaptic Properties in the mPFC by Piccolo Suppression

To examine the synaptic properties of mPFC neurons, electrophysiological recordings of mPFC slices from miPiccolo mice were conducted. Analyses of paired-pulse facilitation, an indicator of presynaptic functions, revealed that miPiccolo mice had significantly lower ratios at an interstimulus interval of 20 and 60 ms than Mock mice (Student's *t*-test, n = 5, Interval 20: $p = 0.0331$, Interval 60: $p = 0.0073$, Interval 100: $p = 0.7503$; Figure 2A).

Next, LTP was examined in the mPFC. The suppression of Piccolo diminished LTP induction (average of 55–60 min, Student's *t*-test, n = 6, $p = 0.0055$; Figure 2B, right panel). Repeated theta-burst stimulation was then used to determine the LTP saturation, which indicated the functional retention of synaptic modification. The Mock mice had greater LTP saturation than the miPiccolo mice (average of 55–60 min, Student's *t*-test, n = 6, $p = 0.0001$; Figure 2C, right panel), suggesting that presynaptic dysfunction diminished the synaptic plasticity in the mPFC of miPiccolo mice.

3.3. Reduction in Depolarization-Evoked Glutamate and Dopamine Elevation in the mPFC by Piccolo Suppression

To clarify the changes in neurotransmission, the high-potassium ion (K^+)-induced elevation of extracellular neurotransmitter levels in the mPFC of miPiccolo mice was assessed using an in vivo microdialysis method. Accordingly, miPiccolo mice were found to have significantly lower basal levels of extracellular Glu in the mPFC than Mock mice (Student's *t*-test, n = 6, $p = 0.0300$; Figure 3A, left panel). In contrast, there was no marked difference in the basal levels of extracellular DA between miPiccolo and Mock mice (Student's *t*-test, n = 5, $p = 0.8845$; Figure 3B, left panel). An increase in the extracellular neurotransmitter levels by high-K^+-induced (100 mM) depolarization was observed in both Mock and miPiccolo mice (Figure 3A,B, right panel). However, there was a significant reduction in the depolarization-evoked Glu and DA elevation in the mPFC of miPiccolo mice (ANOVA with repeated measurement, Glu: n = 6, $F_{(9,90)} = 4.232$, $p = 0.0001$; Figure 3A, right panel and DA: n = 5, $F_{(8,64)} = 6.701$, $p < 0.0001$; Figure 3B, right panel).

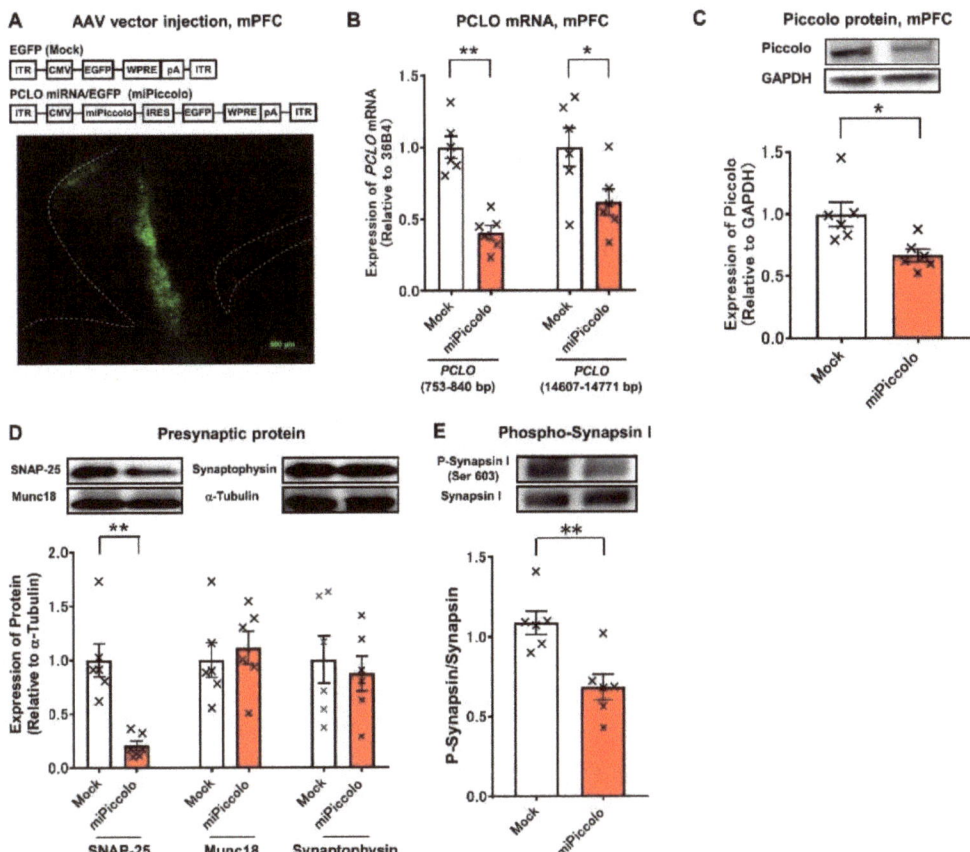

Figure 1. Generation of miPiccolo mice. (**A**) Upper panel, Sequence of AAV-EGFP or AAV- *Pclo* miRNA/EGFP vectors. The AAV vector was constructed using the cytomegalovirus immediate-early promoter (CMV) to drive EGFP or *Pclo* miRNA/EGFP. ITR: inverted terminal repeats, IRES: internal ribosomal entry site, WRPE: woodchuck hepatitis virus post-transcriptional regulatory element, pA: polyadenylation signal sequences. Lower panel, a fluorescent microscopic image of GFP in the mPFC of miPiccolo mouse (sagittal section). (**B**) The expression of *Pclo* mRNA was measured by quantitative real-time RT-PCR and presented as relative to the expression of the housekeeping gene 36B4 (n = 6). * $p < 0.05$, ** $p < 0.01$ vs. Mock (Student's *t*-test). (**C**) The expression of Piccolo was measured by Western blotting and presented as relative to the expression of GAPDH (n = 6). * $p < 0.05$ vs. Mock (Student's *t*-test). (**D**) The expression of presynaptic proteins in the mPFC. The bar graphs show the quantification of the expression of each protein compared with the expression of α-tubulin (n = 6). ** $p < 0.01$ vs. Mock (Student-*t* test). (**E**) The phosphorylation of Synapsin I in the mPFC was measured by Western blotting and presented as relative to the expression of Synapsin I (n = 6). ** $p < 0.01$ vs. Mock (Student's *t*-test).

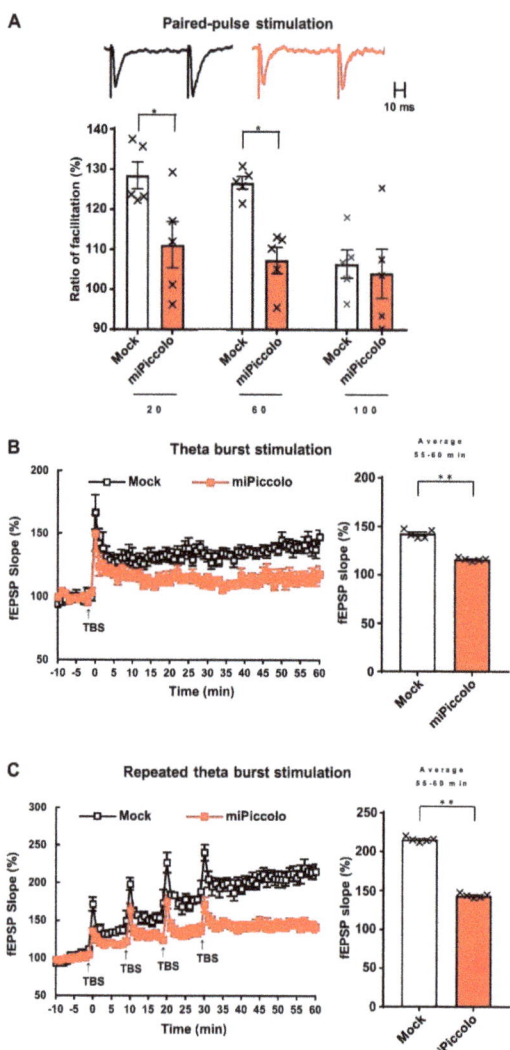

Figure 2. An electrophysiological analysis in the mPFC of miPiccolo mice. (**A**) Ratio of paired-pulse facilitation in the mPFC (n = 5). Representative slope pairs evoked with 60-ms interstimulus intervals are shown for the brain slice acutely prepared from the Mock and miPiccolo mice. * $p < 0.05$ vs. Mock (Student's *t*-test). (**B**) Left panel: Long-term potentiation (LTP) in the mPFC (n = 5). fEPSP: field excitatory postsynaptic potential, TBS: theta burst stimulation (TBS). Right panel: The potentiation rate was calculated by comparing the average slope 55–60 min after the TBS (n = 5). ** $p < 0.01$ vs. Mock (Student's *t*-test). (**C**) Left panel: Saturation of LTP in the mPFC (n = 5). Right panel: The potentiation rate was calculated by comparing the average slope 55–60 min after the first TBS (n = 5). ** $p < 0.01$ vs. Mock (Student's *t*-test).

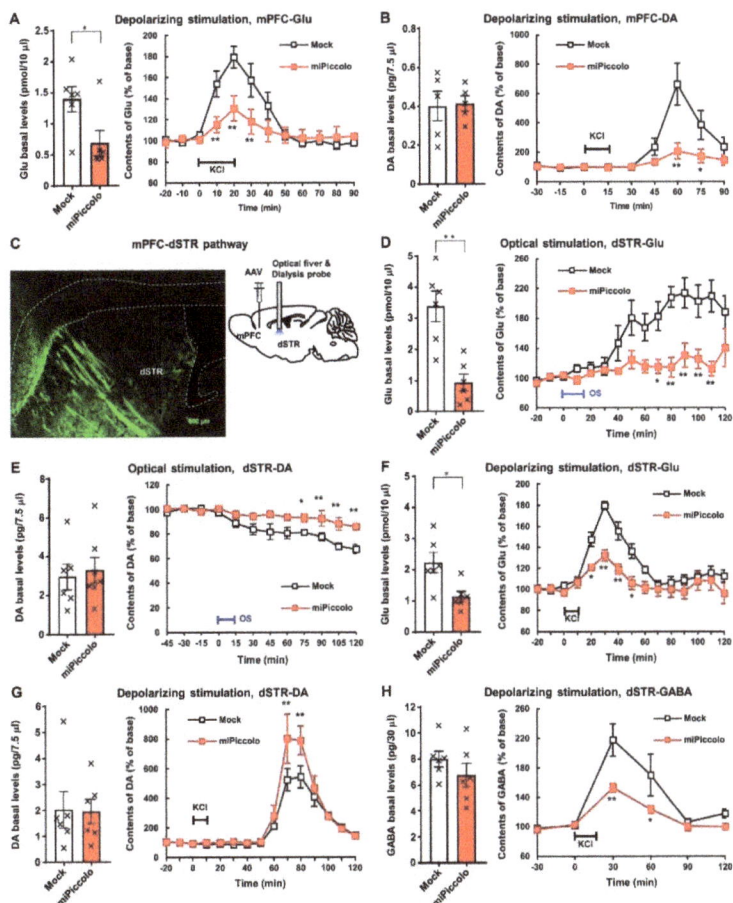

Figure 3. In vivo brain microdialysis in the mPFC and dSTR of miPiccolo mice. (**A**) Left panel: Basal extracellular levels of glutamate (Glu) in the mPFC (n = 6). * $p < 0.05$ vs. Mock (Student's t-test). Right panel: High K$^+$-stimulated (100 mM, 20 min) Glu elevation in the mPFC (n = 6). ** $p < 0.01$ vs. Mock (ANOVA with repeated measurement followed by Bonferroni's *post-hoc* test). (**B**) Left panel: Basal extracellular levels of dopamine (DA) in the mPFC (n = 5). Right panel: High-K$^+$-stimulated (100 mM, 15 min) DA elevation in the mPFC (n = 5). * $p < 0.05$, ** $p < 0.01$ vs. Mock (ANOVA with repeated measurement followed by Bonferroni's *post-hoc* test). (**C**) Left panel: A fluorescence microscopic image of GFP in the dSTR of miPiccolo mouse (sagittal section). Right panel: An image of the AAV vector injection site in the mPFC and the optical fiber and dialysis showing the cannulation site in the dSTR of the mouse. (**D**) Left panel: Basal extracellular levels of Glu in the dSTR (n = 6). ** $p < 0.01$ vs. Mock (Student's t-test). Right panel: Change in the Glu levels by optogenetic stimulation (15 min) in the dSTR (n = 6). * $p < 0.05$, ** $p < 0.01$ vs. Mock (ANOVA with repeated measurement followed by Bonferroni's *post-hoc* test). (**E**) Left panel: Basal extracellular levels of DA in the dSTR (n = 6). Right panel: Change in the DA levels by optogenetic stimulation (15 min) in the dSTR (n = 6). * $p < 0.05$, ** $p < 0.01$ vs. Mock (ANOVA with repeated measurement followed by Bonferroni's *post-hoc* test). (**F**) Left panel: Basal extracellular levels of Glu in the dSTR (n = 6). * $p < 0.05$ vs. Mock (Student's t-test). Right panel: High-K$^+$-stimulated (100 mM, 10 min) Glu elevation in the dSTR (n = 6). * $p < 0.05$, ** $p < 0.01$ vs. Mock (ANOVA with repeated measurement followed by Bonferroni's *post-hoc* test). (**G**) Left panel: Basal extracellular levels of DA in the dSTR (n = 6). Right panel: High-K$^+$-stimulated (100 mM, 10 min) DA elevation in the dSTR (n = 6). ** $p < 0.01$ vs. Mock (ANOVA with repeated measurement followed by Bonferroni's *post-hoc* test). (**H**) Left panel: Basal extracellular levels of GABA in the dSTR (n = 6). Right panel: High-K$^+$-stimulated (100 mM, 10 min) GABA elevation in the dSTR (n = 6). * $p < 0.05$, ** $p < 0.01$ vs. Mock (ANOVA with repeated measurement followed by Bonferroni's *post-hoc* test).

3.4. Diminished Neuronal Responses in the mPFC-dSTR Pathway by Piccolo Suppression

Changes to the neuronal function in the mPFC might significantly influence other brain regions. We therefore examined the brain region projecting from the mPFC by injecting an AAV-EGFP vector to the mPFC in order to visualize neuronal terminus with GFP fluorescence, indicating the projection from mPFC to dSTR (Figure 3C, left panel).

To investigate the neuronal function in the mPFC-dSTR pathway, changes in the extracellular Glu and DA levels in the dSTR were measured in response to optogenetic activation. Optogenetic stimulation of mPFC-dSTR projection was achieved by the local injection of an AAV vector expressing the light-sensitive protein CHIEF and laser stimulation in the dSTR (Figure 3C, right panel). The basal level of Glu without optical stimulation was significantly decreased in the dSTR of miPiccolo mice compared with CHIEF-AAV injection group, while that of DA was not markedly changed (Student's t-test, Glu: n = 6, p = 0.0014; Figure 3D, left panel and DA: n = 6, p = 0.6458; Figure 3E, left panel). Optical stimulation in the dSTR induced an increase in extracellular Glu and a decrease in extracellular DA levels through photosensory protein expression in the mPFC of Mock mice via the AAV-ChIEF vector injection (Figure 3D,E, right panel). However, responses to the optical stimulation of mPFC projections in the dSTR of miPiccolo mice were diminished (ANOVA with repeated measurement, Glu; n = 6, $F_{(14,140)}$ = 3.517, p < 0.0001; Figure 3D, right panel and DA: n = 6; $F_{(11,110)}$ = 5.943, p < 0.0001; Figure 3E, right panel). These results suggest that Piccolo induces abnormal behavior via the regulation of mPFC-dSTR projection in the extracellular Glu and DA levels in the dSTR.

To determine whether decrease of DA in dSTR under optical stimulation is mediated by glutamatergic transmission, NBQX, an antagonist for AMPA type of glutamate receptors, was applied to the microdialysis. The application of NBQX (20 μM) without optical stimulation reduced the extracellular DA in the dSTR (Supplementary Figure S1A). In comparison, NBQX application with optical stimulation induced a transient increase in the extracellular DA in the dSTR, which seems to be a relatively slight change compared to the condition without NBQX (Supplementary Figure S1B). These data suggest that blockade of glutamatergic transmission decreases the extracellular DA increase in the dSTR under optical stimulation.

3.5. Enhanced Depolarization-Evoked Dopamine Elevation Via Disinhibition of GABAergic Regulation in the dSTR by Piccolo Suppression

The high-K^+-induced elevation in extracellular neurotransmitters in the dSTR was measured to confirm the diminished connections in the mPFC-dSTR pathway in miPiccolo mice. miPiccolo mice showed significantly lower basal levels of extracellular Glu in the dSTR than Mock mice (Student's t-test, n = 6, p = 0.0135; Figure 3F, left panel), which is consistent with the results obtained in Figure 3D, left panel. In contrast, there was no observable differences in the basal DA or GABA levels between Mock and miPiccolo mice (Student's t-test, DA: n = 6, p = 0.9375; Figure 3G, left panel and GABA: n = 6, p = 0.2835; Figure 3H, left panel). The miPiccolo mice exhibited a greater reduction in depolarization-evoked Glu and GABA elevation in the dSTR than Mock mice (ANOVA with repeated measurement, Glu: n = 6, $F_{(12,120)}$ = 5.572, p < 0.0001; Figure 3F, right panel and GABA: n = 6; $F_{(5,50)}$ = 2.672, p = 0.0323; Figure 3H, right panel). Conversely, miPiccolo mice exhibited an enhanced depolarization-evoked DA elevation in the dSTR compared with Mock mice (ANOVA with repeated measurement, n = 6; $F_{(14,140)}$ = 2.207, p = 0.0102; Figure 3G, right panel). Taken together, these findings indicate that depolarization due to high-K^+ stimulation induced elevations of extracellular Glu, DA, and GABA levels in the dSTR, and these responses were enhanced in miPiccolo mice.

To investigate the regulation of extracellular DA level by GABAergic transmission, bicuculline, a GABA receptor antagonist, was applied to the microdialysis. Without optical stimulation, bicuculline (50 μM) elevated the extracellular DA levels in the dSTR (Supplementary Figure S1C). The effects of the blockade of the GABAergic transmission with optical stimulation was examined. However, all mice that received the combination of optical stimulation and bicuculline application (10–50 μM) to the dSTR died (n = 3) during or just after the measurement. Mice receiving bicuculline application (20–50 μM) during optical stimulation showed increased extracellular DA levels before death (Supplementary Figure S1D). Collectively, these results suggest blockade of GABAergic transmission elevates the extracellular DA levels in the dSTR.

3.6. Disruption of Locomotor Activity, Sensorimotor Gating, and the Cognitive Function by Piccolo Suppression

The miPiccolo mice showed a significantly increased locomotor activity in a novel environment compared to Mock mice (one-way ANOVA followed by Tukey's *post-hoc* test, n = 12; Mock-Saline vs. miPiccolo-Saline, $p = 0.0117$; Figure 4A, right panel). Significant impairment in the 78-dB prepulse/120-dB pulse trial was observed in miPiccolo mice compared to Mock mice when the acoustic startle response and PPI (psychometric measure of sensorimotor gating) were measured (one-way ANOVA followed by Tukey's *post-hoc* test, n = 11–12, 78–120 db, Mock-Saline vs. miPiccolo-Saline $p = 0.0383$, Figure 4B).

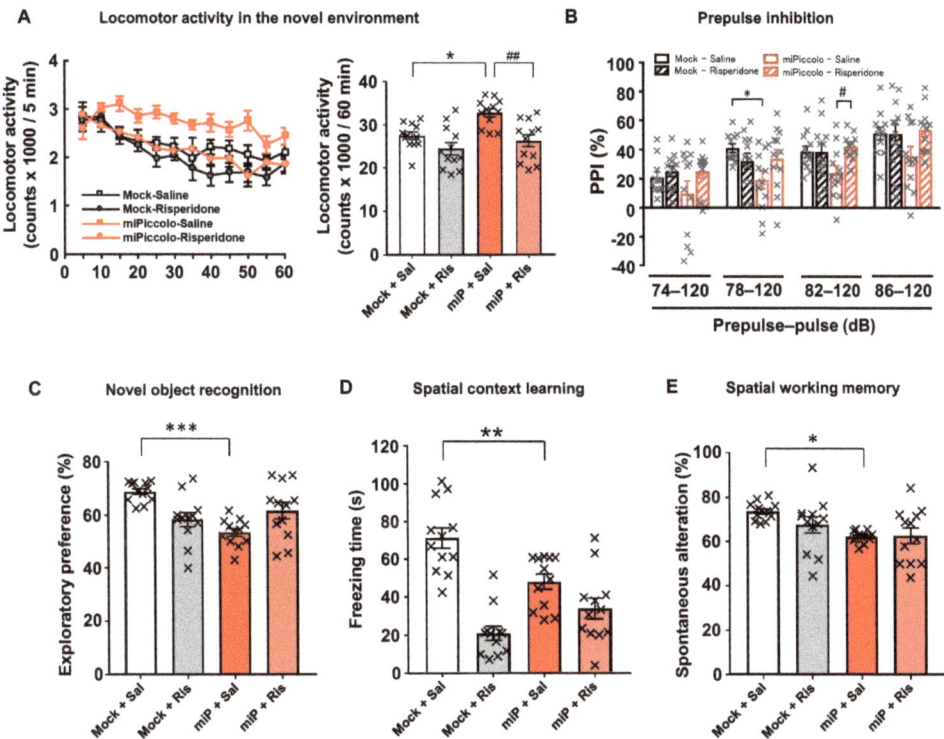

Figure 4. Behavioral analyses of miPiccolo mice. (**A**) The locomotor activity in a novel environment was measured every 5 min for 60 min (n = 12). * $p < 0.05$ vs. Mock-Saline, ## $p < 0.01$ vs. miPiccolo-Saline (one-way ANOVA followed by Tukey's *post-hoc* test). (**B**) Prepulse inhibition (PPI) was measured by presenting a semi-random series of prepulse of various intensities (74, 78, 82, 86 decibels) paired with the acoustic startle stimulus (120 db) to the mice (n = 12). * $p < 0.05$ vs. Mock-Saline, # $p < 0.05$ vs. miPiccolo-Saline (one-way ANOVA followed by Tukey's *post-hoc* test). (**C**) An indication of the time spent approaching the novel object in the trial phase of the novel object recognition test. Risperidone was administered 30 min before the acquisition and test phase (n = 12). *** $p < 0.001$ vs. Mock (one-way ANOVA followed by Tukey's *post-hoc* test). (**D**) Spatial context learning was assessed based on the freezing time at 24 h after a conditioning session. Risperidone was

administered 30 min before the training and test (n = 12). ** $p < 0.01$ vs. Mock (one-way ANOVA followed by Tukey's *post-hoc* test). (E) Spatial working memory was assessed based on spontaneous alterations in the Y-maze test (n = 12). * $p < 0.05$ vs. Mock (one-way ANOVA followed by Tukey's *post-hoc* test). Risperidone (0.01 mg/kg, i.p) was administered 30 min before the behavioral test.

To examine the role of Piccolo in the mPFC on learning and memory, Mock and miPiccolo mice were subjected to behavioral tests requiring precise cognitive control. First, the novel object recognition test was performed to measure the ability of the mice to recognize a familiar object. The Mock mice showed cognitive preference, as indicated by a longer exploration time for the novel object than for a familiar object. However, the miPiccolo mice showed a significantly shorter exploration time for the novel object than did the Mock mice (one-way ANOVA followed by Tukey's *post-hoc* test, n = 12, Mock-Saline vs. miPiccolo-Saline, $p < 0.0001$; Figure 4C).

In the spatial context learning test, we found that the miPiccolo mice exhibited significantly less freezing than Mock mice for context-elicited fear following conditioning (one-way ANOVA followed by Tukey's *post-hoc* test, Mock-Saline vs. miPiccolo-Saline, $p = 0.0064$; Figure 4D).

To determine the performance of immediate spatial working memory, the mice were subjected to the Y-maze test. There was decreased spontaneous alternation in the Y-maze test in the miPiccolo mice (one-way ANOVA followed by Tukey's *post-hoc* test, Mock-Saline vs. miPiccolo-Saline $p = 0.0189$; Figure 4E). As expected, the miPiccolo mice displayed schizophrenia-like behavioral impairments related to positive symptoms and cognitive deficits. Therefore, we evaluated the effect of risperidone (0.01 mg/kg) in Mock and miPiccolo mice. The miPiccolo mice receiving risperidone exhibited a marked reduction in locomotor activity in a novel environment compared to miPiccolo mice receiving saline (one-way ANOVA followed by Tukey's *post-hoc* test, n = 12, miPiccolo-Saline vs. miPiccolo-Risperidone $p = 0.0017$; Figure 4A, right panel). In addition, risperidone treatment reversed the PPI impairment induced by Piccolo suppression in the mPFC (one-way ANOVA followed by Tukey's *post-hoc* test, n = 11–12, 82–120 db, miPicclo-Saline vs. miPiccolo-Risperidone $p = 0.0332$, Figure 4B). In contrast, risperidone treatment did not improve the cognitive deficits in miPiccolo mice at doses effective for alleviating hyperlocomotion and PPI deficit (Figure 4C–E).

3.7. Stress Vulnerability Induced by Piccolo Suppression

To determine changes in stress sensitivity induced by Piccolo suppression in the mPFC, the miPiccolo mice were exposed to mild social defeat stress, after which the behavioral tests were performed. There were no marked differences in the interaction time in the social interaction test or the immobility time in the forced swim test between non-stress- and stress-exposed Mock mice (Figure 5A,B). However, stress-exposed miPiccolo mice had a significantly shorter interaction time in the social interaction test than non-stress-exposed miPiccolo mice (one-way ANOVA followed by Tukey's *post-hoc* test, n = 14, miPiccolo/non-stress vs. miPiccolo/stress $p = 0.0049$; Figure 5A). Similarly, a significant difference in the immobility time in the forced swim test was observed between non-stress- and stress-exposed miPiccolo mice (one-way ANOVA followed by Tukey's *post-hoc* test, n = 13–14, miPiccolo/non-stress vs. miPiccolo/stress $p = 0.0003$; Figure 5B). Thus, miPiccolo mice are suggested to be vulnerable to stress exposure.

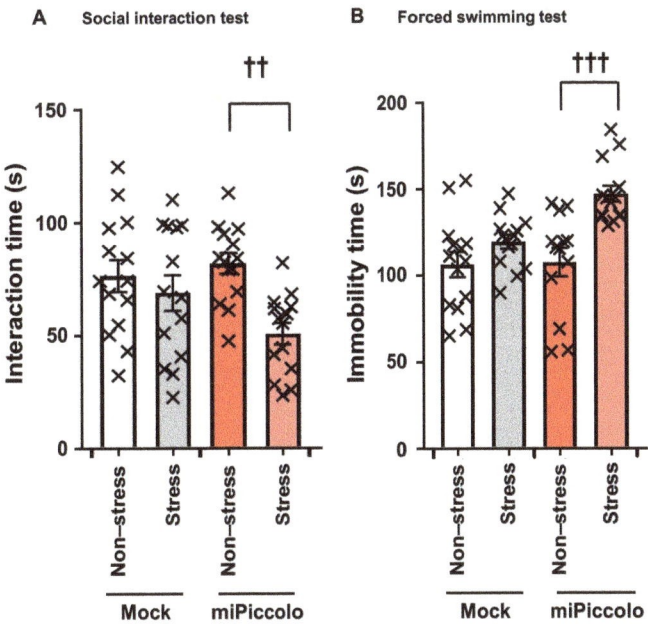

Figure 5. Stress sensitivity in miPiccolo mice. (**A**) After exposure to mild social defeat stress, the time in the interaction zone was measured for 10 min (n = 14). †† $p < 0.01$ vs. miPiccolo/non-stress (one-way ANOVA followed by Tukey's *post-hoc* test). (**B**) After exposure to mild social defeat stress, the immobility time in water was measured for the final 5 min during a 6-min time frame (n = 13–14). ††† $p < 0.001$ vs. miPiccolo/non-stress (one-way ANOVA followed by Tukey's *post-hoc* test).

4. Discussion

In the CNS, the synaptic proteins in the cytomatrix at the active zone (CAZ) in the presynaptic neuron maintain the structural and functional integrity of the synaptic vesicle pools and recruit L-type voltage-dependent Ca^{2+} channels to the presynaptic membrane. This allows the exocytosis of neurotransmitters from the synaptic vesicles [37]. Piccolo, a CAZ protein, can therefore regulate synaptic strength at the presynaptic neurons. In the present study, we showed that local Piccolo suppression in the mPFC resulted in diminished paired-pulse facilitation and LTP in the same brain region. Supporting this result, we observed reductions in the basal levels of extracellular Glu and depolarization-evoked elevations in extracellular Glu levels, which reflects the presynaptic Glu content, in the mPFC of miPiccolo mice. Our observations in electrophysiological and neurochemical analyses suggest that Piccolo suppression causes deficits in synaptic strength due to reduced neurotransmitter exocytosis from synaptic vesicles in the glutamatergic interneuron of the mPFC, whose impairment is related schizophrenia [38]. Furthermore, we observed changes in levels of CAZ proteins associated with the exocytosis of synaptic vesicles (Synapsin I phosphorylation and SNAP-25 expression) in the mPFC of miPiccolo mice, which supports this notion. Thus, Piccolo modulates the synaptic vesicle reserve pool and homeostasis of CAZ protein in vivo. Previously, Yang et al. generated brain-specific SNAP-25 knockout mice by crossbreeding of CaMKIIα-Cre mice of SNAP-25 flox mice [39]. The resultant mice exhibited schizophrenia-like behaviors accompanied by the reduction of SNAP-25 expression in the cortical and hippocampal regions. However, these mice also show the potent increase of glutamate levels in the cortex, which is opposite to the clinical evidence of schizophrenia, that is the glutamatergic dysfunction. In our present study, suppressed expression of Piccolo decreased the extracellular glutamate levels in the prefrontal cortex, following the clinical consensus. Schizophrenia-like behavioral impairments in prefrontal of Science; Japan Agency for Medical Research and Development (AMED) [JP16mk0101076h0001, JP18dm0107087, JP18dk0307081, JP18dm0107108]; Kobayashi Foundation; the SRF Grant for Biomedical Research and Foundation. The funders had no role in study design, data collection and analysis, decision to publish, or preparation of the manuscript.

Institutional Review Board Statement: All experimental procedures used in the present study were approved by the Committee of Animal Experiments at the University of Toyama, Toyama, Japan (approval number for animal experiments: A2018PHA-5; approval number for recombinant DNA experiments: G2015PHA-14). The clinical study was conducted in accordance with the Declaration of Helsinki. The Committee on Medical Ethics of Toyama University approved the present study (No. I2015004).

Informed Consent Statement: Informed consent was not obtained from all subjects inbolved in this study.

Data Availability Statement: Data presented in this manuscript are available upon request from the corresponding authors on reasonable request.

Acknowledgments: We thank Mika Ito and Naomi Takino (Jichi Medical University, Shimotsuke, Japan) for their help with the production of the AAV vectors.

Conflicts of Interest: The authors declare no competing financial interests.

References

Pearlson, G.D. Neurobiology of schizophrenia. *Ann. Neurol.* **2000**, *48*, 556–566. [CrossRef]

Nuechterlein, K.H.; Barch, D.M.; Gold, J.M.; Goldberg, T.E.; Green, M.F.; Heaton, R.K. Identification of separable cognitive factors in schizophrenia. *Schizophr. Res.* **2004**, *72*, 29–39. [CrossRef]

Rössler, W.; Salize, H.J.; van Os, J.; Riecher-Rössler, A. Size of burden of schizophrenia and psychotic disorders. *Eur. Neuropsychopharmacol.* **2005**, *15*, 399–409. [CrossRef] [PubMed]

Kani, A.S.; Shinn, A.K.; Lewandowski, K.E.; Öngür, D. Converging effects of diverse treatment modalities on frontal cortex in schizophrenia: A review of longitudinal functional magnetic resonance imaging studies. *J. Psychiatr. Res.* **2017**, *84*, 256–276. [CrossRef]

van Rossum, J.M. The significance of dopamine receptor blockade for the mechanism of action of neuroleptic drugs. *Arch. Int. Pharmacodyn. Ther.* **1966**, *160*, 492–494. [PubMed]

Weinberger, D.; Laruelle, M. Neurochemical and neuropharmacological imaging in schizophrenia. In *Neuropsychopharmacology—The Fifth Generation of Progress*; Lippincott Williams and Wilkins: Philadelphia, PA, USA, 2001; pp. 833–855.

Benes, F.M.; McSparren, J.; Bird, E.D.; SanGiovanni, J.P.; Vincent, S.L. Deficits in small interneurons in prefrontal and cingulate cortices of schizophrenic and schizoaffective patients. *Arch. Gen. Psychiatry* **1991**, *48*, 996–1001. [CrossRef] [PubMed]

Weinberger, D.R.; Egan, M.F.; Bertolino, A.; Callicott, J.H.; Mattay, V.S.; Lipska, B.K.; Berman, K.F.; Goldberg, T.E. Prefrontal neurons and the genetics of schizophrenia. *Biol. Psychiatry* **2001**, *50*, 825–844. [CrossRef]

Walton, E.; Hibar, D.P.; Van Erp, T.G.M.; Potkin, S.G.; Roiz-Santiañez, R.; Crespo-Facorro, B.; Suarez-Pinilla, P.; Van Haren, N.E.M.; De Zwarte, S.M.C.; Kahn, R.S.; et al. Positive symptoms associate with cortical thinning in the superior temporal gyrus via the ENIGMA schizophrenia consortium. *Acta Psychiatr. Scand.* **2017**, *135*, 439–447. [CrossRef]

Dieck, S.T.; Sanmartí-Vila, L.; Langnaese, K.; Richter, K.; Kindler, S.; Soyke, A.; Wex, H.; Smalla, K.-H.; Kämpf, U.; Fränzer, J.-T.; et al. Bassoon, a novel zinc-finger CAG/glutamine-repeat protein selectively localized at the active zone of presynaptic nerve terminals. *J. Cell Biol.* **1998**, *142*, 499–509. [CrossRef]

Fenster, S.; Chung, W.J.; Zhai, R.; Cases-Langhoff, C.; Voss, B.; Garner, A.M.; Kaempf, U.; Kindler, S.; Gundelfinger, E.D.; Garner, C. Piccolo, a presynaptic zinc finger protein structurally related to Bassoon. *Neuron* **2000**, *25*, 203–214. [CrossRef]

Gerber, S.H.; García, J.; Rizo, J.; Südhof, T.C. An unusual C2-domain in the active-zone protein piccolo: Implications for Ca^{2+} regulation of neurotransmitter release. *EMBO J.* **2001**, *20*, 1605–1619. [CrossRef]

García, J.; Gerber, S.H.; Sugita, S.; Südhof, T.C.; Rizo, J. A conformational switch in the Piccolo C2A domain regulated by alternative splicing. *Nat. Struct. Mol. Biol.* **2003**, *11*, 45–53. [CrossRef]

Shibasaki, T.; Sunaga, Y.; Fujimoto, K.; Kashima, Y.; Seino, S. Interaction of ATP sensor, cAMP sensor, Ca^{2+} sensor, and voltage-dependent Ca^{2+} channel in insulin granule exocytosis. *J. Biol. Chem.* **2004**, *279*, 7956–7961. [CrossRef]

Wang, X.; Kibschull, M.; Laue, M.M.; Lichte, B.; Petrasch-Parwez, E.; Kilimann, M.W. Aczonin, a 550-Kd putative scaffolding protein of presynaptic active zones, shares homology regions with Rim and Bassoon and binds profilin. *J. Cell Biol.* **1999**, *147*, 151–162. [CrossRef] [PubMed]

Südhof, T.C.; Rothman, J.E. Membrane fusion: Grappling with SNARE and SM proteins. *Science* **2009**, *323*, 474–477. [CrossRef]

Wang, X.; Hu, B.; Zieba, A.; Neumann, N.G.; Kasper-Sonnenberg, M.; Honsbein, A.; Hultqvist, G.; Conze, T.; Witt, W.; Limbach, C.; et al. A protein interaction node at the neurotransmitter release site: Domains of Aczonin/Piccolo, Bassoon, CAST, and Rim converge on the N-terminal domain of Munc13-1. *J. Neurosci.* **2009**, *29*, 12584–12596. [CrossRef] [PubMed] between these risk factors plays a potential role in the development of schizophr… The genetic suppression of Piccolo in the mPFC showed the following schizophr… behavioral impairments: enhanced locomotor activity as a positive symptom; d… objective, spatial and working memories as cognitive deficits; and impaired l… accompanying symptom. Such genetic manipulation made the mPFC highly su… to environmental stress. In addition, exposure of the mice to mild social defeat … to social withdrawal and a diminished motivation similar to the negative sym… schizophrenia. Some observed schizophrenia-like behavioral impairments impro… treatment with the atypical antipsychotic drug risperidone. Furthermore, at the r… and cellular levels, Piccolo suppression in the mPFC led to a reduced expressi… presynaptic protein SNAP-25. These findings are consistent with the observation… the postmortem PFC of schizophrenia patients [50–52]. Some brain regions, su… PFC, STR, amygdala, hippocampus, and thalamus, are involved in the pathoph… of schizophrenia. Indeed, neuroimaging studies on the effects of antipsychoti… tions and cognitive remediation therapy have shown that many schizophrenia… exhibit functional, structural, and metabolic abnormalities in the PFC [4]. Theref… been hypothesized that neuronal disconnection between the PFC and other brai… rather than abnormalities in a single brain region, is associated with the pathoph… of schizophrenia [7–9]. As mentioned above, functional disconnection was no… mPFC-dSTR pathway due to the suppression of Piccolo. Thus, miPiccolo mice ha… and predictive validities for schizophrenia. Piccolo-suppressed mice may be usef… models for schizophrenia, suggesting a decline in the expression or function of P… the PFC of schizophrenia patients.

Clinically, SNPs, which reduce the expression of *PCLO*, are related to the hig… of mental disorders [20,22,24]. In contrast, the piccolo levels of the autopsy bra… patients with schizophrenia are controversial (Supporting Figure S2 and [53])… probably because the most patients diagnosed with schizophrenia received the tr… of antipsychotics, which are reported to increase the expression of Piccolo (Su… Figure S2 and [54]). In the present study, mice with the knockdown of *Pclo* ge… mPFC exhibit similarity in the behavioral patterns. Our findings suggest tha… expression decreased in the patients with schizophrenia under the untreated con…

In conclusion, our findings show that the presynaptic cytomatrix protein… plays a functional role in the regulation of neurotransmitter exocytosis from … in vivo. Its suppressed expression in the mPFC affects not only the neuronal activ… mPFC but also the neuronal transmission mediated by Glu, GABA, and DA in t… Such neuronal dysfunction can cause behavioral impairments that resemble schiz… symptoms. Accordingly, the suppressed expression and/or function of Piccolo in… is considered one aspect of the pathophysiological condition in patients with schizo… In addition, these Piccolo-suppressed mice may be useful as a novel animal m… schizophrenia. Further clarification regarding the role of Piccolo in schizophrenia … offer new insight into psychiatry and the therapeutic treatment of schizophrenia.

Supplementary Materials: The following are available online at https://www.mdpi.com/a… .3390/jpm11070607/s1, Figure S1: In vivo antagonism of glutamate and GABA receptor on… lular DA in microdialysis, Figure S2: Piccolo expression in the PFC of schizophrenia patien… antipsychotic drug-treated mice.

Author Contributions: A.N. and Y.M. designed the project; Y.M. conducted all experimen… N.I., K.H., R.I., Y.K. and K.F., carried out the in vivo and in vitro experiments. Y.T., C.H., … and N.O., collected the human postmortem brains. S.-i.M., provided the AAV-Cre vectors. … and Y.M., analyzed the data. Y.M. wrote the manuscript draft. A.N. and N.I., revised and p… the final version of the manuscript. All authors have read and agreed to the published versi… manuscript.

Funding: This work was supported by the grant-in-aid for Scientific Research (KAKEN… [JSPS KAKENHI Grant Number, JP21H02632, 26293213], from the Japan Society for the Pr…

downregulation of Piccolo are probably not mediated by observed reduction of SNAP-25. Piccolo may play a vital role in the regulation of neurotransmitter release.

In combination experiments of microdialysis and optogenetics, we found that optical stimulation of the mPFC-dSTR projection induced the elevation of Glu and reduction of DA. The application of NBQX in the dSTR inhibited the reduction of the extracellular DA level, suggesting that the activation of mPFC-dSTR projection negatively regulated the extracellular DA level in the dSTR mediated by glutamatergic transmission. However, without optical stimulation, the application of NBQX in the dSTR reduced the DA levels, suggesting that the extracellular DA levels in the dSTR receive positive regulation by the local glutamatergic system. Therefore, the relationship between extracellular DA in the dSTR and its regulation by glutamatergic transmission is complicated. In addition, bicuculline application to the dSTR increased the extracellular levels of DA, which suggests that the DA in the dSTR is under the regulation of GABAergic transmission. This does not contradict the elevation of extracellular DA levels observed with the combination of bicuculline application and optical stimulation, although the mice suffered a fatal outcome. Our notion that extracellular DA levels in the dSTR are regulated by glutamatergic and GABAergic transmission is supported by the findings of previous studies. In the neuronal circuits in the STR, glutamatergic projection neurons from the PFC provide excitatory input to GABA neurons in the STR, and GABA neurons in the STR regulate the DA nerve terminals projected from the substantia nigra [40,41]. However, the DA responses in the dSTR under optical and depolarizing stimulation are completely different. This discrepancy may be due to limitations in the methodology, as optogenetic stimulation of the terminals from the mPFC may increase the D2 autoreceptor activity or induce changes in the cholinergic neurotransmission, and depolarizing stimulation may also exert a wide range of mechanisms that could alter DA release. Further analyses of the neuronal composition of the projection from mPFC to dSTR and the relationship between glutamatergic and GABAergic transmissions are necessary. Indeed, our optical stimulation system cannot excite specific neurons, so the auto receptors of D2 and cholinergic neuronal system could be regulated. Many mechanisms potentially underlying the DA release alternation via optical stimulation and depolarization by high K+ should be considered. However, such experiments involve certain technical limitations at present, so no all phenomenon can be explained by knockdown of Piccolo in the mPFC alone.

It is well-known that the glutamatergic and dopaminergic neuronal systems in the PFC control the cognitive functions. Changes in these functions are closely linked to mental disorders, especially schizophrenia. The glutamatergic neuronal system is known to mediate episodic memory. In schizophrenia patients, the PFC exhibits a reduced glutamatergic neuronal activity and NMDA receptor expression compared with that in healthy persons [42,43]. The dopaminergic neuronal system in the PFC is involved in higher-order executive functions and working memory [44–47]. Functional abnormalities of DA receptors have been observed in the PFC of schizophrenia patients [48]. In the present study, a behavioral analysis of Piccolo suppression in the mPFC showed disruptions in episodic memory, such as object recognition and spatial context learning, as well as working memory. These disruptions in the cognitive function were not improved by the administration of the atypical antipsychotic drug risperidone. Similarly, clinically used antipsychotic drugs are not particularly effective in improving cognitive dysfunction in schizophrenia patients. Therefore, the reduced glutamatergic and dopaminergic neuronal responses by Piccolo suppression in the PFC are considered to be similar to the pathophysiological conditions seen in schizophrenia patients.

Current clinical treatments for schizophrenia have proven effective for ameliorating positive symptoms, but only a few treatments have been effective against negative symptoms and cognitive deficits. Therefore, elucidating the pathophysiological conditions related to schizophrenia is crucial for the early development of efficient therapeutic treatments. The two-hit hypothesis has been proposed as an etiology of schizophrenia. Many genetic and environmental risk factors are commonly involved in schizophrenia. The overlap

18. Ibi, D.; Nitta, A.; Ishige, K.; Cen, X.; Ohtakara, T.; Nabeshima, T.; Ito, Y. Piccolo knockdown-induced impairments of spatial learning and long-term potentiation in the hippocampal CA1 region. *Neurochem. Int.* **2010**, *56*, 77–83. [CrossRef] [PubMed]
19. Cen, X.; Nitta, A.; Ibi, D.; Zhao, Y.; Niwa, M.; Taguchi, K.; Hamada, M.; Ito, Y.; Wang, L.; Nabeshima, T. Identification of Piccolo as a regulator of behavioral plasticity and dopamine transporter internalization. *Mol. Psychiatry* **2008**, *13*, 451–463. [CrossRef] [PubMed]
20. Seo, S.; Takayama, K.; Uno, K.; Ohi, K.; Hashimoto, R.; Nishizawa, D.; Ikeda, K.; Ozaki, N.; Nabeshima, T.; Miyamoto, Y.; et al. Functional analysis of deep intronic SNP rs13438494 in intron 24 of PCLO gene. *PLoS ONE* **2013**, *8*, e76960. [CrossRef]
21. Uno, K.; Nishizawa, D.; Seo, S.; Takayama, K.; Matsumura, S.; Sakai, N.; Ohi, K.; Nabeshima, T.; Hashimoto, R.; Ozaki, N.; et al. The Piccolo intronic single nucleotide polymorphism rs13438494 Regulates dopamine and serotonin uptake and shows associations with dependence-like behavior in genomic association study. *Curr. Mol. Med.* **2015**, *15*, 265–274. [CrossRef]
22. Choi, K.H.; Higgs, B.W.; Wendland, J.R.; Song, J.; McMahon, F.J.; Webster, M.J. Gene expression and genetic variation data implicate PCLO in bipolar disorder. *Biol. Psychiatry* **2011**, *69*, 353–359. [CrossRef]
23. Giniatullina, A.; Maroteaux, G.; Geerts, B.; Koopmans, B.; Loos, M.; Klaassen, R.; Chen, N.; Van Der Schors, R.; Van Nierop, P.; Li, K.W.; et al. Functional characterization of the PCLO p. Ser4814Ala variant associated with major depressive disorder reveals cellular but not behavioral differences. *Neuroscience* **2015**, *300*, 518–538. [CrossRef]
24. Sullivan, P.F.; De Geus, E.J.C.; Willemsen, G.; James, M.R.; Smit, J.H.; Zandbelt, T.; Arolt, V.; Baune, B.T.; Blackwood, D.; Cichon, S.; et al. Genome-wide association for major depressive disorder: A possible role for the presynaptic protein Piccolo. *Mol. Psychiatry* **2008**, *14*, 359–375. [CrossRef] [PubMed]
25. Igata, R.; Katsuki, A.; Kakeda, S.; Watanabe, K.; Igata, N.; Hori, H.; Konishi, Y.; Atake, K.; Kawasaki, Y.; Korogi, Y.; et al. PCLO rs2522833-mediated gray matter volume reduction in patients with drug-naive, first-episode major depressive disorder. *Transl. Psychiatry* **2017**, *7*, e1140. [CrossRef] [PubMed]
26. Ryan, J.; Artero, S.; Carrière, I.; Maller, J.J.; Meslin, C.; Ritchie, K.; Ancelin, M.-L. GWAS-identified risk variants for major depressive disorder: Preliminary support for an association with late-life depressive symptoms and brain structural alterations. *Eur. Neuropsychopharmacol.* **2016**, *26*, 113–125. [CrossRef] [PubMed]
27. Schott, B.H.; Assmann, A.; Schmierer, P.; Soch, J.; Erk, S.; Garbusow, M.; Mohnke, S.; Pöhland, L.; Romanczuk-Seiferth, N.; Barman, A.; et al. Epistatic interaction of genetic depression risk variants in the human subgenual cingulate cortex during memory encoding. *Transl. Psychiatry* **2014**, *4*, e372. [CrossRef] [PubMed]
28. Woudstra, S.; Bochdanovits, Z.; Van Tol, M.-J.; Veltman, D.J.; Zitman, F.G.; Van Buchem, M.A.; Van Der Wee, N.J.; Opmeer, E.M.; Demenescu, L.R.; Aleman, A.; et al. Piccolo genotype modulates neural correlates of emotion processing but not executive functioning. *Transl. Psychiatry* **2012**, *2*, e99. [CrossRef] [PubMed]
29. Krzyżosiak, A.; Szyszka-Niagolov, M.; Wietrzych, M.; Gobaille, S.; Muramatsu, S.-I.; Krezel, W. Retinoid X receptor gamma control of affective behaviors involves dopaminergic signaling in mice. *Neuron* **2010**, *66*, 908–920. [CrossRef] [PubMed]
30. Iida, A.; Takino, N.; Miyauchi, H.; Shimazaki, K.; Muramatsu, S.-I. Systemic delivery of tyrosine-mutant AAV vectors results in robust transduction of neurons in adult mice. *BioMed Res. Int.* **2013**, *2013*, 1–8. [CrossRef]
31. Paxinos, G.; Franklin, K. *The Mouse Brain in Stereotaxic Coordinates: Compact*, 3rd ed.; Elsevier: Amsterdam, The Netherlands, 2008; ISBN 9780123742445.
32. Fu, K.; Miyamoto, Y.; Sumi, K.; Saika, E.; Muramatsu, S.-I.; Uno, K.; Nitta, A. Overexpression of transmembrane protein 168 in the mouse nucleus accumbens induces anxiety and sensorimotor gating deficit. *PLoS ONE* **2017**, *12*, e0189006. [CrossRef] [PubMed]
33. Miyamoto, Y.; Iegaki, N.; Fu, K.; Ishikawa, Y.; Sumi, K.; Azuma, S.; Uno, K.; Muramatsu, S.-I.; Nitta, A. Striatal N-acetylaspartate synthetase Shati/Nat8l regulates depression-like behaviors via mGluR3-mediated serotonergic suppression in mice. *Int. J. Neuropsychopharmacol.* **2017**, *20*, 1027–1035. [CrossRef]
34. Niwa, M.; Nitta, A.; Mizoguchi, H.; Ito, Y.; Noda, Y.; Nagai, T.; Nabeshima, T. A novel molecule "Shati" is involved in methamphetamine-induced hyperlocomotion, sensitization, and conditioned place preference. *J. Neurosci.* **2007**, *27*, 7604–7615. [CrossRef] [PubMed]
35. Miyamoto, Y.; Ishikawa, Y.; Iegaki, N.; Sumi, K.; Fu, K.; Sato, K.; Furukawa-Hibi, Y.; Muramatsu, S.-I.; Nabeshima, T.; Uno, K.; et al. Overexpression of Shati/Nat8l, an N-acetyltransferase, in the nucleus accumbens attenuates the response to methamphetamine via activation of group II mGluRs in mice. *Int. J. Neuropsychopharmacol.* **2014**, *17*, 1283–1294. [CrossRef]
36. Lin, J.Y.; Lin, M.Z.; Steinbach, P.; Tsien, R.Y. Characterization of engineered channelrhodopsin variants with improved properties and kinetics. *Biophys. J.* **2009**, *96*, 1803–1814. [CrossRef]
37. Alabi, A.A.; Tsien, R.W. Synaptic vesicle pools and dynamics. *Cold Spring Harb. Perspect. Biol.* **2012**, *4*, a013680. [CrossRef]
38. Wang, H.-X.; Gao, W.-J. Cell type-specific development of NMDA receptors in the interneurons of rat prefrontal cortex. *Neuropsychopharmacology* **2009**, *34*, 2028–2040. [CrossRef] [PubMed]
39. Yang, H.; Zhang, M.; Shi, J.; Zhou, Y.; Wan, Z.; Wang, Y.; Wan, Y.; Li, J.; Wang, Z.; Fei, J. Brain-specific SNAP-25 deletion leads to elevated extracellular glutamate level and schizophrenia-like behavior in mice. *Neural Plast.* **2017**, *2017*, 1–11. [CrossRef] [PubMed]
40. Carlsson, A.; Waters, N.; Holm-Waters, S.; Tedroff, J.; Nilsson, M.; Carlsson, M.L. Interactions between monoamines, glutamate and GABA in schizophrenia: New evidence. *Annu. Rev. Pharmacol. Toxicol.* **2001**, *41*, 237–260. [CrossRef]

41. Meyer-Lindenberg, A.; Miletich, R.S.; Kohn, P.D.; Esposito, G.; Carson, R.E.; Quarantelli, M.; Weinberger, D.R.; Berman, K.F. Reduced prefrontal activity predicts exaggerated striatal dopaminergic function in schizophrenia. *Nat. Neurosci.* **2002**, *5*, 267–271. [CrossRef] [PubMed]
42. Bartha, R.; Williamson, P.C.; Drost, D.J.; Malla, A.; Carr, T.J.; Cortese, L.; Canaran, G.; Rylett, R.J.; Neufeld, R.W.J. Measurement of glutamate and glutamine in the medial prefrontal cortex of never-treated schizophrenic patients and healthy controls by proton magnetic resonance spectroscopy. *Arch. Gen. Psychiatry* **1997**, *54*, 959–965. [CrossRef]
43. Pilowsky, L.S.; Bressan, R.; Stone, J.M.; Erlandsson, K.; Mulligan, R.S.; Krystal, J.H.; Ell, P.J. First in vivo evidence of an NMDA receptor deficit in medication-free schizophrenic patients. *Mol. Psychiatry* **2005**, *11*, 118–119. [CrossRef]
44. Paus, T.; Castro-Alamancos, M.A.; Petrides, M. Cortico-cortical connectivity of the human mid-dorsolateral frontal cortex and its modulation by repetitive transcranial magnetic stimulation. *Eur. J. Neurosci.* **2001**, *14*, 1405–1411. [CrossRef]
45. Strafella, A.P.; Paus, T.; Barrett, J.; Dagher, A. Repetitive transcranial magnetic stimulation of the human prefrontal cortex induces dopamine release in the caudate nucleus. *J. Neurosci.* **2001**, *21*, RC157. [CrossRef]
46. Uylings, H.B.; Groenewegen, H.J.; Kolb, B. Do rats have a prefrontal cortex? *Behav. Brain Res.* **2003**, *146*, 3–17. [CrossRef]
47. Durstewitz, D.; Seamans, J.K. The dual-state theory of prefrontal cortex dopamine function with relevance to catechol-o-methyltransferase genotypes and schizophrenia. *Biol. Psychiatry* **2008**, *64*, 739–749. [CrossRef] [PubMed]
48. Okubo, Y.; Suhara, T.; Suzuki, K.; Kobayashi, K.; Inoue, O.; Terasaki, O.; Someya, Y.; Sassa, T.; Sudo, Y.; Matsushima, E.; et al. Decreased prefrontal dopamine D1 receptors in schizophrenia revealed by PET. *Nat. Cell Biol.* **1997**, *385*, 634–636. [CrossRef]
49. Davis, J.; Eyre, H.; Jacka, F.N.; Dodd, S.; Dean, O.; McEwen, S.; Debnath, M.; McGrath, J.; Maes, M.; Amminger, P.; et al. A review of vulnerability and risks for schizophrenia: Beyond the two hit hypothesis. *Neurosci. Biobehav. Rev.* **2016**, *65*, 185–194. [CrossRef]
50. Thompson, P.M.; Sower, A.C.; Perrone-Bizzozero, N.I. Altered levels of the synaptosomal associated protein SNAP-25 in schizophrenia. *Biol. Psychiatry* **1998**, *43*, 239–243. [CrossRef]
51. Karson, C.N.; Mrak, R.E.; Schluterman, K.O.; Sturner, W.Q.; Sheng, J.G.; Griffin, W.S.T. Alterations in synaptic proteins and their encoding mRNAs in prefrontal cortex in schizophrenia: A possible neurochemical basis for "hypofrontality". *Mol. Psychiatry* **1999**, *4*, 39–45. [CrossRef]
52. Hashimoto, T.; Volk, D.W.; Eggan, S.M.; Mirnics, K.; Pierri, J.N.; Sun, Z.X.; Sampson, A.R.; Lewis, D.A. Gene expression defi-cits in a subclass of GABA neurons in the prefrontal cortex of subjects with schizophrenia. *J. Neurosci.* **2003**, *23*, 6315–6326. [CrossRef] [PubMed]
53. Weidenhofer, J.; Bowden, N.A.; Scott, R.J.; Tooney, P.A. Altered gene expression in the amygdala in schizophrenia: Up-regulation of genes located in the cytomatrix active zone. *Mol. Cell. Neurosci.* **2006**, *31*, 243–250. [CrossRef] [PubMed]
54. Weidenhofer, J.; Scott, R.J.; Tooney, P.A. Investigation of the expression of genes affecting cytomatrix active zone function in the amygdala in schizophrenia: Effects of antipsychotic drugs. *J. Psychiatr. Res.* **2009**, *43*, 282–290. [CrossRef] [PubMed]

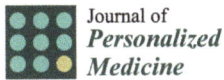

Review

New Insights Regarding Diagnosis and Medication for Schizophrenia Based on Neuronal Synapse–Microglia Interaction

Naotaka Izuo and Atsumi Nitta *

Department of Pharmaceutical Therapy and Neuropharmacology, School of Pharmaceutical Sciences, Graduate School of Pharmaceutical Sciences, University of Toyama, 2630 Sugitani, Toyama 930-0194, Japan; ntk3izuo@pha.u-toyama.ac.jp
* Correspondence: nitta@pha.u-toyama.ac.jp; Tel.: +81-76-415-8822 (ext. 8823); Fax: +81-76-415-8826

Abstract: Schizophrenia is a common psychiatric disorder that usually develops during adolescence and young adulthood. Since genetic and environmental factors are involved in the disease, the molecular status of the pathology of schizophrenia differs across patients. Recent genetic studies have focused on the association between schizophrenia and the immune system, especially microglia–synapse interactions. Microglia physiologically eliminate unnecessary synapses during the developmental period. The overactivation of synaptic pruning by microglia is involved in the pathology of brain disease. This paper focuses on the synaptic pruning function and its molecular machinery and introduces the hypothesis that excessive synaptic pruning plays a role in the development of schizophrenia. Finally, we suggest a strategy for diagnosis and medication based on modulation of the interaction between microglia and synapses. This review provides updated information on the involvement of the immune system in schizophrenia and proposes novel insights regarding diagnostic and therapeutic strategies for this disease.

Keywords: schizophrenia; microglia; synaptic pruning; complement; CX3CR1; medication; diagnosis

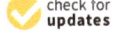

Citation: Izuo, N.; Nitta, A. New Insights Regarding Diagnosis and Medication for Schizophrenia Based on Neuronal Synapse–Microglia Interaction. *J. Pers. Med.* **2021**, *11*, 371. https://doi.org/10.3390/jpm11050371

Academic Editor: Tomiki Sumiyoshi

Received: 13 March 2021
Accepted: 28 April 2021
Published: 3 May 2021

Publisher's Note: MDPI stays neutral with regard to jurisdictional claims in published maps and institutional affiliations.

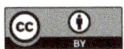

Copyright: © 2021 by the authors. Licensee MDPI, Basel, Switzerland. This article is an open access article distributed under the terms and conditions of the Creative Commons Attribution (CC BY) license (https://creativecommons.org/licenses/by/4.0/).

1. Introduction

Schizophrenia is a severe mental disorder described in the *Diagnostic and Statistical Manual of Mental Disorders, Fifth Edition* and the 11th revision of the International Classification of Diseases, and it develops during adolescence and young adulthood in most cases, with a global prevalence of approximately 1% [1]. Patients with schizophrenia mainly exhibit positive symptoms, such as hallucinations and delusions; negative symptoms, such as decreased motivation and anhedonia; and cognitive dysfunction. Previous twin studies on schizophrenia have estimated heritability at 80% [2]. However, the findings from such twin studies may be exaggerated because of environmental and patient lifestyle factors [3]. The significance of the interaction between genetic and environmental factors has been recognized in the pathogenesis of schizophrenia [3].

Genetic studies are effective for determining the causes and pathogenesis of diseases. Genome-wide association studies (GWASs) are important tools for elucidating the mechanisms underlying schizophrenia, including the formation of diseases. The dopamine hypothesis, the current leading theory of the pathogenesis of schizophrenia [4,5], is supported by genetic studies indicating that single nucleotide variations (SNVs) related to dopaminergic transmission, such as DRD2 [6], COMT [7], DISC1 [8], and PCLO [9–11], are associated with a higher risk of schizophrenia [5,12]. The GWAS conducted by the Schizophrenia Working Group of the Psychiatric Genomics Consortium has had a notable impact on the study of schizophrenia [13]. The study recruited 36,989 patients with schizophrenia and 113,075 controls and revealed 108 genetic loci associated with the pathology of schizophrenia, including *DRD2* and several genes related to neuronal transmission, which supports the conventional pathological theory of schizophrenia. However, 83 of the 108 loci had not been previously reported when the study was conducted, including genes related to the immune system. It is noteworthy that the major histocompatibility complex (MHC) locus located on chromosome 6 displayed a higher association with schizophrenia than any other locus across the genome, which is consistent with the findings of previous reports [14–17]. This region contains genes related to innate immunity. These genetic studies have highlighted immune involvement in the etiology of schizophrenia.

The relationship between schizophrenia and the immune system should be investigated. Human postmortem studies of the brains of patients with schizophrenia have previously reported abnormal morphology and the accumulation of microglia, the resident immune cells in the central nervous system [18,19]. In addition, a number of biomarker studies measuring inflammatory cytokines in the peripheral blood and cerebrospinal fluid (CSF) [20,21], and imaging studies using positron emission tomography (PET) to detect neuroinflammation [22,23] have clarified the immunological characteristics of patients with schizophrenia. Immunological changes modify the pathological state of the neuronal system in the brain of patients with schizophrenia [24]. Therefore, the association between immune dysfunction and schizophrenia depends on the background of each individual. A strategy aiming to modulate the immune system could lead to new medications for schizophrenia, and simultaneously, the treatment should be personalized according to certain criteria based on diagnosis via biomarkers to examine the immunological characteristics of each patient.

Dysfunction of the prefrontal cortex (PFC) is considered to be involved in schizophrenia [25,26]. Patients with schizophrenia exhibit volume loss in the PFC [27,28] and disturbance of cognitive functions related to the PFC, including attention, cognitive flexibility, and working memory [29–32]. For example, in the Wisconsin Card Sorting Test, which assesses the flexibility of thinking associated with the PFC, a higher frequency of perseverative responses has been observed in patients with schizophrenia [31]. Such functional disturbances in the PFC are consistent with the evidence from functional magnetic resonance imaging studies indicating the lower activity of the PFC with respect to episodic encoding and retrieval [33], and in response to consummatory pleasure [34]. In 1982, Feinberg suggested that schizophrenia is caused by a fault in programmed synaptic elimination during adolescence [35]. Thereafter, studies have indicated that synaptic pruning is involved in the development of neuronal circuits, especially in the PFC, in early adulthood, when most individuals are diagnosed with schizophrenia [36]. Furthermore, microglial activations are observed in the PFC of patients with schizophrenia [37]. In a recent decade, synaptic pruning by microglia has been revealed to be involved in psychiatric diseases in addition to normal brain development [38–40]. Thus, Feinberg's suggestion is supported by recent immunological findings in schizophrenia [35].

In the following sections, we introduce microglial functions in synaptic development and maintenance focusing on synaptic pruning, and their relevance to schizophrenia pathology. Afterwards, we provide a novel insight into the diagnosis and treatment of schizophrenia based on microglia–synapse interactions.

2. Microglia–Synapse Interaction

Microglia are brain cells related to innate immunity, and they are involved in various physiological and pathological processes [41]. Similar to peripheral macrophages, the activation of toll-like receptors on the microglial surface mediates their morphological changes and induces phagocytosis and the release of inflammatory cytokines [42,43]. Microglia are activated in disease-specific and aging-specific manners to release inflammatory cytokines and chemokines, and they remove the deposits of pathological proteins by the process of phagocytosis [44]. In recent decades, it has been revealed that the physiological functions of microglia are necessary to construct and maintain healthy neuronal circuits. Microglia dynamically extend their processes to neuronal synapses to survey their conditions [45–48]. The microglia eliminate unnecessary synapses (a process called "synaptic pruning") during the appropriate and specific periods of neuronal development [38,39]. Neuronal circuits then become sophisticated through the selective pruning of synapses with lower activity [39]. The pharmacological depletion of microglia by antagonism of colony-stimulating factor 1 receptor (CSF1R) from postnatal day 2 (P2) to P13 in mice disrupted synaptic pruning and induced poly-innervation of the medial nucleus of the trapezoid body neurons, instead of healthy mono-innervation [49]. CSF1R antagonism from P14 to P28 increased synaptic density due to decreased pruning and disturbed glutamatergic transmission [50]. These findings clearly demonstrated the significance of synaptic pruning by microglia in neuronal development.

Synaptic pruning and phagocytosis share a common machinery mainly regulated by "find-me", "eat-me", and "don't-eat-me" signals [51,52]. The find-me signal is mediated by chemo-attractants and their receptors. Chemokine (C-X3-C motif) ligand 1 (CX3CL1), which is highly expressed in the brain especially in the cerebral cortex and hippocampus [53], is secreted from neurons or synapses to bind to its receptor CX3C chemokine receptor 1 (CX3CR1) and is exclusively expressed in microglia [54]. Each line of *Cx3cl1* and *Cx3cr1* knockout mice exhibited delayed and reduced synaptic pruning during the developmental period [38,39]. The secretion of mature CX3CL1 requires cleavage by a disintegrin and metalloproteinase domain-containing protein 10 (ADAM10) on the plasma membrane [55]. The pharmacological inhibition of ADAM10 further leads to profound deficits in the elimination of sensory synapses [55]. ATP is extracellularly released through the pannexin-1 channel to bind purinergic receptors [56]. P2Y12 mediates microglial recruitment to remove apoptotic cells as well as unnecessary synapses [57–60]. Activity-dependent synaptic pruning during development was shown to be delayed in P2Y12-deficient mice [58–60].

Phosphatidylserine, usually existing on the inner leaflet of the plasma membrane, mediates eat-me signals when exposed on the cellular surface [61,62]. Phospholipid scramblase 1 [62] and transmembrane protein 16F (TMEM16F) [63], which are calcium-activated phosphatidylserine scramblases, reversibly expose phosphatidylserine on the cell surface. Although these scramblases are expressed by neurons and modulate microglia [62], their functions in synaptic pruning are unclear. Among various receptors of phosphatidylserine, triggering receptors expressed on myeloid cells 2 (TREM2) and G protein-coupled receptor 56 modulate microglia to induce synaptic pruning and phagocytosis [64,65].

The complement system, discovered by Bordet and Gengou in 1901, is composed of nine main components (C1–C9), some inhibitory and regulatory substances, and their membrane receptors (Figure 1) [66–68]. They exert their functions, such as the opsonization of antigens, the formation of the membrane attack complex (MAC) to destroy bacteria, and the stimulation of macrophage chemotaxis, via three pathways of enzymatic chain reaction (classical, alternative, and lectin pathways). In addition to the long-studied, immune-activating effects, novel functions of complements of synaptic pruning during development have been revealed [69,70]. C3, expressed in the synaptic regions as a "tag", which allows synapse elimination, mediates synaptic pruning and regulates synaptic density and transmission via its receptor, CR3, on microglia [71,72]. Synaptic C1q and C4 exert a similar tagging function for synaptic pruning [73,74]. The proteomic analysis of the individual synaptosomes conducted using flowcytometry revealed that the local expression of proteins related to neuronal transmission, energy metabolism, and the antioxidant system was altered in the C1q-tagged synaptic fraction [73]. Although it is unclear whether such an alteration is a trigger or consequence of C1q tagging, these proteins altered in C1q-tagged synaptic fractions possibly change the neuronal transmission of synapses.

Cell-surface sugar residues further regulate microglial phagocytosis. Galactose promotes phagocytosis by binding to the galectin family [75], and sialic acid suppresses this function via Siglec [76,77]. The heterozygous mice with glucosamine-2-epimerase/N-acetylmannosamine kinase, a sialic acid synthase, exhibited a decrease in postsynaptic marker PSD-95 accompanied by a decrease in sialic acid in the brain and altered the microglial morphology [78]. The don't-eat-me signal, similar to sialic acid, is mediated by CD47 and its receptor signal-regulatory protein alpha (SIRPα). CD47 suppresses synaptic elimination and phagocytosis by microglia [79].

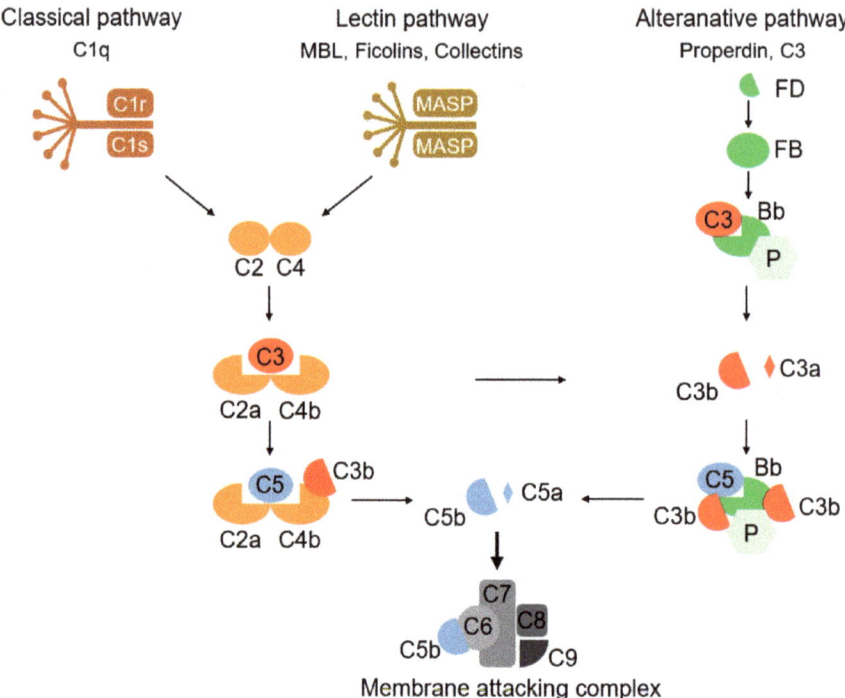

Figure 1. An overview of systemic complement activation. The complement system is composed of nine main components (C1–C9) and regulatory factors. Immunological functions are conducted by three pathways: the classical, alternative, and lectin pathways. In these pathways, enzymatic chain reactions of the complements proceed to finally form a membrane attack complex to destroy bacteria and virus-infected cells. MASP, mannose-binding protein-associated serine protease; FD, factor D; FB, factor B; Bb, factor Bb; P, properdin.

3. Microglia–Synapse Interaction in Schizophrenia

Although synaptic pruning by microglia is essential for the sophistication of neuronal circuits during the developmental stage, excessive elimination is considered to be involved in neurological disorders (Figure 2). As predicted by Feinberg, synaptic pruning might be involved in the pathogenesis of schizophrenia [35], and studies have suggested the presence of excessive synaptic pruning in schizophrenia. Recently, Sekar et al. revealed that an allele of C4 located in the MHC locus increases the risk of schizophrenia [74], which has led to studies searching for a link between the complement system and schizophrenia [80]. The association between C4 and schizophrenia is supported by a study from Sweden that proposed the possibility of predicting the future risk of this disorder by utilizing blood analysis during the neonatal period [81]. Higher C4 levels were likewise detected in the CSF of patients with schizophrenia [82]. The SNVs of the C3 gene with protective or harmful effects regarding schizophrenia onset were identified by a study that recruited more than 2000 Han Chinese individuals [83]. C3 mRNA expression was upregulated in the PFC of those that demonstrated depression followed by suicide [84]. Moreover, the C5 protein levels in the CSF were elevated in patients with schizophrenia [85].

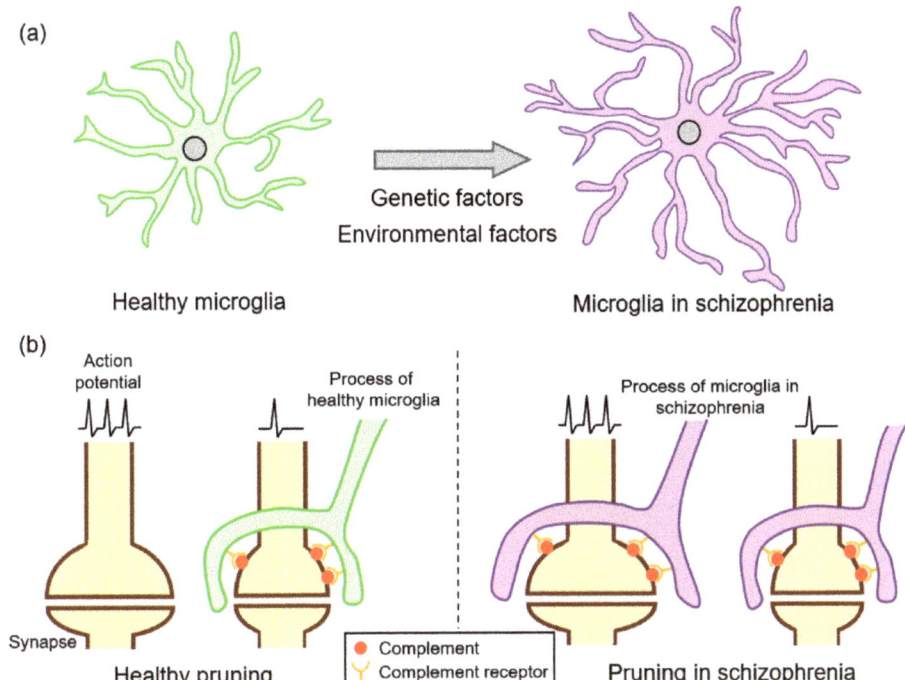

Figure 2. The microglial synaptic pruning in schizophrenia. (**a**) Microglia exhibit hyper-ramified morphology in schizophrenia due to genetic and environmental factors. (**b**) Healthy microglia eliminate complement-tagged synapses with lower activity. In schizophrenia, hyper-ramified microglia prune healthy synapses by the excessive activation of complements.

Since alterations in the complement system of the brain are associated with psychiatric disorders [74,81], identifying their pathological contribution should help clarify the mechanisms underlying these diseases. Mice overexpressing C4 were generated to investigate the pathological significance of C4 upregulation in schizophrenia [86]; the overexpression of C4 in utero in the PFC of the mouse resulted in a reduction in spine density due to abnormal increase in synaptic removal by microglia 21 days after birth and a related decrease in the frequency and amplitude of miniature excitatory postsynaptic potentials [86]. These abnormal neuronal connections caused a decrease in social interaction with the mother at the age of 60 days [86]. Yilmaz et al. generated mice overexpressing human C4A with a knockout of the murine C4 gene [87]. These mice exhibited enhanced microglial synaptic pruning in the PFC and a reduction in spine density at 60 days of age [87]. In addition to decreased social behavior, these mice showed increased anxiety-like behavior and decreased novel environment exploration [87]. Such behavioral alterations observed in both studies are assumed to be equivalent to a part of a schizophrenia symptom. These studies strongly suggest a link between elevated C4 expression associated with this disorder and the pathogenesis of schizophrenia, including spine density reduction in the PFC.

The complement-related synaptic impairment in schizophrenia was revealed by a study with patient-derived induced pluripotent stem cells (iPSCs) [88]. Interestingly, excessive synaptic pruning observed in schizophrenia appears to involve the impairments of both neurons and microglia. The microglia-like cells (iMG) differentiated from the monocytes of patients with schizophrenia exhibited higher phagocytic activity compared to that of synaptosomes prepared from neurons derived from iPSCs of healthy controls and of patients with schizophrenia. Although there were no differences in spine density between the neuronal cultures derived from iPSCs of controls and of patients with schizophrenia, C4 risk variants increased C3 deposition in the latter culture. Furthermore, the co-culture of neurons derived from the iPSCs of patients with schizophrenia with the corresponding iMG showed a reduction in spine density compared to what was prepared from healthy subjects. These results support the notion of excessive synaptic pruning mediated by complements in schizophrenia [88]. The results are expected from the mechanistic analysis on the malignancy of neurons and microglia in schizophrenia.

The deregulation of brain complements, which is closely related to psychiatric disorders including schizophrenia, is derived from genetic and/or environmental factors. Maternal infection during the perinatal period is known to increase the risk of schizophrenia [89,90]. Based on the evidence that maternal infection reduces synaptic density in the brain of the offspring [91,92], such an infection has certain impacts on the brain complement system and possibly increases the risk of schizophrenia. Higher levels of maternal blood C1q have been reported to be associated with the risk of schizophrenia [93]. In this report, adenovirus, herpes simplex virus 2, influenza B virus, and *Toxoplasma gondii* approximately doubled the risk. There was no correlation between C-reactive protein levels and schizophrenia risk [93]. *Toxoplasma* infection in humans is a risk factor for schizophrenia, and it induces behavioral dysfunction in rodent models [94,95]. Severe infection of adult mice with *Toxoplasma* has been reported to greatly upregulate C3 and C4 proteins, and mildly enhance C1q expression [96,97]. In rodent studies, the induction of marked systemic inflammation by lipopolysaccharide administration increased the levels of C3 and C3R in the brain [98,99].

Synaptic pruning is further regulated by signaling other than the complement factors. PolySia is a linear polymer of sialic acid with a degree of polymerization of 8–400, mediating a don't-eat-me signal to microglia [100]. The number of hippocampal and dorsolateral PFC cells with polySia is reduced in the brains of patients with schizophrenia [101,102]. The content of the polisialylated neural cell adhesion molecule (PSA-NCAM) is further reduced in the PFC of patients with schizophrenia [102]. The serum PSA-NCAM is associated with cognitive decline, as evaluated by the Mini-Mental State Examination, and is further associated with the reduction in gray matter volume [103]. Furthermore, the SNVs on *ST8SIA2*, encoding one of the polysialyltransferases, are related to schizophrenia. Associations between rs3759916 and rs3759914 in the promoter regions of *ST8SIA2* and schizophrenia have been identified in the Japanese population [104]. Another association between rs3759915 and schizophrenia has been found in Chinese [105] and Spanish populations [106]. In rodent experiments, *ST8SIA2* knockout mice exhibited disturbed mossy fiber formation and impaired fear-conditioned memory [107]. TREM2, a phosphatidylserine receptor mediating eat-me signaling, is important for adequate neuronal development by modulating microglia [64]. TREM2 mRNA levels are increased in the peripheral leukocytes of patients with schizophrenia [108–110], which is consistent with the results of rodent studies. However, the pathological roles of these sugar residues, phospholipids, and related molecules are not fully understood. Further studies clarifying such molecules will lead to the precise understanding of microglial synaptic pruning in schizophrenia.

4. Potential Diagnosis/Medication for Schizophrenia Based on Microglia–Synapse Interaction

4.1. Perspective for the Diagnosis of Schizophrenia

Although the deficits in synaptic elimination are involved in the pathogenesis of schizophrenia, their contribution will differ among patients because these deficits are derived from the genetic and/or environmental background of the individuals. Obtaining information on patient's brain status is expected to help determine the therapeutic direction for patients with schizophrenia. PET imaging, which visualizes the distribution and behavior of a specific molecule, is generally utilized. Based on the notion that excessive synaptic elimination mediates the pathology of schizophrenia, monitoring the synaptic density or pruning capacity of microglia would help in diagnosis. A small-scale PET study by Howes et al. reported a reduced synaptic density in the PFC of patients with schizophrenia, caused by the reduced binding of the radioactive ligand [^{11}C]UCB-J to its target protein, synaptic vesicle glycoprotein 2A [111,112]. Radio-tracing is strongly expected to be used in the context of schizophrenia to enhance clinical evaluation. With respect to the microglial proteins monitored by PET tracers, the translocator protein 18 kDa (TSPO) has been targeted in neurological diseases, such as Alzheimer's disease and multiple sclerosis [113]. However, TSPO tracers were reported to be unable to discriminate patients with schizophrenia from healthy controls [114]. This is possibly because TSPO is upregulated in the pro-inflammatory context in glial cells [115], while the morphology of microglia with longer processes and more branches observed in schizophrenia are different from those in Alzheimer's disease and multiple sclerosis [18,19]. In order to discriminate patients with schizophrenia, a target that reflects microglial pruning activity is suitable. Scarce radiotracers targeting anti-inflammatory microglia have been developed [116]. Recently, a radioactive ligand that binds to the purinergic receptor P2Y12 was generated and appears to be undergoing structural optimization to enhance blood–brain barrier (BBB) penetration [116]. CX3CR1 and complement receptor CR3 are candidate targets on the cell surface, reflecting phagocytosis and synaptic pruning activity. AZD8797 and SB290157 are selective antagonists of CX3CR1 and CR3 [117,118], respectively, and have the potential to be the lead compounds utilized as radioactive tracers for PET imaging to monitor the synaptic pruning activity of microglia.

The blood biomarkers that reflect the molecular condition of the brain are highly desirable because proteins derived from the brain are mixed with those from peripheral tissues in the circulation and are difficult to discriminate. In schizophrenia, the blood complement levels in patients are not notably altered. In one report, there were no differences in serum C1q, C3, and C4 in patients with first-episode psychosis (FEP) occurring at approximately 20 years of age, but a 20% increase in C4 levels was noted in patients more than seven years after onset [119]. Another study reported a 20% increase in the blood levels of C4 and C9 in drug-free FEP [81]. A meta-analysis of blood complements in patients with schizophrenia revealed no differences compared to the controls [120]. Elevated C4 levels have simultaneously been found in the CSF of patients with schizophrenia [82], and another report further found elevations of C5 in the CSF of patients with this disorder [85], while the blood leukocyte fraction from drug-free FEP showed no change in C4 mRNA [121]. Therefore, complement upregulation specifically occurs in the brain.

The exosome, which is a nano-sized carrier with a lipid bilayer and is secreted into the extracellular space, is attracting attention as a promising tool for disease diagnosis [122,123]. Cells actively enclose proteins and nucleic acids into exosomes to transmit signals to neighboring or distant cells [122,123]. In recent decades, a technique has been developed for extracting cell-type specific exosomes from blood samples via surface markers. Goetzl et al. developed a method to collect neuron-derived exosomes (NDE) using the neuronal surface marker L1CAM [124,125]. Since the proteins and nucleic acids included in the exosome could escape from nonspecific enzymatic degradation in the blood, their methods for collecting NDE made it possible to understand the molecular circumstances in the patient's brain. This method has already been applied to some neurological diseases, including schizophrenia. Goetzl et al. further found a severe reduction in MFN2 and CYPD proteins in the NDE of patients with schizophrenia, suggesting the impairment of mitochondria in the disease [126]. They collected astrocyte-derived exosomes (ADE) to determine the upregulation of complement proteins; this suggests that complement abnormalities occur in astrocytes in schizophrenia [127]. Currently, there are limited reports on the collection of microglia-derived exosomes (MDE) [128] because microglia largely share the surface marker with peripheral macrophages. Thus, targeting microglial-specific surface markers, such as TMEM119 [129], could be beneficial for collecting MDE. Since the complement system functions through cellular interaction, the application of a combination of NDE, ADE, and MDE would be a powerful tool to monitor complement abnormalities in the brain.

4.2. Perspective for Medication Drug Therapy in Schizophrenia

Clinical trials of anti-inflammatory drugs for schizophrenia have been performed. Minocycline, a tetracycline-type antibiotic, suppresses the microglial inflammatory response [130,131]. Minocycline has been reported to rescue cognitive dysfunction and social behavioral impairment in animal models of schizophrenia [132,133]. Minocycline abolished the phagocytosis of patient-derived iMG toward spine density on neurons differentiated by patient-derived iPSCs [88]. In clinical trials, minocycline treatment improved the working memory [134], and verbal and visual learning [135] of patients with schizophrenia. Although minocycline is infrequently prescribed partly because of the increased risk of autoimmune disease [136], these outcomes demonstrate the clinical effectiveness of this strategy targeting microglia in schizophrenia. N-acetylcysteine (NAC), a precursor of antioxidant glutathione, exerts a wide range of protective effects, such as the regulation of oxidative status, inflammation, and monoamine neurotransmission in rodent models and human patients [137,138]. NAC showed a beneficial effect mainly on the negative symptoms of patients with schizophrenia receiving antipsychotic treatment (comprehensively reviewed in [139]). It is possible to achieve these therapeutic effects of NAC by multiple mechanisms, such as modulation of the oxidative and inflammation statuses, and neurotransmission.

The complement components are considered not only as diagnostic biomarkers but also as therapeutic targets. This is partly because the overexpression of C4 in mice induces behavioral impairments related to schizophrenia, which is accompanied by excessive synaptic pruning by microglia and defects in neuronal transmission in the PFC [86,87]. In addition, C3, C4, and C5 are considered to be upregulated in the brains of patients with schizophrenia [81–85]. In 2007, eculizumab, a monoclonal antibody against C5, was approved as a drug for paroxysmal nocturnal hemoglobinuria (PNH) by the FDA [140,141]. However, eculizumab stochastically increases C3 expression in erythrocytes to mediate the formation of MAC leading to de novo extravascular hemolysis in patients with PNH, which reduced the clinical benefits of the treatment [142]. To overcome this side effect, pegcetacoplan, a peptide-based C3 inhibitor, was developed and administered in an open-label, phase Ib, prospective, and non-randomized study [143]. Pegcetacoplan was confirmed to be well-tolerated and resulted in an improved hematological response in patients with PNH who remained anemic during treatment with eculizumab [143]. Another potential modulator of synaptic pruning for schizophrenia treatment targets CX3CL1-CX3CR1 signaling. E6011, a monoclonal antibody that selectively binds to CX3CL1, has been developed for rheumatic diseases [144]. Recently, a phase 2, multicenter, randomized, double-blind, and placebo-controlled study of E6011 for rheumatoid arthritis was conducted after recruiting 190 patients with active rheumatic arthritis (RA) who inadequately responded to methotrexate, the first-choice drug for RA treatment. The administration of E6011 once every two weeks for 24 weeks significantly improved the clinical RA score, which was evaluated using the American College Rheumatology 20% improvement criteria without severe adverse events [145,146]. A clinical trial of E6011 for Crohn's disease has likewise started [147]. Although clinical studies have not been initiated for schizophrenia, modulators of the C3-CR3 and CX3CL1-CX3CR1 pathways could be potential candidates for future medications for the behavioral and cognitive symptoms of schizophrenia mediated by decelerating excessive synaptic pruning.

The activation of the don't-eat-me signal should be effective for schizophrenia medication. The stimulation of this signal by CD47-SIRPα mediates escape from synaptic pruning [148,149]. In preclinical studies, the deficiency of CD47 induced impairment of social behavior [150] and exaggerated cognitive dysfunction in mice [151]. The agonism of SIRPα could be a potential strategy to suppress synaptic pathology in schizophrenia.

Considering that excessive synaptic pruning occurs before the emergence of clinical symptoms in schizophrenia, the strategy to modulate synaptic pruning should start preclinically. Thus, such medication should be combined with the monitoring of the synaptic status in the brain as mentioned above. In addition, there is an increased risk of infection because of the suppression of innate immunity, which could ensue with these medication candidates.

It is necessary for drugs to reach the brain for the treatment of schizophrenia. With respect to recent drug delivery technology into the brain, conjugations by BBB-penetrating peptides [152,153] and intranasal administration have been developed [154,155]. The combination of the synapse-protecting reagent and brain delivery methods could be used to treat schizophrenia.

5. Conclusions

Microglia have been suggested to play a significant role in excessive synaptic elimination with respect to the pathology of schizophrenia. Various molecules, such as CX3CL1-CX3CR1, CD47-SIRPα, and lectins, are physiologically and pathologically involved in this process. Recent publications indicating the contribution of complement components to schizophrenia are attracting attention with respect to this relationship. The monitoring and modulation of microglial synaptic pruning based on the complement system would be powerful tools for diagnosis and medication in schizophrenia. Further investigation on synapse–microglia interaction could reveal other molecular targets for diagnosis and medication. Considering that schizophrenia is a polygenic disease, such medication and diagnosis should be combined to find excessive pruning in the preclinical stage, and early medication could maximize the therapeutic effects for schizophrenia. Developments of the medication and diagnosis focusing on synapse–microglia interaction and its clinical application to schizophrenia are desired.

Author Contributions: N.I. drafted the manuscript. N.I. and A.N. revised and approved the final version of the manuscript. Both authors have read and agreed to the published version of the manuscript.

Funding: This study was supported by JSPS KAKENHI Grant-in Aid for Young Scientists (JP20K16006) and Scientific Research (JP21H02632). Kobayashi Foundation; and Smoking Research Foundation partially supported the review.

Conflicts of Interest: The authors declare no competing financial interest.

References

1. Janoutova, J.; Janackova, P.; Sery, O.; Zeman, T.; Ambroz, P.; Kovalova, M.; Varechova, K.; Hosak, L.; Jirik, V.; Janout, V. Epidemiology and risk factors of schizophrenia. *Neuroendocrinol. Lett.* **2016**, *37*, 1–8. [PubMed]
2. Besteher, B.; Brambilla, P.; Nenadic, I. Twin studies of brain structure and cognition in schizophrenia. *Neurosci. Biobehav. Rev.* **2020**, *109*, 103–113. [CrossRef] [PubMed]
3. Torrey, E.F.; Yolken, R.H. Schizophrenia as a pseudogenetic disease: A call for more gene-environmental studies. *Psychiatry Res.* **2019**, *278*, 146–150. [CrossRef] [PubMed]
4. Devor, A.; Andreassen, O.A.; Wang, Y.; Maki-Marttunen, T.; Smeland, O.B.; Fan, C.C.; Schork, A.J.; Holland, D.; Thompson, W.K.; Witoelar, A.; et al. Genetic evidence for role of integration of fast and slow neurotransmission in schizophrenia. *Mol. Psychiatry* **2017**, *22*, 792–801. [CrossRef]
5. Howes, O.D.; McCutcheon, R.; Owen, M.J.; Murray, R.M. The Role of Genes, Stress, and Dopamine in the Development of Schizophrenia. *Biol. Psychiatry* **2017**, *81*, 9–20. [CrossRef]
6. Hanif, F.; Amir, Q.U.; Washdev, W.; Bilwani, F.; Simjee, S.U.; Haque, Z. A Novel Variant in Dopamine Receptor Type 2 Gene is Associated with Schizophrenia. *Arch. Med. Res.* **2020**, *52*, 348–353. [CrossRef]
7. Bassett, A.S.; Marshall, C.R.; Lionel, A.C.; Chow, E.W.C.; Scherer, S.W. Copy number variations and risk for schizophrenia in 22q11.2 deletion syndrome. *Hum. Mol. Genet.* **2008**, *17*, 4045–4053. [CrossRef]
8. Wang, H.Y.; Liu, Y.; Yan, J.W.; Hu, X.L.; Zhu, D.M.; Xu, X.T.; Li, X.S. Gene polymorphisms of DISC1 is associated with schizophrenia: Evidence from a meta-analysis. *Prog. Neuropsychopharmacol. Biol. Psychiatry* **2018**, *81*, 64–73. [CrossRef]
9. Inoue, K.; Ando, N.; Suzuki, E.; Hayashi, H.; Tsuji, D.; Itoh, K. Genotype distributions and allele frequencies of possible major depressive disorder-associated single nucleotide polymorphisms, cyclic adenosine monophosphate response element binding protein 1 rs4675690 and Piccolo rs2522833, in a Japanese population. *Biol. Pharm. Bull.* **2012**, *35*, 265–268. [CrossRef]
10. Cen, X.; Nitta, A.; Ibi, D.; Zhao, Y.; Niwa, M.; Taguchi, K.; Hamada, M.; Ito, Y.; Ito, Y.; Wang, L.; et al. Identification of Piccolo as a regulator of behavioral plasticity and dopamine transporter internalization. *Mol. Psychiatry* **2008**, *13*, 451–463. [CrossRef]
11. Seo, S.; Takayama, K.; Uno, K.; Ohi, K.; Hashimoto, R.; Nishizawa, D.; Ikeda, K.; Ozaki, N.; Nabeshima, T.; Miyamoto, Y.; et al. Functional Analysis of Deep Intronic SNP rs13438494 in Intron 24 of PCLO Gene. *PLoS ONE* **2013**, *8*, e76960. [CrossRef]

12. Farrell, M.S.; Werge, T.; Sklar, P.; Owen, M.J.; Ophoff, R.A.; O'Donovan, M.C.; Corvin, A.; Cichon, S.; Sullivan, P.F. Evaluating historical candidate genes for schizophrenia. *Mol. Psychiatry* **2015**, *20*, 555–562. [CrossRef]
13. Schizophrenia Working Group of the Psychiatric Genomics Consortium. Biological insights from 108 schizophrenia-associated genetic loci. *Nature* **2014**, *511*, 421–427. [CrossRef]
14. International Schizophrenia Consortium. Common polygenic variation contributes to risk of schizophrenia and bipolar disorder. *Nature* **2009**, *460*, 748–752. [CrossRef]
15. Shi, J.X.; Levinson, D.F.; Duan, J.B.; Sanders, A.R.; Zheng, Y.L.; Pe'er, I.; Dudbridge, F.; Holmans, P.A.; Whittemore, A.S.; Mowry, B.J.; et al. Common variants on chromosome 6p22.1 are associated with schizophrenia. *Nature* **2009**, *460*, 753–757. [CrossRef] [PubMed]
16. Stefansson, H.; Ophoff, R.A.; Steinberg, S.; Andreassen, O.A.; Cichon, S.; Rujescu, D.; Werge, T.; Pietilainen, O.P.H.; Mors, O.; Mortensen, P.B.; et al. Common variants conferring risk of schizophrenia. *Nature* **2009**, *460*, 744–747. [CrossRef] [PubMed]
17. Mokhtari, R.; Lachman, H.M. The Major Histocompatibility Complex (MHC) in Schizophrenia: A Review. *J. Clin. Cell. Immunol.* **2016**, *7*, 479. [CrossRef] [PubMed]
18. Radewicz, K.; Garey, L.J.; Gentleman, S.M.; Reynolds, R. Increase in HLA-DR immunoreactive microglia in frontal and temporal cortex of chronic schizophrenics. *J. Neuropathol. Exp. Neurol.* **2000**, *59*, 137–150. [CrossRef]
19. Steiner, J.; Bielau, H.; Brisch, R.; Danos, P.; Ullrich, O.; Mawrin, C.; Bernstein, H.G.; Bogerts, B. Immunological aspects in the neurobiology of suicide: Elevated microglial density in schizophrenia and depression is associated with suicide. *J. Psychiatr. Res.* **2008**, *42*, 151–157. [CrossRef]
20. Goldsmith, D.R.; Rapaport, M.H.; Miller, B.J. A meta-analysis of blood cytokine network alterations in psychiatric patients: Comparisons between schizophrenia, bipolar disorder and depression. *Mol. Psychiatry* **2016**, *21*, 1696–1709. [CrossRef] [PubMed]
21. Orlovska-Waast, S.; Kohler-Forsberg, O.; Brix, S.W.; Nordentoft, M.; Kondziella, D.; Krogh, J.; Benros, M.E. Cerebrospinal fluid markers of inflammation and infections in schizophrenia and affective disorders: A systematic review and meta-analysis. *Mol. Psychiatry* **2019**, *24*, 869–887. [CrossRef] [PubMed]
22. Bloomfield, P.S.; Selvaraj, S.; Veronese, M.; Rizzo, G.; Bertoldo, A.; Owen, D.R.; Bloomfield, M.A.P.; Bonoldi, I.; Kalk, N.; Turkheimer, F.; et al. Microglial Activity in People at Ultra High Risk of Psychosis and in Schizophrenia: An [(11)C]PBR28 PET Brain Imaging Study. *Am. J. Psychiatry* **2016**, *173*, 44–52. [CrossRef] [PubMed]
23. Van Berckel, B.N.; Bossong, M.G.; Boellaard, R.; Kloet, R.; Schuitemaker, A.; Caspers, E.; Luurtsema, G.; Windhorst, A.D.; Cahn, W.; Lammertsma, A.A.; et al. Microglia activation in recent-onset schizophrenia: A quantitative (R)-[11C]PK11195 positron emission tomography study. *Biol. Psychiatry* **2008**, *64*, 820–822. [CrossRef] [PubMed]
24. Almulla, A.F.; Al-Rawi, K.F.; Maes, M.; Al-Hakeim, H.K. In schizophrenia, immune-inflammatory pathways are strongly associated with depressive and anxiety symptoms, which are part of a latent trait which comprises neurocognitive impairments and schizophrenia symptoms. *J. Affect. Disord.* **2021**, *287*, 316–326. [CrossRef]
25. Stuss, D.T.; Kaplan, E.F.; Benson, D.F.; Weir, W.S.; Steven, C.; Sarazin, F.F. Evidence for the involvement of orbitofrontal cortex in memory functions: An interference effect. *J. Comp. Physiol. Psychol.* **1982**, *96*, 913–925. [CrossRef]
26. Müller, H.F. Prefrontal cortex dysfunction as a common factor in psychosis. *Acta Psychiatr. Scand.* **1985**, *71*, 431–440. [CrossRef]
27. Walton, E.; Hibar, D.P.; van Erp, T.G.M.; Potkin, S.G.; Roiz-Santianez, R.; Crespo-Facorro, B.; Suarez-Pinilla, P.; van Haren, N.E.M.; de Zwarte, S.M.C.; Kahn, R.S.; et al. Prefrontal cortical thinning links to negative symptoms in schizophrenia via the ENIGMA consortium. *Psychol. Med.* **2018**, *48*, 82–94. [CrossRef]
28. Kuo, S.S.; Pogue-Geile, M.F. Variation in fourteen brain structure volumes in schizophrenia: A comprehensive meta-analysis of 246 studies. *Neurosci. Biobehav. Rev.* **2019**, *98*, 85–94. [CrossRef]
29. Buchsbaum, M.S.; Nuechterlein, K.H.; Haier, R.J.; Wu, J.; Sicotte, N.; Hazlett, E.; Asarnow, R.; Potkin, S.; Guich, S. Glucose metabolic rate in normals and schizophrenics during the Continuous Performance Test assessed by positron emission tomography. *Br. J. Psychiatry* **1990**, *156*, 216–227. [CrossRef] [PubMed]
30. Hommer, D.W.; Clem, T.; Litman, R.; Pickar, D. Maladaptive anticipatory saccades in schizophrenia. *Biol. Psychiatry* **1991**, *30*, 779–794. [CrossRef]
31. Franke, P.; Maier, W.; Hain, C.; Klingler, T. Wisconsin Card Sorting Test: An indicator of vulnerability to schizophrenia? *Schizophr. Res.* **1992**, *6*, 243–249. [CrossRef]
32. GoldmanRakic, P.S.; Selemon, L.D. Functional and anatomical aspects of prefrontal pathology in schizophrenia. *Schizophr. Bull.* **1997**, *23*, 437–458. [CrossRef] [PubMed]
33. Ragland, J.D.; Laird, A.R.; Ranganath, C.; Blumenfeld, R.S.; Gonzales, S.M.; Glahn, D.C. Prefrontal activation deficits during episodic memory in schizophrenia. *Am. J. Psychiatry* **2009**, *166*, 863–874. [CrossRef] [PubMed]
34. Yan, C.; Yang, T.; Yu, Q.J.; Jin, Z.; Cheung, E.F.C.; Liu, X.; Chan, R.C.K. Rostral medial prefrontal dysfunctions and consummatory pleasure in schizophrenia: A meta-analysis of functional imaging studies. *Psychiatry Res.* **2015**, *231*, 187–196. [CrossRef]
35. Feinberg, I. Schizophrenia: Caused by a fault in programmed synaptic elimination during adolescence? *J. Psychiatr. Res.* **1982**, *17*, 319–334. [CrossRef]
36. Selemon, L.D.; Zecevic, N. Schizophrenia: A tale of two critical periods for prefrontal cortical development. *Transl. Psychiatry* **2015**, *5*, e623. [CrossRef]

37. Fillman, S.G.; Cloonan, N.; Catts, V.S.; Miller, L.C.; Wong, J.; McCrossin, T.; Cairns, M.; Weickert, C.S. Increased inflammatory markers identified in the dorsolateral prefrontal cortex of individuals with schizophrenia. *Mol. Psychiatry* **2013**, *18*, 206–214. [CrossRef]
38. Paolicelli, R.C.; Bolasco, G.; Pagani, F.; Maggi, L.; Scianni, M.; Panzanelli, P.; Giustetto, M.; Ferreira, T.A.; Guiducci, E.; Dumas, L.; et al. Synaptic pruning by microglia is necessary for normal brain development. *Science* **2011**, *333*, 1456–1458. [CrossRef] [PubMed]
39. Kettenmann, H.; Kirchhoff, F.; Verkhratsky, A. Microglia: New roles for the synaptic stripper. *Neuron* **2013**, *77*, 10–18. [CrossRef]
40. Wilton, D.K.; Dissing-Olesen, L.; Stevens, B. Neuron-Glia Signaling in Synapse Elimination. *Annu. Rev. Neurosci.* **2019**, *42*, 107–127. [CrossRef]
41. Bright, F.; Werry, E.L.; Dobson-Stone, C.; Piguet, O.; Ittner, L.M.; Halliday, G.M.; Hodges, J.R.; Kiernan, M.C.; Loy, C.T.; Kassiou, M.; et al. Neuroinflammation in frontotemporal dementia. *Nat. Rev. Neurol.* **2019**, *15*, 540–555. [CrossRef] [PubMed]
42. Akiyama, H.; Barger, S.; Barnum, S.; Bradt, B.; Bauer, J.; Cole, G.M.; Cooper, N.R.; Eikelenboom, P.; Emmerling, M.; Fiebich, B.L.; et al. Inflammation and Alzheimer's disease. *Neurobiol. Aging* **2000**, *21*, 383–421. [CrossRef]
43. Izuo, N.; Kasahara, C.; Murakami, K.; Kume, T.; Maeda, M.; Irie, K.; Yokote, K.; Shimizu, T. Toxic Conformer of Aβ42 with a Turn at 22–23 is a Novel Therapeutic Target for Alzheimer's Disease. *Sci. Rep.* **2017**, *7*, 11811. [CrossRef] [PubMed]
44. Dubbelaar, M.L.; Kracht, L.; Eggen, B.J.L.; Boddeke, E.W.G.M. The Kaleidoscope of Microglial Phenotypes. *Front. Immunol.* **2018**, *9*, 1753. [CrossRef]
45. Davalos, D.; Grutzendler, J.; Yang, G.; Kim, J.V.; Zuo, Y.; Jung, S.; Littman, D.R.; Dustin, M.L.; Gan, W.B. ATP mediates rapid microglial response to local brain injury in vivo. *Nat. Neurosci.* **2005**, *8*, 752–758. [CrossRef] [PubMed]
46. Nimmerjahn, A.; Kirchhoff, F.; Helmchen, F. Resting microglial cells are highly dynamic surveillants of brain parenchyma in vivo. *Science* **2005**, *308*, 1314–1318. [CrossRef]
47. Tremblay, M.E.; Lowery, R.L.; Majewska, A.K. Microglial interactions with synapses are modulated by visual experience. *PLoS Biol.* **2010**, *8*, e1000527. [CrossRef]
48. Wake, H.; Moorhouse, A.J.; Jinno, S.; Kohsaka, S.; Nabekura, J. Resting microglia directly monitor the functional state of synapses in vivo and determine the fate of ischemic terminals. *J. Neurosci.* **2009**, *29*, 3974–3980. [CrossRef]
49. Milinkeviciute, G.; Henningfield, C.M.; Muniakz, M.A.; Chokr, S.M.; Green, K.N.; Cramer, K.S. Microglia Regulate Pruning of Specialized Synapses in the Auditory Brainstem. *Front. Neural. Circuits* **2019**, *13*, 55. [CrossRef]
50. Ma, X.K.; Chen, K.; Cui, Y.H.; Huang, G.N.; Nehme, A.; Zhang, L.; Li, H.D.; Wei, J.; Liong, K.; Liu, Q.; et al. Depletion of microglia in developing cortical circuits reveals its critical role in glutamatergic synapse development, functional connectivity, and critical period plasticity. *J. Neurosci. Res.* **2020**, *98*, 1968–1986. [CrossRef]
51. Brown, G.C.; Neher, J.J. Eaten alive! Cell death by primary phagocytosis: 'phagoptosis'. *Trends Biochem. Sci.* **2012**, *37*, 325–332. [CrossRef] [PubMed]
52. Vilalta, A.; Brown, G.C. Neurophagy, the phagocytosis of live neurons and synapses by glia, contributes to brain development and disease. *FEBS J.* **2018**, *285*, 3566–3575. [CrossRef] [PubMed]
53. Harrison, J.K.; Jiang, Y.; Chen, S.Z.; Xia, Y.Y.; Maciejewski, D.; McNamara, R.K.; Streit, W.J.; Salafranca, M.N.; Adhikari, S.; Thompson, D.A.; et al. Role for neuronally derived fractalkine in mediating interactions between neurons and CX3CR1-expressing microglia. *Proc. Natl. Acad. Sci. USA* **1998**, *95*, 10896–10901. [CrossRef] [PubMed]
54. Jung, S.; Aliberti, J.; Graemmel, P.; Sunshine, M.J.; Kreutzberg, G.W.; Sher, A.; Littman, D.R. Analysis of fractalkine receptor CX(3)CR1 function by targeted deletion and green fluorescent protein reporter gene insertion. *Mol. Cell. Biol.* **2000**, *20*, 4106–4114. [CrossRef]
55. Gunner, G.; Cheadle, L.; Johnson, K.M.; Ayata, P.; Badimon, A.; Mondo, E.; Nagy, M.A.; Liu, L.W.; Bemiller, S.M.; Kim, K.W.; et al. Sensory lesioning induces microglial synapse elimination via ADAM10 and fractalkine signaling. *Nat. Neurosci.* **2019**, *22*, 1075–1088. [CrossRef]
56. Chekeni, F.B.; Elliott, M.R.; Sandilos, J.K.; Walk, S.F.; Kinchen, J.M.; Lazarowski, E.R.; Armstrong, A.J.; Penuela, S.; Laird, D.W.; Salvesen, G.S.; et al. Pannexin 1 channels mediate 'find-me' signal release and membrane permeability during apoptosis. *Nature* **2010**, *467*, 863–867. [CrossRef]
57. Haynes, S.E.; Hollopeter, G.; Yang, G.; Kurpius, D.; Dailey, M.E.; Gan, W.B.; Julius, D. The P2Y12 receptor regulates microglial activation by extracellular nucleotides. *Nat. Neurosci.* **2006**, *9*, 1512–1519. [CrossRef]
58. Maeda, M.; Tsuda, M.; Tozaki-Saitoh, H.; Inoue, K.; Kiyama, H. Nerve injury-activated microglia engulf myelinated axons in a P2Y12 signaling-dependent manner in the dorsal horn. *Glia* **2010**, *58*, 1838–1846. [CrossRef]
59. Sipe, G.O.; Lowery, R.L.; Tremblay, M.E.; Kelly, E.A.; Lamantia, C.E.; Majewska, A.K. Microglial P2Y12 is necessary for synaptic plasticity in mouse visual cortex. *Nat. Commun.* **2016**, *7*, 10905. [CrossRef]
60. Cserep, C.; Posfai, B.; Lenart, N.; Fekete, R.; Laszlo, Z.I.; Lele, Z.; Orsolits, B.; Molnar, G.; Heindl, S.; Schwarcz, A.D.; et al. Microglia monitor and protect neuronal function through specialized somatic purinergic junctions. *Science* **2020**, *367*, 528–537. [CrossRef]
61. Arandjelovic, S.; Ravichandran, K.S. Phagocytosis of apoptotic cells in homeostasis. *Nat. Immunol.* **2015**, *16*, 907–917. [CrossRef]
62. Tufail, Y.; Cook, D.; Fourgeaud, L.; Powers, C.J.; Merten, K.; Clark, C.L.; Hoffman, E.; Ngo, A.; Sekiguchi, K.J.; O'Shea, C.C.; et al. Phosphatidylserine Exposure Controls Viral Innate Immune Responses by Microglia. *Neuron* **2017**, *93*, 574–586. [CrossRef] [PubMed]

63. Soulard, C.; Salsac, C.; Mouzat, K.; Hilaire, C.; Roussel, J.; Mezghrani, A.; Lumbroso, S.; Raoul, C.; Scamps, F. Spinal Motoneuron TMEM16F Acts at C-boutons to Modulate Motor Resistance and Contributes to ALS Pathogenesis. *Cell Rep.* **2020**, *30*, 2581–2593. [CrossRef] [PubMed]
64. Filipello, F.; Morini, R.; Corradini, I.; Zerbi, V.; Canzi, A.; Michalski, B.; Erreni, M.; Markicevic, M.; Starvaggi-Cucuzza, C.; Otero, K.; et al. The Microglial Innate Immune Receptor TREM2 Is Required for Synapse Elimination and Normal Brain Connectivity. *Immunity* **2018**, *48*, 979–991. [CrossRef] [PubMed]
65. Li, T.; Chiou, B.; Gilman, C.K.; Luo, R.; Koshi, T.; Yu, D.K.; Oak, H.C.; Giera, S.; Johnson-Venkatesh, E.; Muthukumar, A.K.; et al. A splicing isoform of GPR56 mediates microglial synaptic refinement via phosphatidylserine binding. *EMBO J.* **2020**, *39*, e104136. [CrossRef] [PubMed]
66. Biatynicki-Birula, R. The 100th anniversary of Wassermann-Neisser-Bruck reaction. *Clin. Dermatol.* **2008**, *26*, 79–88. [CrossRef]
67. Carroll, M.C. The role of complement and complement receptors in induction and regulation of immunity. *Annu. Rev. Immunol.* **1998**, *16*, 545–568. [CrossRef]
68. Dunkelberger, J.R.; Song, W.C. Complement and its role in innate and adaptive immune responses. *Cell Res.* **2010**, *20*, 34–50. [CrossRef]
69. Stevens, B.; Allen, N.J.; Vazquez, L.E.; Howell, G.R.; Christopherson, K.S.; Nouri, N.; Micheva, K.D.; Mehalow, A.K.; Huberman, A.D.; Stafford, B.; et al. The classical complement cascade mediates CNS synapse elimination. *Cell* **2007**, *131*, 1164–1178. [CrossRef]
70. Schartz, N.D.; Tenner, A.J. The good, the bad, and the opportunities of the complement system in neurodegenerative disease. *J. Neuroinflammation* **2020**, *17*, 354. [CrossRef]
71. Shi, Q.Q.; Colodner, K.J.; Matousek, S.B.; Merry, K.; Hong, S.Y.; Kenison, J.E.; Frost, J.L.; Le, K.X.; Li, S.M.; Dodart, J.C.; et al. Complement C3-Deficient Mice Fail to Display Age-Related Hippocampal Decline. *J. Neurosci.* **2015**, *35*, 13029–13042. [CrossRef] [PubMed]
72. Anderson, S.R.; Zhang, J.M.; Steele, M.R.; Romero, C.O.; Kautzman, A.G.; Schafer, D.P.; Vetter, M.L. Complement Targets Newborn Retinal Ganglion Cells for Phagocytic Elimination by Microglia. *J. Neurosci.* **2019**, *39*, 2025–2040. [CrossRef] [PubMed]
73. Gyorffy, B.A.; Kun, J.; Torok, G.; Bulyaki, E.; Borhegyi, Z.; Gulyassy, P.; Kis, V.; Szocsics, P.; Micsonai, A.; Matko, J. Local apoptotic-like mechanisms underlie complement-mediated synaptic pruning. *Proc. Natl. Acad. Sci. USA* **2018**, *115*, 6303–6308. [CrossRef] [PubMed]
74. Sekar, A.; Bialas, A.R.; de Rivera, H.; Davis, A.; Hammond, T.R.; Kamitaki, N.; Tooley, K.; Presumey, J.; Baum, M.; Van Doren, V.; et al. Schizophrenia risk from complex variation of complement component 4. *Nature* **2016**, *530*, 177–183. [CrossRef]
75. Nomura, K.; Vilalta, A.; Allendorf, D.H.; Hornik, T.C.; Brown, G.C. Activated Microglia Desialylate and Phagocytose Cells via Neuraminidase, Galectin-3, and Mer Tyrosine Kinase. *J. Immunol.* **2017**, *198*, 4792–4801. [CrossRef]
76. Angata, T.; Kerr, S.C.; Greaves, D.R.; Varki, N.M.; Crocker, P.R.; Varki, A. Cloning and characterization of human Siglec-11—A recently evolved signaling molecule that can interact with SHP-1 and SHP-2 and is expressed by tissue macrophages, including brain microglia. *J. Biol. Chem.* **2002**, *277*, 24466–24474. [CrossRef]
77. Puigdellivol, M.; Allendorf, D.H.; Brown, G.C. Sialylation and Galectin-3 in Microglia-Mediated Neuroinflammation and Neurodegeneration. *Front. Cell. Neurosci.* **2020**, *14*, 162. [CrossRef]
78. Klaus, C.; Hansen, J.N.; Ginolhac, A.; Gerard, D.; Gnanapragassam, V.S.; Horstkorte, R.; Rossdam, C.; Buettner, F.F.R.; Sauter, T.; Sinkkonen, L.; et al. Reduced sialylation triggers homeostatic synapse and neuronal loss in middle-aged mice. *Neurobiol. Aging* **2020**, *88*, 91–107. [CrossRef]
79. Lehrman, E.K.; Wilton, D.K.; Litvina, E.Y.; Welsh, C.A.; Chang, S.T.; Frouin, A.; Walker, A.J.; Heller, M.D.; Umemori, H.; Chen, C.F.; et al. CD47 Protects Synapses from Excess Microglia-Mediated Pruning during Development. *Neuron* **2018**, *100*, 120–134. [CrossRef]
80. Lee, J.D.; Coulthard, L.G.; Woodruff, T.M. Complement dysregulation in the central nervous system during development and disease. *Semin. Immunol.* **2019**, *45*, 101340. [CrossRef]
81. Cooper, J.D.; Ozcan, S.; Gardner, R.M.; Rustogi, N.; Wicks, S.; van Rees, G.F.; Leweke, F.M.; Dalman, C.; Karlsson, H.; Bahn, S. Schizophrenia-risk and urban birth are associated with proteomic changes in neonatal dried blood spots. *Transl. Psychiatry* **2017**, *7*, 1290. [CrossRef]
82. Gallego, J.A.; Blanco, E.A.; Morell, C.; Lencz, T.; Malhotra, A.K. Complement component C4 levels in the cerebrospinal fluid and plasma of patients with schizophrenia. *Neuropsychopharmacology* **2020**, *46*. [CrossRef] [PubMed]
83. Zhang, S.C.; Zhou, N.; Liu, R.; Rao, W.W.; Yang, M.J.; Cao, B.N.; Kang, G.J.; Kang, Q.; Zhu, X.J.; Li, R.X.; et al. Association Between Polymorphisms of the Complement 3 Gene and Schizophrenia in a Han Chinese Population. *Cell. Physiol. Biochem.* **2018**, *46*, 2480–2486. [CrossRef]
84. Crider, A.; Feng, T.; Pandya, C.D.; Davis, T.; Nair, A.; Ahmed, A.O.; Baban, B.; Turecki, G.; Pillai, A. Complement component 3a receptor deficiency attenuates chronic stress-induced monocyte infiltration and depressive-like behavior. *Brain Behav. Immun.* **2018**, *70*, 246–256. [CrossRef]
85. Ishii, T.; Hattori, K.; Miyakawa, T.; Watanabe, K.; Hidese, S.; Sasayama, D.; Ota, M.; Teraishi, T.; Hori, H.; Yoshida, S.; et al. Increased cerebrospinal fluid complement C5 levels in major depressive disorder and schizophrenia. *Biochem. Biophys. Res. Commun.* **2018**, *497*, 683–688. [CrossRef]

86. Comer, A.L.; Jinadasa, T.; Sriram, B.; Phadke, R.A.; Kretsge, L.N.; Nguyen, T.P.H.; Antognetti, G.; Gilbert, J.P.; Lee, J.; Newmark, E.R.; et al. Increased expression of schizophrenia-associated gene C4 leads to hypoconnectivity of prefrontal cortex and reduced social interaction. *PLoS Biol.* **2020**, *18*, e3000604. [CrossRef]
87. Yilmaz, M.; Yalcin, E.; Presumey, J.; Aw, E.; Ma, M.H.; Whelan, C.W.; Stevens, B.; McCarroll, S.A.; Carroll, M.C. Overexpression of schizophrenia susceptibility factor human complement C4A promotes excessive synaptic loss and behavioral changes in mice. *Nat. Neurosci.* **2021**, *24*, 214–224. [CrossRef]
88. Sellgren, C.M.; Gracias, J.; Watmuff, B.; Biag, J.D.; Thanos, J.M.; Whittredge, P.B.; Fu, T.; Worringer, K.; Brown, H.E.; Wang, J.; et al. Increased synapse elimination by microglia in schizophrenia patient-derived models of synaptic pruning. *Nat. Neurosci.* **2019**, *22*, 374–385. [CrossRef] [PubMed]
89. Davies, C.; Segre, G.; Estrade, A.; Radua, J.; De Micheli, A.; Provenzani, U.; Oliver, D.; de Pablo, G.S.; Ramella-Cravaro, V.; Besozzi, M.; et al. Prenatal and perinatal risk and protective factors for psychosis: A systematic review and meta-analysis. *Lancet Psychiatry* **2020**, *7*, 399–410. [CrossRef]
90. Zimmer, A.; Youngblood, A.; Adnane, A.; Miller, B.J.; Goldsmith, D.R. Prenatal exposure to viral infection and neuropsychiatric disorders in offspring: A review of the literature and recommendations for the COVID-19 pandemic. *Brain Behav. Immun.* **2021**, *91*, 756–770. [CrossRef]
91. Glynn, M.W.; Elmer, B.M.; Garay, P.A.; Liu, X.B.; Needleman, L.A.; El-Sabeawy, F.; McAllister, A.K. MHCI negatively regulates synapse density during the establishment of cortical connections. *Nat. Neurosci.* **2011**, *14*, 442–451. [CrossRef] [PubMed]
92. Elmer, B.M.; Estes, M.L.; Barrow, S.L.; McAllister, A.K. MHCI requires MEF2 transcription factors to negatively regulate synapse density during development and in disease. *J. Neurosci.* **2013**, *33*, 13791–13804. [CrossRef] [PubMed]
93. Severance, E.G.; Gressitt, K.L.; Buka, S.L.; Cannon, T.D.; Yolken, R.H. Maternal complement C1q and increased odds for psychosis in adult offspring. *Schizophr. Res.* **2014**, *159*, 14–19. [CrossRef]
94. Flegr, J. Effects of toxoplasma on human behavior. *Schizophr. Bull.* **2007**, *33*, 757–760. [CrossRef]
95. Kannan, G.; Pletnikov, M.V. *Toxoplasma Gondii* and Cognitive Deficits in Schizophrenia: An Animal Model Perspective. *Schizophr. Bull.* **2012**, *38*, 1155–1161. [CrossRef] [PubMed]
96. Xiao, J.C.; Li, Y.; Gressitt, K.L.; He, H.; Kannan, G.; Schultz, T.L.; Svezhova, N.; Carruthers, V.B.; Pletnikov, M.V.; Yolken, R.H.; et al. Cerebral complement C1q activation in chronic *Toxoplasma* infection. *Brain Behav. Immun.* **2016**, *58*, 52–56. [CrossRef]
97. Li, Y.; Severance, E.G.; Viscidi, R.P.; Yolken, R.H.; Xiao, J. Persistent *Toxoplasma* Infection of the Brain Induced Neurodegeneration Associated with Activation of Complement and Microglia. *Infect. Immun.* **2019**, *87*, e00139-19. [CrossRef]
98. Xin, Y.R.; Jiang, J.X.; Hu, Y.; Pan, J.P.; Mi, X.N.; Gao, Q.; Xiao, F.; Zhang, W.; Luo, H.M. The Immune System Drives Synapse Loss During Lipopolysaccharide-Induced Learning and Memory Impairment in Mice. *Front. Aging Neurosci.* **2019**, *11*, 279. [CrossRef]
99. Li, S.M.; Li, B.; Zhang, L.; Zhang, G.F.; Sun, J.; Ji, M.H.; Yang, J.J. A complement-microglial axis driving inhibitory synapse related protein loss might contribute to systemic inflammation-induced cognitive impairment. *Int. Immunopharmacol.* **2020**, *87*, 106814. [CrossRef]
100. Sato, C.; Kitajima, K. Disialic, oligosialic and polysialic acids: Distribution, functions and related disease. *J. Biochem.* **2013**, *154*, 115–136. [CrossRef]
101. Barbeau, D.; Liang, J.; Robitalille, Y.; Quirion, R.; Srivastava, L. Decreased expression of the embryonic form of the neural cell adhesion molecule in schizophrenic brains. *Proc. Natl. Acad. Sci. USA* **1995**, *92*, 2785–2789. [CrossRef]
102. Gilabert-Juan, J.; Varea, E.; Guirado, R.; Blasco-Ibanez, J.M.; Crespo, C.; Nacher, J. Alterations in the expression of PSA-NCAM and synaptic proteins in the dorsolateral prefrontal cortex of psychiatric disorder patients. *Neurosci. Lett.* **2012**, *530*, 97–102. [CrossRef] [PubMed]
103. Piras, F.; Schiff, M.; Chiapponi, C.; Bossu, P.; Muhlenhoff, M.; Caltagirone, C.; Gerardy-Schahn, R.; Hildebrandt, H.; Spalletta, G. Brain structure, cognition and negative symptoms in schizophrenia are associated with serum levels of polysialic acid-modified NCAM. *Transl. Psychiatry* **2015**, *5*, e658. [CrossRef]
104. Arai, M.; Yamada, K.; Toyota, T.; Obata, N.; Haga, S.; Yoshida, Y.; Nakamura, K.; Minabe, Y.; Ujike, H.; Sora, I.; et al. Association between polymorphisms in the promoter region of the sialyltransferase 8B (SIAT8B) gene and schizophrenia. *Biol. Psychiatry* **2006**, *59*, 652–659. [CrossRef]
105. Tao, R.; Li, C.; Zheng, Y.L.; Qin, W.; Zhang, J.; Li, X.W.; Xu, Y.F.; Shi, Y.Y.; Feng, G.Y.; He, L. Positive association between SIAT8B and schizophrenia in the Chinese Han population. *Schizophr. Res.* **2007**, *90*, 108–114. [CrossRef] [PubMed]
106. Gilabert-Juan, J.; Nacher, J.; Sanjuan, J.; Molto, M.D. Sex-specific association of the ST8SIAII gene with schizophrenia in a Spanish population. *Psychiatry Res.* **2013**, *210*, 1293–1295. [CrossRef]
107. Angata, K.; Long, J.M.; Bukalo, O.; Lee, W.; Dityatev, A.; Wynshaw-Boris, A.; Schachner, M.; Fukuda, M.; Marth, J.D. Sialyltransferase ST8Sia-II assembles a subset of polysialic acid that directs hippocampal axonal targeting and promotes fear behavior. *J. Biol. Chem.* **2004**, *279*, 32603–32613. [CrossRef]
108. Mori, Y.; Yoshino, Y.; Ochi, S.; Yamazaki, K.; Kawabe, K.; Abe, M.; Kitano, T.; Ozaki, Y.; Yoshida, T.; Numata, S.; et al. TREM2 mRNA Expression in Leukocytes Is Increased in Alzheimer's Disease and Schizophrenia. *PLoS ONE* **2015**, *10*, e0136835. [CrossRef] [PubMed]
109. Yoshino, Y.; Kawabe, K.; Yamazaki, K.; Watanabe, S.; Numata, S.; Mori, Y.; Yoshida, T.; Iga, J.; Ohmori, T.; Ueno, S.I. Elevated TREM2 mRNA expression in leukocytes in schizophrenia but not major depressive disorder. *J. Neural Transm.* **2016**, *123*, 637–641. [CrossRef] [PubMed]

110. Yoshino, Y.; Ozaki, Y.; Yamazaki, K.; Sao, T.; Mori, Y.; Ochi, S.; Iga, J.; Ueno, S. DNA Methylation Changes in Intron 1 of Triggering Receptor Expressed on Myeloid Cell 2 in Japanese Schizophrenia Subjects. *Front. Neurosci.* **2017**, *11*, 275. [CrossRef]
111. Onwordi, E.C.; Halff, E.F.; Whitehurst, T.; Mansur, A.; Cotel, M.C.; Wells, L.; Creeney, H.; Bonsall, D.; Rogdaki, M.; Shatalina, E.; et al. Synaptic density marker SV2A is reduced in schizophrenia patients and unaffected by antipsychotics in rats. *Nat. Commun.* **2020**, *11*, 246. [CrossRef] [PubMed]
112. Germann, M.; Brederoo, S.G.; Sommer, I.E.C. Abnormal synaptic pruning during adolescence underlying the development of psychotic disorders. *Curr. Opin. Psychiatry* **2021**, *34*, 222–227. [CrossRef] [PubMed]
113. Zhang, L.L.; Hu, K.; Shao, T.; Hou, L.; Zhang, S.J.; Ye, W.J.; Josephson, L.; Meyer, J.H.; Zhang, M.R.; Vasdev, N.; et al. Recent developments on PET radiotracers for TSPO and their applications in neuroimaging. *Acta Pharm. Sin. B* **2021**, *11*, 373–393. [CrossRef] [PubMed]
114. Marques, T.R.; Ashok, A.H.; Pillinger, T.; Veronese, M.; Turkheimer, F.E.; Dazzan, P.; Sommer, I.E.C.; Howes, O.D. Neuroinflammation in schizophrenia: Meta-analysis of in vivo microglial imaging studies. *Psychol. Med.* **2019**, *49*, 2186–2196. [CrossRef]
115. Sneeboer, M.A.M.; van der Doef, T.; Litjens, M.; Psy, N.B.B.; Melief, J.; Hol, E.M.; Kahn, R.S.; de Witte, L.D. Microglial activation in schizophrenia: Is translocator 18 kDa protein (TSPO) the right marker? *Schizophr. Res.* **2020**, *215*, 167–172. [CrossRef]
116. Narayanaswami, V.; Dahl, K.; Bernard-Gauthier, V.; Josephson, L.; Cumming, P.; Vasdev, N. Emerging PET Radiotracers and Targets for Imaging of Neuroinflammation in Neurodegenerative Diseases: Outlook Beyond TSPO. *Mol. Imaging* **2018**, *17*. [CrossRef]
117. Karlstrom, S.; Nordvall, G.; Sohn, D.; Hettman, A.; Turek, D.; Ahlin, K.; Kers, A.; Claesson, M.; Slivo, C.; Lo-Alfredsson, Y.; et al. Substituted 7-amino-5-thio-thiazolo[4,5-d]pyrimidines as potent and selective antagonists of the fractalkine receptor (CX3CR1). *J. Med. Chem.* **2013**, *56*, 3177–3190. [CrossRef] [PubMed]
118. Zhang, Y.; Yan, X.; Zhao, T.; Xu, Q.; Peng, Q.; Hu, R.; Quan, S.; Zhou, Y.; Xing, G. Targeting C3a/C5a receptors inhibits human mesangial cell proliferation and alleviates immunoglobulin A nephropathy in mice. *Clin. Exp. Immunol.* **2017**, *189*, 60–70. [CrossRef]
119. Laskaris, L.; Zalesky, A.; Weickert, C.S.; Di Biase, M.A.; Chana, G.; Baune, B.T.; Bousman, C.; Nelson, B.; McGorry, P.; Everall, I.; et al. Investigation of peripheral complement factors across stages of psychosis. *Schizophr. Res.* **2019**, *204*, 30–37. [CrossRef]
120. Mongan, D.; Sabherwal, S.; Susai, S.R.; Focking, M.; Cannon, M.; Cotter, D.R. Peripheral complement proteins in schizophrenia: A systematic review and meta-analysis of serological studies. *Schizophr. Res.* **2020**, *222*, 58–72. [CrossRef]
121. Zhang, T.; Tang, Y.; Yang, X.; Wang, X.; Ding, S.; Huang, K.; Liu, Y.; Lang, B. Expression of GSK3β, PICK1, NEFL, C4, NKCC1 and Synaptophysin in peripheral blood mononuclear cells of the first-episode schizophrenia patients. *Asian J. Psychiatry* **2021**, *55*, 102520. [CrossRef]
122. Hill, A.F. Extracellular Vesicles and Neurodegenerative Diseases. *J. Neurosci.* **2019**, *39*, 9269–9273. [CrossRef]
123. Vassileff, N.; Cheng, L.; Hill, A.F. Extracellular vesicles—Propagators of neuropathology and sources of potential biomarkers and therapeutics for neurodegenerative diseases. *J. Cell Sci.* **2020**, *133*, jcs243139. [CrossRef] [PubMed]
124. Fiandaca, M.S.; Kapogiannis, D.; Mapstone, M.; Boxer, A.; Eitan, E.; Schwartz, J.B.; Abner, E.L.; Petersen, R.C.; Federoff, H.J.; Miller, B.L.; et al. Identification of preclinical Alzheimer's disease by a profile of pathogenic proteins in neurally derived blood exosomes: A case-control study. *Alzheimers Dement.* **2015**, *11*, 600–607. [CrossRef] [PubMed]
125. Goetzl, E.J.; Boxer, A.; Schwartz, J.B.; Abner, E.L.; Petersen, R.C.; Miller, B.L.; Kapogiannis, D. Altered lysosomal proteins in neural-derived plasma exosomes in preclinical Alzheimer disease. *Neurology* **2015**, *85*, 40–47. [CrossRef]
126. Goetzl, E.J.; Srihari, V.H.; Guloksuz, S.; Ferrara, M.; Tek, C.; Heninger, G.R. Neural cell-derived plasma exosome protein abnormalities implicate mitochondrial impairment in first episodes of psychosis. *FASEB J.* **2021**, *35*, e21339. [CrossRef] [PubMed]
127. Goetzl, E.J.; Srihari, V.H.; Guloksuz, S.; Ferrara, M.; Tek, C.; Heninger, G.R. Decreased mitochondrial electron transport proteins and increased complement mediators in plasma neural-derived exosomes of early psychosis. *Transl. Psychiatry* **2020**, *10*, 361. [CrossRef]
128. Kawata, K.; Mitsuhashi, M.; Aldret, R. A Preliminary Report on Brain-Derived Extracellular Vesicle as Novel Blood Biomarkers for Sport-Related Concussions. *Front. Neurol.* **2018**, *9*, 239. [CrossRef] [PubMed]
129. Bennett, M.L.; Bennett, F.C.; Liddelow, S.A.; Ajami, B.; Zamanian, J.L.; Fernhoff, N.B.; Mulinyawe, S.B.; Bohlen, C.J.; Adil, A.; Tucker, A.; et al. New tools for studying microglia in the mouse and human CNS. *Proc. Natl. Acad. Sci. USA* **2016**, *113*, E1738–E1746. [CrossRef]
130. Miyanohara, J.; Kakae, M.; Nagayasu, K.; Nakagawa, T.; Mori, Y.; Arai, K.; Shirakawa, H.; Kaneko, S. TRPM2 Channel Aggravates CNS Inflammation and Cognitive Impairment via Activation of Microglia in Chronic Cerebral Hypoperfusion. *J. Neurosci.* **2018**, *38*, 3520–3533. [CrossRef]
131. Shin, D.A.; Kim, T.U.; Chang, M.C. Minocycline for Controlling Neuropathic Pain: A Systematic Narrative Review of Studies in Humans. *J. Pain Res.* **2021**, *14*, 139–145. [CrossRef]
132. Mizoguchi, H.; Takuma, K.; Fukakusa, A.; Ito, Y.; Nakatani, A.; Ibi, D.; Kim, H.C.; Yamada, K. Improvement by minocycline of methamphetamine-induced impairment of recognition memory in mice. *Psychopharmacology* **2008**, *196*, 233–241. [CrossRef]
133. Zhu, F.; Liu, Y.; Zhao, J.; Zheng, Y. Minocycline alleviates behavioral deficits and inhibits microglial activation induced by intrahippocampal administration of Granulocyte-Macrophage Colony-Stimulating Factor in adult rats. *Neuroscience* **2014**, *266*, 275–281. [CrossRef] [PubMed]

134. Kelly, D.L.; Sullivan, K.M.; McEvoy, J.P.; McMahon, R.P.; Wehring, H.J.; Gold, J.M.; Liu, F.; Warfel, D.; Vyas, G.; Richardson, C.M.; et al. Adjunctive Minocycline in Clozapine-Treated Schizophrenia Patients With Persistent Symptoms. *J. Clin. Psychopharmacol.* **2015**, *35*, 374–381. [CrossRef] [PubMed]
135. Zhang, L.L.; Zheng, H.B.; Wu, R.R.; Kosten, T.R.; Zhang, X.Y.; Zhao, J.P. The effect of minocycline on amelioration of cognitive deficits and pro-inflammatory cytokines levels in patients with schizophrenia. *Schizophr. Res.* **2019**, *212*, 92–98. [CrossRef]
136. Dominic, M.R. Adverse Reactions Induced by Minocycline: A Review of Literature. *Curr. Drug Saf.* **2021**, *16*. [CrossRef] [PubMed]
137. Fan, C.Q.; Long, Y.F.; Wang, L.Y.; Liu, X.H.; Liu, Z.C.; Lan, T.; Li, Y.; Yu, S.Y. N-Acetylcysteine Rescues Hippocampal Oxidative Stress-Induced Neuronal Injury via Suppression of p38/JNK Signaling in Depressed Rats. *Front. Cell. Neurosci.* **2020**, *14*, 554613. [CrossRef]
138. Steullet, P.; Cabungcal, J.H.; Monin, A.; Dwir, D.; O'Donnell, P.; Cuenod, M.; Do, K.Q. Redox dysregulation, neuroinflammation, and NMDA receptor hypofunction: A "central hub" in schizophrenia pathophysiology? *Schizophr. Res.* **2016**, *176*, 41–51. [CrossRef]
139. Smaga, I.; Frankowska, M.; Filip, M. N-acetylcysteine as a new prominent approach for treating psychiatric disorders. *Br. J. Pharmacol.* **2021**. [CrossRef]
140. Hillmen, P.; Hall, C.; Marsh, J.C.W.; Elebute, M.; Bombara, M.P.; Petro, B.E.; Cullen, M.J.; Richards, S.J.; Rollins, S.A.; Mojcik, C.F.; et al. Effect of eculizumab on hemolysis and transfusion requirements in patients with paroxysmal nocturnal hemoglobinuria. *N. Engl. J. Med.* **2004**, *350*, 552–559. [CrossRef]
141. Hillmen, P.; Young, N.S.; Schubert, J.; Brodsky, R.A.; Socie, G.; Muus, P.; Roth, A.; Szer, J.; Elebute, M.O.; Nakamura, R.; et al. The complement inhibitor eculizumab in paroxysmal nocturnal hemoglobinuria. *N. Engl. J. Med.* **2006**, *355*, 1233–1243. [CrossRef]
142. Notaro, R.; Sica, M. C3-mediated extravascular hemolysis in PNH on eculizumab: Mechanism and clinical implications. *Semin. Hematol.* **2018**, *55*, 130–135. [CrossRef]
143. De Castro, C.; Grossi, F.; Weitz, I.C.; Maciejewski, J.; Sharma, V.; Roman, E.; Brodsky, R.A.; Tan, L.; Casoli, C.D.; Mehdi, D.E.; et al. C. C3 inhibition with pegcetacoplan in subjects with paroxysmal nocturnal hemoglobinuria treated with eculizumab. *Am. J. Hematol.* **2020**, *95*, 1334–1343. [CrossRef]
144. Tanaka, Y.; Takeuchi, T.; Umehara, H.; Nanki, T.; Yasuda, N.; Tago, F.; Kawakubo, M.; Kitahara, Y.; Hojo, S.; Kawano, T.; et al. Safety, pharmacokinetics, and efficacy of E6011, an antifractalkine monoclonal antibody, in a first-in-patient phase 1/2 study on rheumatoid arthritis. *Mod. Rheumatol.* **2018**, *28*, 58–65. [CrossRef] [PubMed]
145. Tanaka, Y.; Hoshino-Negishi, K.; Kuboi, Y.; Tago, F.; Yasuda, N.; Imai, T. Emerging Role of Fractalkine in the Treatment of Rheumatic Diseases. *Immunotargets Ther.* **2020**, *9*, 241–253. [CrossRef] [PubMed]
146. Tanaka, Y.; Takeuchi, T.; Yamanaka, H.; Nanki, T.; Umehara, H.; Yasuda, N.; Tago, F.; Kitahara, Y.; Kawakubo, M.; Torii, K.; et al. Efficacy and Safety of E6011, an Anti-Fractalkine Monoclonal Antibody, in Patients With Active Rheumatoid Arthritis With Inadequate Response to Methotrexate: Results of a Randomized, Double-Blind, Placebo-Controlled Phase II Study. *Arthritis Rheumatol.* **2021**, *73*, 587–595. [CrossRef] [PubMed]
147. Matsuoka, K.; Naganuma, M.; Hibi, T.; Tsubouchi, H.; Oketani, K.; Katsurabara, T.; Hojo, S.; Takenaka, O.; Kawano, T.; Imai, T.; et al. Phase 1 study on the safety and efficacy of E6011, antifractalkine antibody, in patients with Crohn's disease. *J. Gastroenterol. Hepatol.* **2021**. [CrossRef]
148. Yates, D. Stop, don't prune me! *Nat. Rev. Neurosci.* **2018**, *19*, 712–713. [CrossRef]
149. Butler, C.A.; Popescu, A.; Kitchener, E.; Allendorf, D.H.; Puigdellívol, M.; Brown, G.C. Microglial phagocytosis of neurons in neurodegeneration, and its regulation. *J. Neurochem.* **2021**. [CrossRef]
150. Koshimizu, H.; Takao, K.; Matozaki, T.; Ohnishi, H.; Miyakawa, T. Comprehensive behavioral analysis of cluster of differentiation 47 knockout mice. *PLoS ONE* **2014**, *9*, e89584. [CrossRef]
151. Ding, X.; Wang, J.; Huang, M.; Chen, Z.; Liu, J.; Zhang, Q.; Zhang, C.; Xiang, Y.; Zen, K.; Li, L. Loss of microglial SIRPα promotes synaptic pruning in preclinical models of neurodegeneration. *Nat. Commun.* **2021**, *12*, 2030. [CrossRef] [PubMed]
152. Reissmann, S.; Filatova, M.P. New generation of cell-penetrating peptides: Functionality and potential clinical application. *J. Pept. Sci.* **2021**, *27*, e3300. [CrossRef]
153. Tashima, T. Smart Strategies for Therapeutic Agent Delivery into Brain across the Blood-Brain Barrier Using Receptor-Mediated Transcytosis. *Chem. Pharm. Bull.* **2020**, *68*, 316–325. [CrossRef] [PubMed]
154. Mignani, S.; Shi, X.Y.; Karpus, A.; Majoral, J.P. Non-invasive intranasal administration route directly to the brain using dendrimer nanoplatforms: An opportunity to develop new CNS drugs. *Eur. J. Med. Chem.* **2021**, *209*, 112905. [CrossRef]
155. Hallschmid, M. Intranasal Insulin for Alzheimer's Disease. *CNS Drugs* **2021**, *35*, 21–37. [CrossRef] [PubMed]

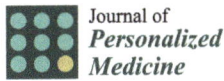

Article

Cognitive Insight in First-Episode Psychosis: Changes during Metacognitive Training

Irene Birulés [1,2], Raquel López-Carrilero [1,3,4,5], Daniel Cuadras [1,4], Esther Pousa [6,7], Maria Luisa Barrigón [8,9], Ana Barajas [10,11], Ester Lorente-Rovira [3,12], Fermín González-Higueras [13], Eva Grasa [3,6,14], Isabel Ruiz-Delgado [15], Jordi Cid [16], Ana de Apraiz [1], Roger Montserrat [1,2], Trinidad Pélaez [1,3], Steffen Moritz [17], the Spanish Metacognition Study Group [18,†] and Susana Ochoa [1,3,5,*]

1. Parc Sanitari Sant Joan de Déu, Sant Boi de Llobregat, 08830 Barcelona, Spain; i.birules@pssjd.org (I.B.); raquellopez@pssjd.org (R.L.-C.); d.cuadras@pssjd.org (D.C.); aapraiz@pssjd.org (A.d.A.); rm.jovellar@pssjd.org (R.M.); tpelaez@pssjd.org (T.P.)
2. Department of Cognition, Development and Educational Psychology, Universitat de Barcelona, 08035 Barcelona, Spain
3. Investigación Biomédica en Red de Salud Mental (CIBERSAM) Instituto de Salud Carlos III C/Monforte de Lemos 3-5, Pabellón 11, Planta 0, 28029 Madrid, Spain; esterlorente@hotmail.com (E.L.-R.); egrasa@santpau.cat (E.G.)
4. Fundació Sant Joan de Déu, Esplugues de Llobregat, Santa Rosa, 39-57, 3a planta 08950 Esplugues de Llobregat, Barcelona, Spain
5. Institut de Recerca en Salut Mental Sant Joan de Déu, Parc Sanitari Sant Joan de Déu, Sant Boi de Llobregat, 08830 Barcelona, Spain
6. Department of Psychiatry, Hospital de la Santa Creu i Sant Pau, 08041 Barcelona, Spain; epousa@santpau.cat
7. Consorci Corporació Sanitària Parc Taulí de Sabadell, Parc Taulí, 1, 08208 Sabadell, Barcelona, Spain
8. Psychiatry Service, Area de Gestión Sanitaria Sur Granada, Motril, 18600 Granada, Spain; marisabe@gmail.com
9. Department of Psychiatry, IIS-Fundación Jiménez Díaz Hospital, 28040 Madrid, Spain
10. Centre d'Higiene Mental Les Corts, 08029 Barcelona, Spain; ana.barajas@chmcorts.com or ana.barajas@uab.cat
11. Departament de Psicologia Clínica i de la Salut, Facultat de Psicologia, Universitat Autònoma de Barcelona, Bellaterra, 08193 Barcelona, Spain
12. Psychiatry Service, Hospital Clínico Universitario de Valencia, 46010 Valencia, Spain
13. UGC Salud Mental de Jaén, Servicio Andaluz de Salud, 23007 Jaen, Spain; pablofermingh78@gmail.com
14. Institut d'Investigació Biomèdica-Sant Pau (IIB-Sant Pau), Universitat Autònoma de Barcelona, 08193 Barcelona, Spain
15. Unidad de Salud Mental Comunitaria Málaga Norte, UGC Salud Mental Carlos Haya, Servicio Andaluz de Salud Psychiatry Service, Antequera, 29200 Málaga, Spain; isabelruizdelgado@hotmail.com
16. Mental Health & Addiction Research Group, IdiBGi, Institut d'Assistència Sanitària, 17190 Girona, Spain; jordi.cid@ias.cat
17. Department of Psychiatry and Psychotherapy, University Medical Center Hamburg, 20251 Hamburg, Germany; moritz@uke.uni-hamburg.de
18. Sant Boi de Llobregat, 08830 Barcelona, Spain
* Correspondence: sochoa@pssjd.org; Tel.: +34-936-406-350 (ext. 12538)
† Membership of the Spanish Metacognition Study Group is provided in the Acknowledgments.

Received: 22 October 2020; Accepted: 24 November 2020; Published: 27 November 2020

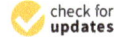

Abstract: Background: Metacognitive training (MCT) has demonstrated its efficacy in psychosis. However, the effect of each MCT session has not been studied. The aim of the study was to assess changes in cognitive insight after MCT: (a) between baseline, post-treatment, and follow-up; (b) after each session of the MCT controlled for intellectual quotient (IQ) and educational level. Method: A total of 65 patients with first-episode psychosis were included in the MCT group from nine centers of Spain. Patients were assessed at baseline, post-treatment, and 6 months follow-up, as well as after each session of MCT with the Beck Cognitive Insight Scale (BCIS). The BCIS contains two subscales: self-reflectiveness and self-certainty, and the Composite Index. Statistical analysis was performed using linear mixed models with repeated measures at different time points. Results: Self-certainty decreased significantly ($p = 0.03$) over time and the effect of IQ was negative and significant ($p = 0.02$). From session 4 to session 8, all sessions improved cognitive insight by significantly reducing self-certainty and the Composite Index. Conclusions: MCT intervention appears to have beneficial effects on cognitive insight by reducing self-certainty, especially after four sessions. Moreover, a minimum IQ is required to ensure benefits from MCT group intervention.

Keywords: first-episode psychosis; metacognitive training; cognitive insight; sessions; experiment

1. Introduction

Schizophrenia and first-episode psychosis represent one of the most invalidating disorders. It concurs with high psychosocial disability and is associated with stigma and discrimination. Although it has a strong genetic basis, psychosocial protective aspects must always be considered to ensure their acceptance and integration in the community [1,2]. In this line, psychological aspects in relation to symptoms should be explored. The relationship between cognitive biases and psychotic symptoms has been well studied. People with psychosis are more likely to present some characteristic cognitive biases such as personal attributional style [3,4], self-serving bias [5], bias against disconfirmatory evidence [6], and jumping to conclusions [7,8]. Apart from cognitive distortions, it has also been found that people suffering from psychosis have more difficulties in social cognition, in particular in theory of mind (ToM) [9] and emotional recognition [10].

Metacognitive training (MCT) was developed in order to deal with the problems related to cognitive biases and social cognition in psychosis [11]. Metacognition is broadly defined as cognition about one's own cognitions [12]. MCT consists of a manualized group training program of eight sessions addressed to reduce cognitive biases that are putatively involved in the formation and maintenance of psychotic symptoms such as jumping to conclusions and overconfidence in errors; hence, MCT is designed to improve social cognition. Previous research indicates that MCT is an effective psychological intervention for people with schizophrenia [13]. Specifically, in recent-onset of psychosis, MCT is an effective treatment for improving psychotic symptoms, cognitive insight, and attributional style, as well as for reducing irrational beliefs [14]. Moreover, people who attend MCT deemed it positive in terms of entertainment and usefulness in everyday life, and most of them will recommend it [11,15,16].

The present study builds on a previously published controlled trial assessing the efficacy of MCT in a recent-onset of psychosis sample. A remarkable observation from this study was that the MCT group had a significantly higher improvement in cognitive insight when compared with the psycho-educational group [14]. Cognitive insight refers to the cognitive processes involved in the metacognitive ability to examine and question one's beliefs and appraisals and to re-evaluate anomalous experiences and misinterpretations. It should be differed from clinical insight (or unawareness of insight) and anosognosia, considering these concepts as a lack of awareness of symptoms, their need for treatment, and its consequences in daily life or problems in basic cognitive processes [17]. The absence of insight occurs by a failure of objectivity, a loss of ability to put this into perspective, a resistance to correct information from the other opinions, and an excess of confidence in the conclusions. Cognitive insight, usually assessed with the Beck Cognitive Insight Scale (BCIS), includes two subscales: self-certainty and self-reflectiveness [18,19]. Higher self-certainty scores reflect greater confidence about being right and more resistance to correction, while higher self-reflectiveness scores indicate the willingness to question one's thoughts and greater capacity to analyze them with perspective. Increasing cognitive insight is associated with higher levels of metacognition and fewer symptoms in people with first-episode psychosis [20]. Moreover, a positive relationship between cognitive insight and premorbid intelligence quotient (IQ) and educational level has been described in several studies [21]. MCT enhances the ability to distance oneself from one's own thoughts and misinterpretations and to reappraise them. Reducing self-certainty is one of the core aims of MCT. By reducing this attitude, the overconfidence bias in one's own thoughts is reduced and, presumably, the risk of emergence of new delusions is also decreased [22]. Furthermore, a recent study shows cognitive insight training can improve meaning-making in patients and help them come to terms with their diagnosis [23].

As MCT is known to improve cognitive insight, it would be of interest to analyze the results of each subcomponent separately and the effect of each session on self-reflectiveness and self-certainty. To the best of our knowledge, there is no published study analyzing the effects of each MCT session in cognitive insight. Therefore, the aim of this study was to assess the changes in cognitive insight before and after treatment, and then after the follow-up measures and after each session of the MCT intervention, controlling for IQ and educational level.

Our hypothesis is that the aforementioned changes will progressively increase throughout treatment and will be maintained at follow-up. We expect that significant changes will be detectable after two or three sessions because of the complexity of the nuclear construct in the formation of delusions.

2. Materials and Methods

2.1. Participants

Patients with recent-onset of psychosis were recruited by staff members of the nine participating Spanish mental health centers. A total of 126 patients were recruited and 122 cases were finally analyzed, as 4 patients did not continue the study after enrollment.

Patients were randomized during inclusion into the experimental or psycho-educational group by blocks of four from the list of random numbers in each center's MCT group. In the present study, the data from the 65 patients belonging to the experimental group (44 men and 21 women) were analyzed. Of this group, 48 completed the treatment and were evaluated in the post-treatment, and 17 were lost during the intervention, declining to participate. Forty-one patients completed the study, as 7 patients discontinued the treatment.

The inclusion criteria were as follows: (1) presence of one of the following diagnoses (according to DSM-IV-TR): schizophrenia, psychotic disorder not otherwise specified, delusional disorder, schizoaffective disorder, brief psychotic disorder, schizophreniform disorder; (2) less than five years from the onset of symptoms; (3) score during the previous year ≥ 3 in item delusions, grandiosity, or suspicions of Positive and Negative Syndrome Scale (PANSS) positive subscale; and (4) age between 17 and 45. The exclusion criteria were as follows: (1) traumatic brain injury, dementia, or intellectual disabilities (premorbid IQ ≤ 70); (2) substance dependence; and (3) scores on the PANSS ≥ 5 in hostility and uncooperative and ≥ 6 in suspiciousness, in order to avoid altering the dynamics of the group.

2.2. Instruments

Patients were assessed by a blinded evaluator at baseline, after each session, post-treatment, and at six months follow-up. The evaluators were trained in the scales of the study, scoring > 0.70 in inter-rater reliability. Assessment included clinical, meta-cognitive, social, and neuropsychological functioning [14]. For the present study, only the data from the Beck Cognitive Insight Scale were analyzed. By administering the BCIS scale [18,19] after each session, at baseline, at post-treatment, and at 6 months follow-up, the correction of distorted beliefs and misinterpretations through scores in the self-reflectiveness and self-certainty subscales could be evaluated.

Beck Cognitive Insight Scale (BCIS) is a self-administered scale assessing cognitive insight yielding a nine-item self-reflectiveness subscale and a six-item self-certainty subscale, as well as a Composite Index score. The Composite Index is calculated by subtracting the score for the self-certainty scale from that of the self-reflectiveness scale. Higher scores in self-reflectiveness and the Composite Index indicate higher cognitive insight, while low scores in self-certainty indicate better cognitive insight. Sensibility and specificity values of the scale are described by Martin et al. [24]. Respondents are asked to rate how much they agree with each statement using a four-point scale that ranges from 0 (do not agree at all) to 3 (agree completely). Self-report instrument was constructed to contain two sets of items. The first set included items relevant to objectivity, reflectiveness, and openness to feedback. The questions were written to capture patients' recognition that they could be wrong even when they felt strongly that they were right, that other people could be more objective than they were, and that they were willing to consider other people pointing out that their beliefs were wrong. An item was included to evaluate the patients' acceptance of the notion of alternative explanations. There were also items about patients being receptive to feedback, being able to make more adaptive attributions, and being able to admit to inadequate cognitive strategies. Perspective was based on the recognition that patients had misconstrued peoples' attitudes towards themselves, that they had jumped to conclusions too fast, that certain experiences that had seemed real were due to their imagination, that some of the ideas they believed to be true were false, and that some of their unusual experiences were due to their being upset or stressed. The second set of items in the BCIS was written to address decision-making regarding mental products: jumping to conclusions, certainty about being right, and resistance to correction. These six items addressed patient's certainty about their beliefs and conclusions, such as doing something if it feels right, dogmatic rightness, and resistance to feedback from others [18]. The internal consistency coefficients (Cronbach's alpha) of the Spanish adaptation of BCIS for schizophrenia were 0.59 for self-reflectiveness and 0.62 for self-certainty [19].

Premorbid intelligence quotient (IQ) was estimated with the Vocabulary Subtest of the Spanish adaptation of the Wechsler Adult Intelligence Scale (WAIS-III) [25,26].

Patients were assessed with a sociodemographic and clinical questionnaire created ad hoc at baseline. We collected data on gender, academic background, cohabitants, and age of onset of the disease.

2.3. Procedure

As mentioned above, this study builds on a previous multicenter randomized clinical trial in which one group received MCT, while the control group was a psycho-educational group matched in frequency and duration. Both interventions were applied in a group setting.

The current study focused on the results of insight scores only in the metacognitive group. The research process flow-chart is shown in Figure 1.

The project was evaluated by the research and ethics committees of each participating center in the study. The first evaluation was performed by Sant Joan de Déu Ethics Committee (PIC-73-11). The participants were informed about the aims of the study and signed informed consent for participation in the study. The main study was registered in the Clinical Trials registry (Identifier: NCT02340559).

The intervention consisted of eight weekly group sessions of MCT. All therapists were trained by Steffen Moritz, author of MCT, and Lisa Schilling. The MCT program included eight modules (one for each session): module 1: Avoid the only causes and uncontrolled; modules 2 and 7: Jumping to conclusions; module 3: Cognitive flexibility; modules 4 and 6: Theory of mind; module 5: Overconfidence in memory errors; and module 8: Depression and low self-esteem.

The software used was R 3.0 (R Foundation for Statistical Computing, Vienna, Austria). Statistical analysis was performed using linear mixed models with repeated measures at different time points, with the baseline evaluation as the reference. The dependent variables are the two BCIS subscales and the Composite Index (a model is estimated for each of them individually), and the IQ and educational level were included as covariates.

Two analyses were performed. First, three time points were used: the baseline assessment, the post-treatment assessment, and the six months follow-up. Secondly, the results after each session and at the end of the treatment were used in order to determine whether there were MCT sessions that were more effective than others in improving cognitive insight.

Empirical size effects (Cohen's d) were also calculated, comparing each evaluation with the baseline. These analyses used all the available data without the need to impute missing values.

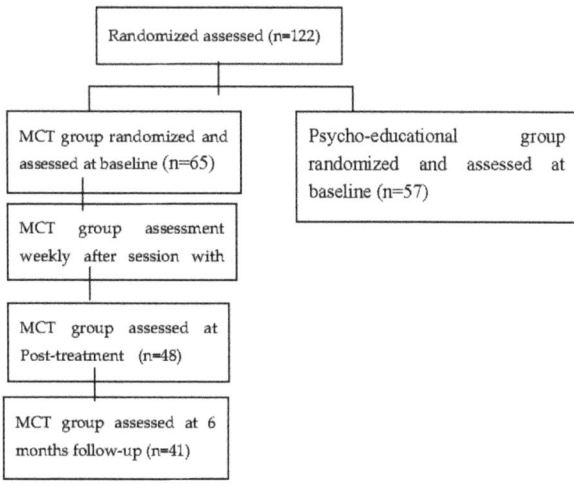

Figure 1. Research process flow-chart. MCT, metacognitive training.

3. Results

Table 1 shows the sociodemographic characteristics of the sample.

Table 1. Socio-demographic characteristics of the sample. MCT, metacognitive training.

		MCT Group	
		N	%
Gender	Men	44	67.7
	Women	21	32.3
Marital status	Single	53	81.5
	Married	8	12.3
	Divorced	4	6.2
Level of education	Primary	26	40.0
	Secondary	25	38.5
	University	14	21.5
Employment status	Working	14	21.5
	Student	12	18.5
	Incapacity	13	20.0
	Unemployed	19	29.3
	Other	7	10.7
		Mean	SD *
Age		27.05	7.94
Age at onset		25.16	7.79
Years of psychosis duration		2.15	2.01
Number of hospitalizations		1.16	1.54
Antipsychotic dose mg/d **		472.53	703.89

* SD = Standard Deviation. ** Antipsychotic drug doses are expressed as chlorpromazine equivalence.

Average attendance in the training program was 5.53/8 sessions (SD = 2.46) in session 1: 50 patients, session 2: 42, session 3: 28, session 4: 37, session 5: 41, session 6: 36, session 6: 36, and session 8: 40. No differences were found in the linear mixed model regarding the number of sessions attended and educational level, so these variables were not controlled for. The results were controlled for intellectual quotient as a significant influence on insight was found.

Self-certainty decreased significantly ($p = 0.03$) over time and the effect of IQ was negative and significant ($p = 0.02$) (patients with higher IQ obtained lower scores in self-certainty). Changes in self-reflectiveness throughout the treatment and at the six months follow-up were far from significant ($p = 0.99$), but IQ had a positive effect. Those with a higher IQ obtained better results in self-reflectiveness ($p < 0.01$). The Composite Index increased over time, but the coefficient was not significant ($p = 0.36$). The effect of IQ was significantly positive ($p < 0.01$), so that patients with higher IQ obtained better results in the Composite Index.

Figures 2–4 show the scores of BCIS subscales in each session.

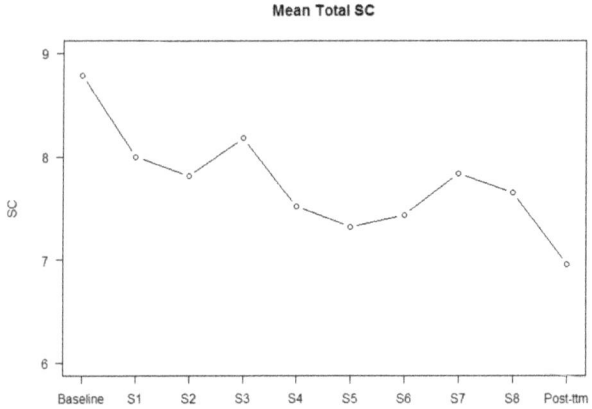

Figure 2. Changes in self-certainty (SC) in every session and in the post-treatment.

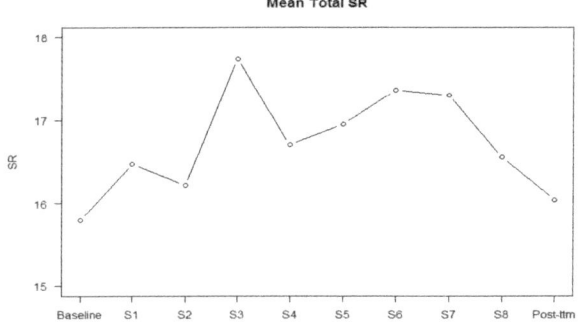

Figure 3. Mean of self-reflectiveness (SR) in each session and in the post-treatment.

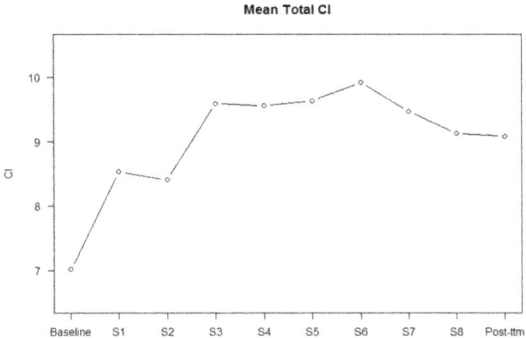

Figure 4. Mean of the Composite Index (CI) in each session and in the post-treatment.

Table 2 shows the results regarding the effect of changes in self-certainty, self-reflectiveness, and the Composite Index in each session. From session 4 to session 8 (ToM, overconfidence in memory errors, jumping to conclusions, and depression and self-esteem), all sessions improved cognitive insight by significantly reducing self-certainty. In the post-treatment assessment, changes in cognitive insight were maintained. No differences by session were found regarding the self-reflectiveness BCIS subscale. However, a trend towards significance was found regarding the influence of IQ. Regarding the Composite Index, from session 4 to session 7 (theory of mind, overconfidence in memory errors, and jumping to conclusions), significant improvements in cognitive insight were found. In session 8 (depression and self-esteem), a trend towards significance was found. These improvements were maintained post-treatment. IQ was significant in the analysis.

Table 2. Effects of each session and at the post-treatment in self-certainty, self-reflectiveness, and the Composite Index and influence of intelligence quotient (IQ).

	Self-Certainty					Self-Reflectiveness					Composite Index			
	Value	Std. Error	t-Value	p-Value	Effect Size	Value	Std. Error	t-Value	p-Value	Effect Size	Value	Std. Error	t-Value	p-Value	Effect Size
Intercept	12.181	2.448	4.976	<0.001		10.280	3.108	3.308	0.001		−1.432	4.276	−0.335	0.738	
S1	−0.606	0.395	−1.532	0.127	0.126	0.216	0.534	0.405	0.685	0.064	0.853	0.655	1.303	0.194	0.147
S2	−0.771	0.421	−1.832	0.068	0.112	0.027	0.564	0.048	0.962	0.046	0.832	0.693	1.201	0.231	0.116
S3	−0.785	0.488	−1.608	0.109	0.111	0.311	0.664	0.468	0.640	0.283	1.260	0.815	1.546	0.123	0.326
S4	−1.404	0.449	−3.124	0.002	0.380	0.020	0.591	0.034	0.973	0.013	1.621	0.747	2.170	0.031	0.265
S5	−1.294	0.419	−3.091	0.002	0.364	0.630	0.561	1.123	0.262	0.036	1.956	0.689	2.839	0.005	0.251
S6	−1.357	0.449	−3.020	0.003	0.309	0.657	0.596	1.101	0.272	0.146	2.156	0.739	2.916	0.004	0.321
S7	−1.181	0.441	−2.678	0.008	0.210	0.567	0.591	0.961	0.338	0.085	1.778	0.725	2.451	0.015	0.202
S8	−0.946	0.425	−2.225	0.027	0.242	0.237	0.580	0.410	0.682	0.016	1.346	0.712	1.891	0.060	0.279
Post-treatment	−1.564	0.399	−3.920	0.000	0.460	−0.031	0.535	−0.059	0.953	0.062	1.570	0.656	2.392	0.017	0.189
IQ	−0.035	0.025	−1.404	0.166		0.062	0.032	1.949	0.056		0.092	0.044	2.107	0.039	

4. Discussion

As expected, the results revealed that cognitive insight improved with the MCT, in particular regarding the self-certainty subscale. These results were maintained at the six months follow-up. Regarding the effect of each session in changing cognitive insight, the results indicated that, after the fourth session, there was an improvement in cognitive insight, particularly in the self-certainty subscale and in the Composite Index. Moreover, it was found that IQ could have an effect on insight changes, revealing that people with a higher IQ improved more in insight.

Patients included in the MCT improved their cognitive insight over the course of treatment, in particular in the self-certainty domain, coinciding with other studies [27]. It is likely that different mechanisms are involved. Analysing the effect of each session, the results show a significant improvement in cognitive insight after session 4 (ToM). These results suggest that there is a cumulative effect over the sessions. Despite this suggestion, not all the sessions seemed to be equally efficient; some of them had a bigger effect size: ToM (session 4), memory (session 5), and empathy (session 6) are the sessions with the greatest contribution to reducing self-certainty. Considering that self-certainty is intended to reduce dogmatic rightness and resistance to feedback from others, these sessions were the ones that best achieved this aim. Session 4 (ToM) and session 6 (empathy) were the two sessions focused on working on relationships with the others and the idea that others can have a different point of view from us, facilitating patients to have more doubt about the certainty of their own thoughts. Session 5 (memory) tackled the memory errors that everyone can experience in everyday life such as rebuilding memories with mistakes. The results of the Composite Index coincide with the self-certainty results, except for the eighth session, where a trend towards significance was found. These results have some clinical implications. Benoit et al. found that better scores in self-certainty were related to improvement in speed processing and visual memory in people attending a remediation cognitive program [28]. Other studies have related self-certainty insight with premorbid IQ, premorbid academic adjustment, and clinical insight in patients with first-episode psychosis [21], as well as with jumping to conclusion and weaknesses in cognitive flexibility, assessed with the Wisconsin Card Sorting Test (WSCT), in At Risk of Mental State subjects [29,30].

Overall, no significant improvements were found regarding self-reflectiveness during the course of the MCT group. Our results are contradictory to those found by Lam et al. performed in Chinese people with schizophrenia, which found significant improvements in cognitive insight and increasing self-reflectiveness, but not self-certainty in those patients included in the MCT condition [15]. There are some differences with our study; Lam's study was done with people with schizophrenia, included inpatients and outpatients, compared with treatment as usual (TAU), was performed twice a week, and was delivered by occupational therapists. On the other hand, patients from our sample scored higher in self-reflectiveness at baseline compared with other studies of validation of the instrument and of intervention [15,31], which suggests a ceiling effect for the self-reflectiveness subscale. Moreover, it should be taken into account that other authors have not found differences in the self-reflectiveness subscale between healthy and psychotic populations [22,24]. Additionally, the Composite Index improved in the same sessions as self-certainty did. Moreover, it should be considered that the biggest effect size was found in session 3 (cognitive flexibility), although it was not statistically significant, probably because of the small number of participants in this session.

Considering the different studies regarding this issue, the results obtained are different in both dimensions of the cognitive insight. In this line, this finding suggests separately studying the sub-components of cognitive insight because higher cognitive insight does not always lead to the same psychological functioning. For instance, higher levels of self-reflectiveness are often associated with depressive mood [32] and with functional capacity [33], while self-certainty has been related to cognitive function [21,23]. Considering the different effect of each dimension, it should be taken independently and assessed at baseline in order to better fit the intervention. Moreover, the Composite Index has been related to social functioning [34]. In this line, it would be useful to implement the MCT intervention in first-episode patients before psychosocial therapies.

In the main part of our study, the results suggest that self-reflectiveness was significantly better in the follow-up regarding the MCT group than in the control group. Self-reflectiveness scores decreased, while in the MCT group, they were stable [14], considering a possible sleeper effect of the MCT intervention as suggested by Moritz, Veckenstedt, et al. in a 3-year follow-up study [35] and Sarin et al. in Cognitive Behavioral Therapy [36]. In the present study, no differences were found in self-reflectiveness over time, but it did not decrease as it did in the control group. The increase in self-reflectiveness and consequently in cognitive insight could act as a protective factor against future psychotic episodes and as a better functioning response, as suggested by Benoit et al. [33].

Intellectual quotient (IQ) is related to cognitive insight changes; patients with a higher IQ are more likely to improve their cognitive insight (concretely in the Composite Index and a tendency in self-reflectiveness). These results are in concordance with those of González-Blanch et al. [21] and with the meta-analysis of Nair et al. [37]. So, taking into consideration this result, it is recommended to guarantee a minimum IQ before considering patients for MCT intervention in order to maximize benefit.

Some limitations should be considered in the present study. The effect size of the results could be conditioned by the size of the sample included in each session. Not all the patients attended every session and some of them had lower attendance rates. Another limitation is that the cumulative effect of treatment is not controlled because all the patients received the sessions in the same order. However, there was no progressive increase in the effect size, suggesting that some sessions are more useful than others. Future studies should consider a randomization of the sessions in order to avoid the learning effect and to control the real effect of each session independently. The main study was performed before the launch of the DSM V. Therefore, patients were diagnosed according to DSM-IV-TR criteria. Of note, the remarkable difference between the two editions concerns subtypes of schizophrenia. Subtypes of schizophrenia was not a variable of our study. Furthermore, although the main project compared the effectiveness of MCT over a psychoeducational group, the BCIS in each session was assessed only in the MCT group. Future researchers should assess BCIS in both groups in order to compare them in terms of cognitive insight.

A first clear implication of our results is the importance of psychological interventions, such as metacognitive training, in addressing cognitive biases in first-episode psychosis. In daily clinical practice, it is sometimes unrealistic to administer complete interventions to all the patients. Therefore, we believe that the following sessions of the MCT should be a priority: attributional style, memory mistakes, and stimulating empathy and theory of mind. These modules are more implicated in reducing self-certainty and in increasing thought flexibility. In turn, improvements in these areas could prevent the formation of delusions and a new relapse. Considering the present health emergency due to the COVID-19 pandemic, adapting its application on virtual settings emerges as a new challenge.

In conclusion, MCT could be considered an appropriate psychological intervention to improve cognitive insight. The study has demonstrated that, after the fourth session, improvements in insight are evident in those patients who received the MCT intervention. Moreover, IQ is an important component to take into account before initiating the MCT intervention.

Author Contributions: All the authors of the study have participated in the design, the assessment of patients, and the drafting and revising of the manuscript. I.B., S.O., and S.M. have participated in conceptualization of the manuscript; I.B., R.L.-C., E.P., M.L.B., A.B., E.L.-R., F.G.-H., E.G., I.R.-D., J.C., A.d.A., R.M., T.P., and S.O. have participated in data acquisition; D.C. has performed formal analysis; I.B., R.L.-C., S.O., and D.C. have participated in writing—original draft preparation; R.M. has performed the review and editing of the manuscript. All authors have read and agreed to the published version of the manuscript.

Funding: The project has been funded by the Instituto de Salud Carlos III (Spanish Government), research grant number PI11/01347 and PI14/00044; by the Fondo Europeo de Desarrollo Regional (FEDER), Progress and Health Foundation of the Andalusian Regional Ministry of Health, grant PI-0634/2011; Obra Social La Caixa (RecerCaixa call 2013); and Obra Social Sant Joan de Déu (BML).

Acknowledgments: We thank González-Blanch C., clinical pshycologist in Hospital Universitario Marqués de Valdecilla (Santander, Spain); Birulés J., researcher in Universitat de Barcelona, Department of Cognition, Development, and Educational Psychology (Barcelona, Spain), Marta Ferrer-Quintero from Parc Sanitari Sant Joan de Déu and Mabel Romero Rius from the University of Barcelona for their collaboration. Spanish Metacognition

Study Group (SMSG): Acevedo A., Anglès J., Argany M.A., Barajas A., Barrigón M.L., Beltrán M., Birulés I., Bogas J.L., Camprubí N., Carbonero M., Carmona Farrés C., Carrasco E., Casañas R., Cid J., Conesa E., Corripio I., Cortes P., Crosas J.M., de Apraiz A., Delgado M., Domínguez L., Escartí M.J., Escudero A., Esteban Pinos I., Figueras M., Franco C., García C., Gil V., Giménez-Díaz D., Gonzalez-Casares R., González Higueras F., González-MontoroMªL, González E., Grasa Bello E., Guasp A., Huerta-Ramos Mª E., Huertas P., Jiménez-Díaz A., Lalucat L.L., LLacer B., López-Alcayada R., López-Carrilero R., Lorente E., Luengo A., Mantecón N., Mas-Expósito L., Montes M., Moritz S., Murgui E., Nuñez M., Ochoa S., Palomer E., Paniego E., Peláez T., Pérez V., Planell K., Planellas C., Pleguezuelo-Garrote P., Pousa E., Rabella M., Renovell M., Rubio R., Ruiz-Delgado I., San Emeterio M., Sánchez E., Sanjuán J., Sans B., Schilling L., Sió H., Teixidó M., Torres P., Vila M.A., Vila-Badia R., Villegas F., Villellas R.

Conflicts of Interest: The authors declare no conflict of interest. The funders had no role in the design of the study; in the collection, analyses, or interpretation of data; in the writing of the manuscript; or in the decision to publish the results.

References

1. Serafini, G.; Pompili, M.; Haghighat, R.; Pucci, D.; Pastina, M.; Lester, D.; Angeletti, G.; Tatarelli, R.; Girardi, P. Stigmatization of schizophrenia as perceived by nurses, medical doctors, medical students and patients. *J. Psychiatr. Ment. Health Nurs.* **2011**, *18*, 576–585. [CrossRef] [PubMed]
2. Fusar-Poli, P.; Smieskova, R.; Serafini, G.; Politi, P.; Borgwardt, S. Neuroanatomical markers of genetic liability to psychosis and first episode psychosis: A voxelwise meta-analytical comparison. *World J. Biol. Psychiatry* **2014**, *15*, 219–228. [CrossRef] [PubMed]
3. Fornells-Ambrojo, M.; Garety, P.A. Understanding attributional biases, emotions and self-esteem in "poor me" paranoia: Findings from an early psychosis sample. *Br. J. Clin. Psychol.* **2009**, *48*, 141–162. [CrossRef] [PubMed]
4. Langdon, R.; Still, M.; Connors, M.H.; Ward, P.B.; Catts, S.V. Attributional biases, paranoia, and depression in early psychosis. *Br. J. Clin. Psychol.* **2013**, *52*, 408–423. [CrossRef]
5. Kaney, S.; Bentall, R.P. Persecutory delusions and the self-serving bias: Evidence from a contingency judgment task. *J. Nerv. Ment. Dis.* **1992**, *180*, 773–780. [CrossRef]
6. Moritz, S.; Woodward, T.S. A generalized bias against disconfirmatory evidence in schizophrenia. *Psychiatry Res.* **2006**, *142*, 157–165. [CrossRef]
7. Dudley, R.; Taylor, P.; Wickham, S.; Hutton, P. Psychosis, delusions and the "Jumping to Conclusions" reasoning bias: A systematic review and meta-analysis. *Schizophr. Bull.* **2016**, *42*, 652–665. [CrossRef]
8. So, S.H.; Siu, N.Y.; Wong, H.-I.; Chan, W.; Garety, P.A. 'Jumping to conclusions' data-gathering bias in psychosis and other psychiatric disorders—Two meta-analyses of comparisons between patients and healthy individuals. *Clin. Psychol. Rev.* **2016**, *46*, 151–167. [CrossRef]
9. Brüne, M. "Theory of mind" in schizophrenia: A review of the literature. *Schizophr. Bull.* **2005**, *31*, 21–42. [CrossRef]
10. Healey, K.M.; Bartholomeusz, C.F.; Penn, D.L. Deficits in social cognition in first episode psychosis: A review of the literature. *Clin. Psychol. Rev.* **2016**, *50*, 108–137. [CrossRef]
11. Moritz, S.; Woodward, T.S. Metacognitive training for schizophrenia patients (MCT): A pilot study on feasibility, treatment adherence, and subjective efficacy. *Ger. J. Psychiatry* **2007**, *10*, 69–78.
12. Moritz, S.; Lysaker, P.H. Metacognition—What did James H. Flavell really say and the implications for the conceptualization and design of metacognitive interventions. *Schizophr. Res.* **2018**, *201*, 20–26. [CrossRef] [PubMed]
13. Moritz, S.; Andreou, C.; Schneider, B.C.; Wittekind, C.E.; Menon, M.; Balzan, R.P.; Woodward, T.S. Sowing the seeds of doubt: A narrative review on metacognitive training in schizophrenia. *Clin. Psychol. Rev.* **2014**, *34*, 358–366. [CrossRef] [PubMed]
14. Ochoa, S.; López-Carrilero, R.; Barrigón, M.L.; Pousa, E.; Barajas, A.; Lorente-Rovira, E.; González-Higueras, F.; Grasa, E.; Ruiz-Delgado, I.; Cid, J.; et al. Randomized control trial to assess the efficacy of metacognitive training compared with a psycho-educational group in people with a recent-onset psychosis. *Psychol. Med.* **2017**, *47*, 1573–1584. [CrossRef] [PubMed]
15. Lam, K.C.K.; Ho, C.P.S.; Wa, J.C.; Chan, S.M.Y.; Yam, K.K.N.; Yeung, O.S.F.; Wong, W.C.H.; Balzan, R.P. Metacognitive training (MCT) for schizophrenia improves cognitive insight: A randomized controlled trial in a Chinese sample with schizophrenia spectrum disorders. *Behav. Res. Ther.* **2015**, *64*, 38–42. [CrossRef] [PubMed]

16. Pos, K.; Meijer, C.J.; Verkerk, O.; Ackema, O.; Krabbendam, L.; de Haan, L. Metacognitive training in patients recovering from a first psychosis: An experience sampling study testing treatment effects. *Eur. Arch. Psychiatry Clin. Neurosci.* **2018**, *268*, 57–64. [CrossRef] [PubMed]
17. Lysaker, P.H.; Pattison, M.L.; Leonhardt, B.L.; Phelps, S.; Vohs, J.L. Insight in schizophrenia spectrum disorders: Relationship with behavior, mood and perceived quality of life, underlying causes and emerging treatments. *World Psychiatry* **2018**, *17*, 12–23. [CrossRef]
18. Beck, A.T.; Baruch, E.; Balter, J.M.; Steer, R.A.; Warman, D.M. A new instrument for measuring insight: The Beck Cognitive Insight Scale. *Schizophr. Res.* **2004**, *68*, 319–329. [CrossRef]
19. Gutiérrez-Zotes, J.A.; Valero, J.; Cortés, M.J.; Labad, A.; Ochoa, S.; Ahuir, M.; Carlson, J.; Bernardo, M.; Cañizares, S.; Escartin, G.; et al. Spanish adaptation of the Beck Cognitive Insight Scale (BCIS) for schizophrenia. *Actas Esp. Psiquiatr.* **2012**, *40*, 2–9.
20. Vohs, J.L.; Lysaker, P.H.; Liffick, E.; Francis, M.M.; Leonhardt, B.L.; James, A.; Buck, K.D.; Hamm, J.A.; Minor, K.S.; Mehdiyoun, N.; et al. Metacognitive capacity as a predictor of insight in first-episode psychosis. *J. Nerv. Ment. Dis.* **2015**, *203*, 372–378. [CrossRef]
21. González-Blanch, C.; Álvarez-Jiménez, M.; Ayesa-Arriola, R.; Martínez-García, O.; Pardo-García, G.; Balanzá-Martínez, V.; Suárez-Pinilla, P.; Crespo-Facorro, B. Differential associations of cognitive insight components with pretreatment characteristics in first-episode psychosis. *Psychiatry Res.* **2014**, *215*, 308–313. [CrossRef] [PubMed]
22. Engh, J.A.; Friis, S.; Birkenaes, A.B.; Jónsdóttir, H.; Klungsøyr, O.; Ringen, P.A.; Simonsen, C.; Vaskinn, A.; Opjordsmoen, S.; Andreassen, O.A. Delusions are associated with poor cognitive insight in schizophrenia. *Schizophr. Bull.* **2010**, *36*, 830–835. [CrossRef] [PubMed]
23. Moritz, S.; Mahlke, C.I.; Westermann, S.; Ruppelt, F.; Lysaker, P.H.; Bock, T.; Andreou, C. Embracing Psychosis: A Cognitive Insight Intervention Improves Personal Narratives and Meaning-Making in Patients with Schizophrenia. *Schizophr. Bull.* **2018**, *44*, 307–316. [CrossRef]
24. Martin, J.M.; Warman, D.M.; Lysaker, P.H. Cognitive insight in non-psychiatric individuals and individuals with psychosis: An examination using the Beck Cognitive Insight Scale. *Schizophr. Res.* **2010**, *121*, 39–45. [CrossRef] [PubMed]
25. Seisdedos, N.; Corral, S.; Cordero, A.; de la Cruz, M.V.; Hernández, M.V.; Pereña, J. *WAIS-III. Escala de Inteligencia de Wechsler para Adultos-III: Manual Técnico.*; TEA Ediciones: Madrid, Spain, 1999.
26. Wechsler, D. *Wechsler Adult Intelligence Scale-Third Edition (WAIS-III)*; Psychological Corporation: San Antonio, TX, USA, 1997; pp. 1–3.
27. Köther, U.; Vettorazzi, E.; Veckenstedt, R.; Hottenrott, B.; Bohn, F.; Scheu, F.; Pfueller, U.; Roesch-Ely, D.; Moritz, S. Bayesian Analyses of the Effect of Metacognitive Training on Social Cognition Deficits and Overconfidence in Errors. *J. Exp. Psychopathol.* **2017**, *8*, 158–174. [CrossRef]
28. Benoit, A.; Harvey, P.O.; Bherer, L.; Lepage, M. Does the Beck Cognitive Insight Scale Predict Response to Cognitive Remediation in Schizophrenia? *Schizophr. Res. Treat.* **2016**, *2016*, 1–6. [CrossRef] [PubMed]
29. O'Connor, J.A.; Ellett, L.; Ajnakina, O.; Schoeler, T.; Kollliakou, A.; Trotta, A.; Wiffen, B.D.; Falcone, A.M.; Di Forti, M.; Murray, R.M.; et al. Can cognitive insight predict symptom remission in a first episode psychosis cohort? *BMC Psychiatry* **2017**, *17*, 1–8. [CrossRef]
30. Ohmuro, N.; Katsura, M.; Obara, C.; Kikuchi, T.; Hamaie, Y.; Sakuma, A.; Iizuka, K.; Ito, F.; Matsuoka, H.; Matsumoto, K. The relationship between cognitive insight and cognitive performance among individuals with at-risk mental state for developing psychosis. *Schizophr. Res.* **2018**, *192*, 281–286. [CrossRef]
31. Warman, D.M.; Lysaker, P.H.; Martin, J.M. Cognitive insight and psychotic disorder: The impact of active delusions. *Schizophr. Res.* **2007**, *90*, 325–333. [CrossRef]
32. Van Camp, L.S.C.; Sabbe, B.G.C.; Oldenburg, J.F.E. Cognitive insight: A systematic review. *Clin. Psychol. Rev.* **2017**, *55*, 12–24. [CrossRef]
33. Benoit, A.; Bowie, C.R.; Lepage, M. Is cognitive insight relevant to functional capacity in schizophrenia? *Schizophr. Res.* **2017**, *184*, 150–151. [CrossRef] [PubMed]
34. Sumiyoshi, T.; Nishida, K.; Niimura, H.; Toyomaki, A.; Morimoto, T.; Tani, M.; Inada, K.; Ninomiya, T.; Hori, H.; Manabe, J.; et al. Cognitive insight and functional outcome in schizophrenia; a multi-center collaborative study with the specific level of functioning scale–Japanese version. *Schizophr. Res. Cogn.* **2016**, *6*, 9–14. [CrossRef] [PubMed]

35. Moritz, S.; Veckenstedt, R.; Andreou, C.; Bohn, F.; Hottenrott, B.; Leighton, L.; Köther, U.; Woodward, T.S.; Treszl, A.; Menon, M.; et al. Sustained and "sleeper" effects of group metacognitive training for schizophrenia a randomized clinical trial. *JAMA Psychiatry* **2014**, *71*, 1103–1111. [CrossRef] [PubMed]
36. Sarin, F.; Wallin, L.; Widerlöv, B. Cognitive behavior therapy for schizophrenia: A meta-analytical review of randomized controlled trials. *Nord. J. Psychiatry* **2011**, *65*, 162–174. [CrossRef] [PubMed]
37. Nair, A.; Palmer, E.C.; Aleman, A.; David, A.S. Relationship between cognition, clinical and cognitive insight in psychotic disorders: A review and meta-analysis. *Schizophr. Res.* **2014**, *152*, 191–200. [CrossRef]

Publisher's Note: MDPI stays neutral with regard to jurisdictional claims in published maps and institutional affiliations.

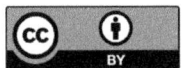

© 2020 by the authors. Licensee MDPI, Basel, Switzerland. This article is an open access article distributed under the terms and conditions of the Creative Commons Attribution (CC BY) license (http://creativecommons.org/licenses/by/4.0/).

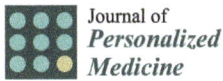

Article

Evaluation of Social Cognition Measures for Japanese Patients with Schizophrenia Using an Expert Panel and Modified Delphi Method

Hiroki Okano [1], Ryotaro Kubota [1], Ryo Okubo [1,2,*], Naoki Hashimoto [3], Satoru Ikezawa [4], Atsuhito Toyomaki [3], Akane Miyazaki [3], Yohei Sasaki [2], Yuji Yamada [1], Takahiro Nemoto [5] and Masafumi Mizuno [5]

1. Department of Psychiatry, National Center of Neurology and Psychiatry Hospital, Tokyo 187-8551, Japan; hokano@ncnp.go.jp (H.O.); kubotar@ncnp.go.jp (R.K.); yujiyamada@ncnp.go.jp (Y.Y.)
2. Translational Medical Center, National Center of Neurology and Psychiatry, Department of Clinical Epidemiology, Tokyo 187-8551, Japan; ysasaki@ncnp.go.jp
3. Department of Psychiatry, Hokkaido University Graduate School of Medicine, Sapporo 060-8638, Japan; hashinao@med.hokudai.ac.jp (N.H.); toyomaki@gmail.com (A.T.); a-miyazaki@med.hokudai.ac.jp (A.M.)
4. Endowed Institute for Empowering Gifted Minds, University of Tokyo Graduate School of Arts and Sciences, Tokyo 153-0041, Japan; satoru-ikezawa@g.ecc.u-tokyo.ac.jp
5. Department of Neuropsychiatry, Toho University Faculty of Medicine, Tokyo 143-8541, Japan; takahiro.nemoto@med.toho-u.ac.jp (T.N.); mizuno@med.toho-u.ac.jp (M.M.)
* Correspondence: ryo-okubo@ncnp.go.jp; Tel.: +81-42-341-2712 (ext. 5843)

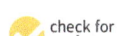

Citation: Okano, H.; Kubota, R.; Okubo, R.; Hashimoto, N.; Ikezawa, S.; Toyomaki, A.; Miyazaki, A.; Sasaki, Y.; Yamada, Y.; Nemoto, T.; et al. Evaluation of Social Cognition Measures for Japanese Patients with Schizophrenia Using an Expert Panel and Modified Delphi Method. *J. Pers. Med.* **2021**, *11*, 275. https://doi.org/10.3390/jpm11040275

Academic Editor: Tomiki Sumiyoshi

Received: 9 February 2021
Accepted: 4 April 2021
Published: 6 April 2021

Publisher's Note: MDPI stays neutral with regard to jurisdictional claims in published maps and institutional affiliations.

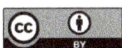

Copyright: © 2021 by the authors. Licensee MDPI, Basel, Switzerland. This article is an open access article distributed under the terms and conditions of the Creative Commons Attribution (CC BY) license (https://creativecommons.org/licenses/by/4.0/).

Abstract: Social cognition is strongly linked to social functioning outcomes, making it a promising treatment target. Because social cognition measures tend to be sensitive to linguistic and cultural differences, existing measures should be evaluated based on their relevance for Japanese populations. We aimed to establish an expert consensus on the use of social cognition measures in Japanese populations to provide grounds for clinical use and future treatment development. We assembled a panel of experts in the fields of schizophrenia, social psychology, social neuroscience, and developmental disorders. The panel engaged in a modified Delphi process to (1) affirm expert consensus on the definition of social cognition and its constituent domains, (2) determine criteria to evaluate measures, and (3) identify measures appropriate for Japanese patients with a view toward future quantitative research. Through two online voting rounds and two online video conferences, the panel agreed upon a definition and four-domain framework for social cognition consistent with recent literature. Evaluation criteria for measures included feasibility and tolerability, reliability, clinical effectiveness, validity, and international comparability. The panel finally identified nine promising measures, including one task originally developed in Japan. In conclusion, we established an expert consensus on key discussion points in social cognition and arrived at an expert-selected set of measures. We hope that this work facilitates the use of these measures in Japanese clinical scenarios. We plan to further examine these measures in a psychometric evaluation study.

Keywords: mental disorders; schizophrenia; developmental disorders; social cognition; social function; facial expression recognition; test battery; quality of life; systematic review; needs survey

1. Introduction

Schizophrenia is a severe mental disorder, and many patients with schizophrenia experience some degree of long-lasting functional impairment. One area that is impaired throughout the course of the disease is social cognition, which is defined as "the mental operations that underlie social interactions, including perceiving, interpreting, and generating responses to the intentions, dispositions, and behaviors of others" [1]. Social cognitive impairments directly affect patients' social participation and capacity to build and maintain social relationships, thereby profoundly decreasing quality of life. This area has garnered considerable interest in recent years because the social cognition construct is believed to be more strongly linked to social functioning outcomes than traditional neurocognition [2], making it a promising treatment target.

With the emergence of social cognition as a major focus of schizophrenia research, numerous measures have been developed to assess its various aspects. However, the complexity and breadth of the social cognition construct, together with a lack of consensus regarding its constituent subdomains, has resulted in an overwhelming variety of measures based on differing theories and interpretations. Paradoxically, there is a dearth of widely accepted and standardized measures available for practical use. The Social Cognition Psychometric Evaluation (SCOPE) study aimed to establish a consensus on the theoretical structure of social cognition in schizophrenia and to systematically evaluate the psychometric properties of existing measures [3–5]. Four core theoretical domains of social cognition were established through expert surveys and RAND expert panel discussions: emotion processing, attributional style/bias, social perception, and theory of mind (ToM) [3]. Experts further identified the existing measures best suited to assess these domains. Two large-scale studies of schizophrenia patients and healthy control groups were subsequently conducted to examine the psychometric properties of 11 measures. Three measures showing particularly strong psychometric properties and associations with functional outcomes were recommended for use in clinical trials: the Hinting task [6], the Bell Lysaker Emotion Recognition Task (BLERT) [7], and the Penn Emotion Recognition Task (ER-40) [8].

The SCOPE study represents a significant step forward by providing a provisional battery of measures and a springboard for future endeavors. However, these results were based on data collected exclusively in the United States and may not be generalizable to different cultural contexts. Social cognition tasks are more sensitive to cultural and linguistic differences than neurocognitive tasks [9]. Stimuli for social cognition tasks often require the participant to understand social interactions. The "correct" interpretation of a social situation may be less obvious or even entirely different for people from a different culture. Stimuli may also include words or ambiguous dialogue with meanings that are not fully replicable across languages. Furthermore, there are believed to be baseline cultural differences in social cognitive ability and tendencies [10]. In short, the same measures established in the United States may not be suitable for assessing social cognition in other, particularly non-English-speaking, cultures. Thus, the cultural relevance and translatability of tasks must be individually considered for each culture [11].

Until recently, social cognition research in Asian populations has been limited to specific domains or been inconsistent in its choice of measures [12–14]. Following the SCOPE study, Lim et al. conducted a psychometric evaluation study examining a similar array of social cognition tasks with Singaporean schizophrenia patients and healthy controls [15]. All participants were fluent in English, and tasks were registered verbatim, without any modifications to the original English versions. The results were consistent with those of the SCOPE study in that the BLERT and ER-40 showed the strongest psychometric properties. However, contrary to the SCOPE study, the Hinting task showed less favorable characteristics. A possible explanation offered by the authors was that some of the vignettes used in the task could be culturally sensitive. These results suggest that, even with a shared language, social cognition tasks may show differing psychometric properties among populations with different cultural backgrounds. However, this study did not examine associations with neurocognitive and social functioning measures.

To our knowledge, no comprehensive psychometric evaluation studies in non-English-speaking populations have been conducted using either translated or originally non-English tasks. Such an attempt would face several new challenges. First, many social cognition tasks include ambiguous phrases or dialogue, which may be difficult to translate fully. Another factor is the anticipated correlation between familiarity with a culture and fluency in its language and its effect on task performance. In other words, in a typically non-English speaking country or cultural group, individuals fluent in English would be expected to have more insight into Western culture and thus may perform better on certain Western-developed tasks. The presence of such factors dictates the need to consider alternative social cognition measures than those originally developed in the Anglosphere.

The present study aimed to identify social cognition measures suitable for use in Japanese schizophrenia patients. It represents a pioneering attempt to systematically investigate the utility of social cognition measures for a non-English-speaking population. An expert panel was assembled and tasked with selecting a comprehensive group of measures that are relevant for the target population while also consistent with the abovementioned related studies.

2. Materials and Methods

2.1. Expert Panel Members

Expert panel members were recruited using a reputation-based snowball sampling procedure. Panel members were chosen from Japanese researchers performing psychological, neurobiological, psychophysiological, or neuroimaging research in the area of social cognition, broadly defined. Experts from fields other than schizophrenia were included to incorporate important concepts from closely related areas. Ultimately, nine experts in the areas of social psychology, social neuroscience, schizophrenia, and developmental disorders agreed to serve as panelists (Table S1). No panelists reported financial conflicts of interest.

2.2. Key Discussion Points and Candidate Social Cognition Measures

We prepared a draft of items comprising key discussion points for establishing an expert consensus. This list included the definition and core domains of social cognition, the target population for the social cognition measures selected in this study, objectives for their use, and evaluation criteria for final recommendations following a psychometric evaluation study.

The definition of social cognition was quoted from the NIMH Workshop on Social Cognition in Schizophrenia [1], as this definition that had already garnered consensus from several experts in the SCOPE study [3]. We prepared a preliminary list of candidate social cognition measures to be considered by the expert panel. Measures were selected based on similar studies examining the psychometric properties of social cognition measures. The SCOPE study recommendations were given particular importance, although measures cited as promising but ultimately excluded were also reconsidered. In addition, the authors inspected the literature for relevant or promising social cognition measures that were originally developed in Japan or with pre-existing Japanese versions. The resulting list comprised 15 preliminary candidate measures, including all six measures recommended by the SCOPE study and two measures developed in Japan. The remaining measures were selected based on history of use in Japanese populations (Table 1). The principal investigators and secretariat then prepared a database listing the results of previous studies that examined the psychometric properties for each measure (Table S3).

Table 1. Candidate social cognition measures.

Domain/Measure	Original Citation	Total Citations (PubMed)	Citations Per Year (PubMed)
Emotion Processing			
Bell Lysaker Emotion Recognition Task (BLERT)	Bryson et al., 1997 [7]	44	1.91
Face Emotion Identification Test (FEIT)	Kerr and Neale, 1993 [16]	94	3.48
Noh Mask Test	Minoshita et al., 2005 [17]	2	0.13
Penn Emotion Recognition Test (ER-40)	Kohler et al., 2003 [8]	174	10.24
Theory of Mind			
Faux Pas Test	Stone et al., 1998 [18]	212	9.64
Hinting Task	Corcoran et al., 1995 [6]	145	5.8
Metaphor and Sarcasm Scenario Test (MSST)	Adachi et al., 2004 [19]	9	0.56
Reading the Mind in the Eyes Test (Eyes)	Baron-Cohen et al., 2001 [20]	864	45.47
The Awareness of Social Inference Test (TASIT)	McDonald et al., 2003 [21]	100	5.88
Attributional Style/Bias			
Ambiguous Intentions and Hostility Questionnaire (AIHQ)	Combs et al., 2007 [22]	59	4.54
Intentionality Bias Task (IBT)	Rosset, 2008 [23]	23	1.92
Social Cognition Screening Questionnaire (SCSQ) *	Roberts et al., 2011 [24]	(N/A)	(N/A)
Social Perception			
Biological Motion (BM) Task	Hashimoto et al., 2014 [25]	5	0.83
Social Attribution Task-Multiple Choice (SAT-MC)	Bell et al., 2010 [26]	20	2
Situational Feature Recognition Test (SFRT)	Corrigan and Green, 1993 [27]	(N/A)	(N/A)

* Also measures Theory of Mind.

2.3. The Modified Delphi Process

This study used a modified Delphi process (RAND/UCLA appropriateness method) to (1) reaffirm consensus on the definition of the social cognition construct and its key domains, (2) establish criteria for evaluating the appropriateness of social cognition measures for use in Japanese populations, and (3) rate and select measures based on the established criteria with a view toward future psychometric evaluation studies (see Figure 1) [28,29]. This method was also chosen for the SCOPE study as a proven method to develop consensus-based test batteries, having been successfully used in the development of the MATRICS battery [30] and VALERO initiative [31] in the field of schizophrenia research [3]. We defined consensus as when the compilation of item statements reached approval of 80% or higher [32] in online voting sessions conducted via the *Google Forms* website. Panelists had approximately 2 weeks to complete each of the online surveys. Voting was repeated until consensus was reached on all items. After each round, iterative refinements were made to the item compilation based on participant feedback.

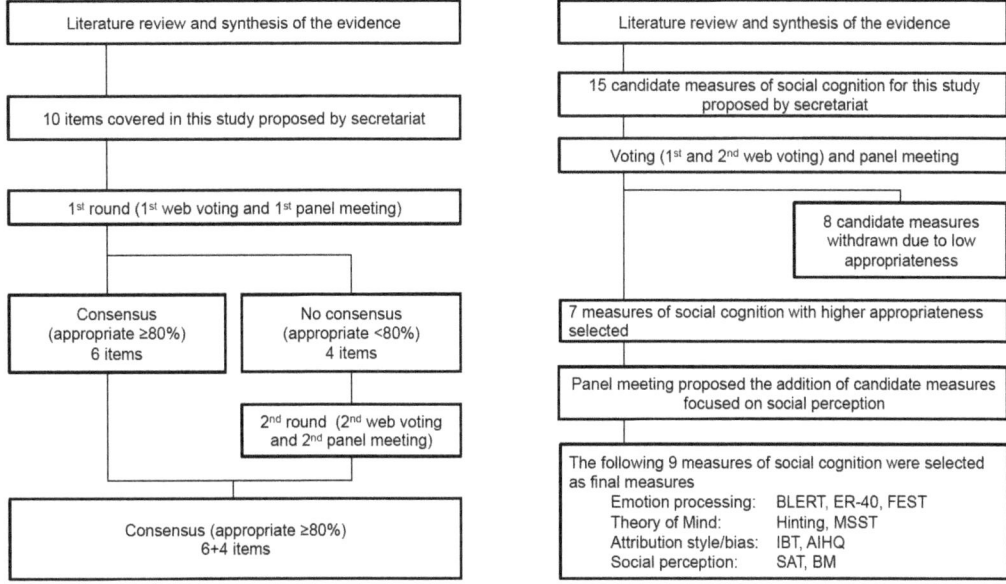

Figure 1. Overview of voting process.

Panelists rated the appropriateness of each measure for use in Japanese schizophrenia patients based on the following criteria: (1) practicality of administration and tolerability for participants, (2) reliability, (3) utility, (4) convergent and criterion validity, and (5) international comparability. Panel members were provided with detailed descriptions of each measure, including psychometric data from the SCOPE study if available, along with a supplementary database of psychometric indicators for each measure that we compiled from the literature (Table S3). Ratings were given on a 9-point scale, where 1 was "extremely inappropriate" and 9 was "extremely appropriate." Panel members were also encouraged to provide feedback on individual items through a free form comment section. After each round, the results were compiled to prepare a summary document that presented the raw rating, mean, and median scores in histograms, together with individual comments gathered from each panel member. These documents were shared and used as a basis for the discussion rounds, where individual rating discrepancies were addressed. Certain points were agreed upon beforehand; 7 measures were to be selected from the 15 candidates for inclusion in a subsequent psychometric evaluation study, and the selected measures were to, as a whole, address as wide a range of social cognition domains as possible. Discussions were held in the form of online video conferences because of the COVID-19 pandemic and precautions regarding face-to-face group meetings and traveling.

3. Results

The final list of items agreed upon by the expert panel is shown in Table S2.

3.1. Definition and Core Domains of Social Cognition

The panel agreed to maintain the well-known NIMH Workshop definition [1] and the four-domain structure of emotion processing, attribution style/bias, social perception, and ToM for social cognition in schizophrenia.

3.2. Target Population, Purpose of Use, and Evaluation Criteria of Social Cognition Measures

The target population for the social cognition measures selected in this study was Japanese schizophrenia patients. It was further specified in the panel discussions that the subsequent psychometric study would target "patients with schizophrenia whose symptoms have stabilized following the medication adjustment period in the acute phase and who are undergoing rehabilitation to improve social function."

The initial focus of this study was to select measures that could be widely used in clinical practice. However, following discussion, the objectives were expanded to also consider the suitability of the measures for clinical trials.

A set of criteria to assess social cognition measures following the psychometric study was discussed and agreed upon among the panel. Feasibility and tolerability criteria were established in terms of administration time and participant ratings, respectively. Test–retest reliability would be considered acceptable with correlation coefficients greater than or equal to 0.6. Utility as a measure would be assessed in terms of floor and ceiling effects, with emphasis being placed particularly on the absence of floor effects because a task showing ceiling effects may still be useful for clinical purposes such as screening and aiding diagnosis. However, if a task is to be used as an outcome for interventional studies, the absence of both floor and ceiling effects across administration times was agreed to be favorable. Measures showing clear group differences between patients and healthy controls would be favored. Correlation with social function outcomes would also be emphasized. Incremental validity, or, in this case, increased predictive ability of social function outcomes beyond neurocognition, would also be given consideration. Finally, tasks recommended in the SCOPE study were agreed to be favorable in terms of international comparability. Grading criteria were modified so that grades would be considered for each purpose of use. Specific advantages and precautions for the use of each test would be described in the final article.

3.3. Panel Ratings and Selection of Social Cognition Measures

Descriptive statistics for the two rounds of panel ratings are provided in Table 2. A set of consensus measures was selected based on the final ratings. Seven tasks with the highest mean appropriateness ratings were selected: three tasks representing the emotion processing domain (the BLERT, ER-40, and Facial Emotion Selection Test (FEST)) and two tasks each for the domains of attributional style/bias (the Ambiguous Intentions and Hostility Questionnaire (AIHQ) and the Intentionality Bias Task (IBT)) and ToM (the Hinting Task and the Metaphor and Sarcasm Scenario Test (MSST)) (Table 3). No social perception tasks were included in the initially planned selection of seven tasks, prompting an additional discussion regarding whether the omission of a previously established core domain was acceptable. Ultimately, it was unanimously agreed to include two tasks representing social perception: The Social Attribution Task-Multiple Choice (SAT-MC) and the Biological Motion (BM) task. Thus, a total of nine measures representing each of the four established core domains comprised the final selection.

Table 2. Results of the expert panel ratings.

Domain/Measure	Median, Mean (SD)	
	1st Round	2nd Round
Emotion Processing		
ER-40	8, 7.1 (1.8)	8, 7.1 (1.7)
FEST *	7, 7.2 (0.8)	8, 7.1 (1.9)
BLERT-J	7, 7.1 (1.6)	7, 7.3 (0.9)
Noh Mask Test	4, 4.2 (1.7)	3, 3.1 (0.9)

Table 2. Cont.

Domain/Measure	Median, Mean (SD)	
	1st Round	2nd Round
Theory of Mind		
MSST	8, 6.9 (1.9)	8, 6.8 (1.9)
Hinting	8, 7.2 (1.6)	7, 7.1 (1.6)
Eyes	5, 5.2 (2.4)	5, 5.0 (1.6)
Faux Pas	5, 5.0 (2.1)	5, 4.8 (1.8)
TASIT	5, 4.6 (2.8)	5, 4.3 (1.5)
Attributional Style/Bias		
AIHQ	7, 6.4 (1.8)	7, 6.2 (1.7)
IBT	6, 6.0 (1.9)	6, 5.8 (0.9)
SCSQ **	7, 7.2 (1.1)	5, 5.2 (2.0)
Social Perception		
SAT	6, 5.7 (2.4)	4, 5.1 (2.3)
SFRT	6, 5.6 (2.1)	4, 4.1 (1.7)
Biological Motion	5, 4.6 (2.0)	4, 4.0 (1.3)

* Japanese version of the FEIT, ** Also measures Theory of Mind.

Table 3. List and descriptions of the final measures.

Domain/Measure	Description
Emotion Processing	
Penn Emotion Recognition Test (ER-40)	Measures the ability to identify emotional state from facial expressions. Participants view 40 still photographs of people's faces, each expressing a particular emotion (joy, sadness, anger, fear, or no emotion). Participants are then asked to answer, which emotion is expressed in each photograph. Performance is indexed as the number of correct answers. The estimated time required is 3–7 min.
Facial Emotion Selection Test (FEST)	Japanese version of the FEIT. Measures ability to infer emotions from the facial expressions of others. Participants view 21 photographs and answer which emotion (joy, sadness, anger, fear, surprise, disgust, or no emotion) it corresponds to. Performance is indexed as the total number of correct answers. The estimated time required is about 10 min.
Bell Lysaker Emotion Recognition Task-Japanese Version (BLERT-J)	Japanese version of the BLERT. Measures the ability to identify emotional state from facial expression, tone of speech, and body language. Participants view 21 short videos in which an actor portrays different emotional states (happiness, sadness, fear, disgust, surprise, anger, or no emotion) and must answer which emotion was portrayed in each video. Performance is indexed as the number of correct answers. The estimated time required is 7–10 min.
Theory of Mind	
Metaphor and Sarcasm Scenario Test (MSST)	Measures ability to understand metaphorical and sarcastic expressions in dialogue. Participants read short passages that provide context for a figurative or sarcastic statement and then choose what they think it means. There are five figurative and five sarcastic statements. The number of correct answers for each type is summed to produce metaphor and sarcasm scores. For each of the sarcasm scenarios, one of the incorrect answers is a "landmine answer" representing the statement's meaning when taken at face value. The number of times the landmine answer was avoided is tallied as "the landmine avoidance score." The estimated time required is 5–10 min.
Hinting Task	Measures the ability to detect sarcasm and indirect requests from others' statements. Participants are read passages of dialogue between two characters in 10 different scenarios. In each conversation, one of the characters tries to indirectly convey a certain intention or request to the other. Participants are asked what the intention or request is. If the answer is incorrect, the participant is provided with additional dialogue that further clarifies the intention. First-time correct answers are awarded two points, and second-time correct answers are awarded one point. Performance is indexed as the total number of points. The estimated time required is about 7 min.

Table 3. *Cont.*

Domain/Measure	Description
Attributional Style/Bias	
Ambiguous Intentions and Hostility Questionnaire (AIHQ)	Assesses hostile social cognitive biases. Participants read passages describing hypothetical, negative scenarios and answer why they think the situation occurred. Participants then rate the degree to which they perceived the action to be intentional, how angry it would make them feel, and how much they would blame the other person on separate Likert scales. Finally, participants answer how they would respond to the situation. Responses to the open-ended questions are coded by independent raters to compute Hostility Bias and Aggression Bias indexes, whereas the Likert ratings are averaged and summed to produce a Blame Score. The estimated time required is 5–10 min.
Intentionality Bias Task (IBT)	Assesses tendency to assign intentionality to the actions of others. Up to 80 short sentences (fewer in some versions) depicting another person's action (such as "He broke the window") are presented on a screen. Participants answer whether the behavior is "intentional" or "accidental" within a short time limit. Performance is indexed as the number of questions answered "intentional" to the total number of questions. The estimated time required is about 5 min.
Social Perception	
Social Attribution Task-Multiple Choice (SAT-MC)	Assesses implicit social attribution formation. Participants view a 64-s, animated video of anthropomorphized geometric shapes enacting a social drama. The video does not include dialogue. After viewing the video twice, participants answer 19 multiple-choice questions about what happens or how the shapes feel. Performance is indexed as the total number of correct answers. The estimated time required is about 10 min.
Biological Motion (BM) Task	Measures capacity to perceive human body motion at high speed. Participants are presented with images of moving light spots, either moving in coordination to mimic human body movements (Biological Motion) or at random (Scrambled Motion). Participants view multiple images and answer whether each is either Biological Motion or Scrambled Motion. In later parts of the task, random light spots are added/removed in response to correct/incorrect responses to adjust difficulty and determine participants' level of performance.

4. Discussion

Our primary aim was to identify social cognition measures appropriate for Japanese schizophrenia patients based on the opinions of experts in related fields, with a view toward future quantitative research. After establishing grounds for measure selection, the panel rated and discussed the suitability of 15 candidate measures (Table 2), ultimately arriving at nine measures representing all four domains (Table 3).

We first sought to obtain an expert consensus on the definition and theoretical framework of the social cognition construct. Our proposal of using the same four core domains established in the SCOPE study was met with some debate in the initial round of surveys. Several experts questioned the inclusion of the social perception domain, with concerns about the lack of clarity surrounding its definition and scope and an absence of well-established tasks. However, it was agreed that such shortcomings underscore the need for inclusion and further investigation of the construct. Other experts were concerned about the omission of metacognitive aspects. Nonetheless, the panel ultimately agreed to adopt the proposed four-domain structure, citing the importance of consistency and international comparability.

Initially, the target population was not specified to any stage of schizophrenia. However, it was pointed out that performance on social cognition tasks would vary significantly depending on what stage the patient was in and that such variance would make it difficult to adequately evaluate tasks' psychometric properties. The panel agreed to narrow the target population to more stable patients, as they would also be the main targets for treatments to improve social functioning. The initial target population also included outpatients only. However, the panel discussed the need to address social cognitive dysfunctions in chronic patients hospitalized for reasons other than pure severity of symptoms, such as those in forensic psychiatric wards or patients with problematic behaviors not directly related to psychosis. Thus, the phrasing was modified to include such patients.

Two of the selected measures, the MSST and BM, are novel tasks that have yet to be systematically examined in the context of social cognition in schizophrenia. Furthermore, the MSST is a task that was developed in Japan. The panel unanimously agreed that the nature of this study as one of the first attempts to examine social cognition tasks in a non-English context dictates the need to consider tasks already established as suitable for Japanese populations. Although originally intended to evaluate autism spectrum disorder tendencies in children, it was agreed that the MSST could be applied to assess ToM in schizophrenia populations. The BM task has been mentioned in the literature in the context of incorporating social neuroscience paradigms into the field of social cognition [33,34] and specifically as a promising measure to explore the social perception domain [5]. The panel deemed the BM suitable for the particular objectives of this study due to its low dependence on cultural and linguistic factors, which suggests a high level of international comparability.

The AIHQ and SAT-MC were included despite being classified as "not recommended" in the SCOPE study [4,5]. The AIHQ comprises both open-ended, scorer-rated items and self-report Likert scales assessing participants' responses to negative social situations. Answers for the open-ended questions are coded by two independent raters, which has been speculated to negatively affect psychometrics such as test–retest reliability. Buck et al. suggested that the psychometric properties of the AIHQ could be improved by expanding self-report items and removing the open-ended questions [35]. The Singaporean psychometric evaluation study conducted by Lim et al. showed more favorable results for the AIHQ, further suggesting its utility [15]. The SAT-MC was not included in the initially planned selection of seven tasks but was chosen as the highest rated among candidate social perception tasks. In the SCOPE study, the SAT-MC showed sub-par results in basic psychometrics such as test–retest reliability, owing largely to the use of two independent forms across the two administration times. The use of consistent test forms across administration times may produce more favorable results. In addition, given that the SCOPE study evaluated tasks based on suitability for clinical trials, the SAT-MC may potentially receive more favorable gradings when viewed through the lens of utility in clinical practice. Furthermore, the SAT-MC has long been considered less affected by linguistic and cultural differences than other social cognition tasks because it is non-verbal and less culturally loaded [26,36,37]. A recent cross-cultural study with South Korean and North American schizophrenia patients and healthy controls showed the SAT-MC to be consistent across groups and supported its utility across language and cultures [13], making it a strong candidate for our current study.

Notable omissions included the Eyes test and The Awareness of Social Inference Test (TASIT), which were both included in the SCOPE recommendations. The Eyes test was seen as possibly not suitable for Japanese populations due to cultural differences; in Japan, it is considered rude to stare at someone's face and it is therefore not customary to read others' emotions through their eyes. There was also further concern that the Eyes test significantly overlaps with emotion processing, despite being classified as a measure of ToM. The TASIT, which uses short but relatively complex video vignettes of actors enacting various social interactions, received lower ratings mainly due to concerns over translatability. Many experts also shared the opinion that certain task structures, such as the TASIT, are inherently more dependent on working memory, with performance on these tasks at risk of reflecting neurocognitive ability more strongly than social cognitive function.

This study is not without its limitations. First, it was largely influenced by the SCOPE study, and measures indicated in the SCOPE study therefore received more attention than others. We attempted to reduce these limitations by reconsidering measures not recommended by the SCOPE study and conducting a search of literature for Japanese-developed social cognition measures. Furthermore, our reliance on the SCOPE study for guidance meant inheriting its limitations regarding the social perception domain and lack of strong candidate measures to represent it. The expert rating results and ensuing discussions also suggested that the objectives of the present study may have inadvertently led to emotion processing tasks being favored because their simpler structures seemingly make them less vulnerable to changes in psychometrics caused by translation to Japanese. These observations were addressed in the panel discussions and ultimately influenced the decision to include a roughly equal number of measures from each of the four core domains. Another limitation is the relatively small number of experts recruited. Diversity regarding fields of expertise may have been somewhat limited, with relatively high weight on the field of schizophrenia and only one expert representing another clinical population (developmental disorders). Furthermore, this study may have benefited from including experts from other academic fields, such as cultural anthropology, to provide a more rigid examination of which tasks may or may not be appropriate for Japanese people.

The present study established an expert consensus on key discussion points and promising measures for assessing social cognition in Japanese schizophrenia patients. There is currently a lack of available information regarding the use of social cognition measures in a non-English-speaking cultural context. We hope that our research will inform and facilitate future endeavors in other countries. Subsequent phases of this study will involve a multi-center psychometric evaluation study in Japanese schizophrenia and healthy control populations using the expert-selected measures. However, a considerable portion of the selected tasks has yet to be validated in Japanese schizophrenia populations (BLERT, BM, and MSST) or even translated to Japanese (SAT-MC and IBT). A pilot study may be warranted to preliminarily confirm the utility and structural validity of the tasks and to identify any need for modifications. Cross-cultural studies comparing results among groups of different cultural and linguistic backgrounds may shed further light on which measures are more suitable for international comparison and collaborative research.

Supplementary Materials: The following are available online at https://www.mdpi.com/article/10.3390/jpm11040275/s1, Table S1: Expert panel members, Table S2: List of items agreed upon by the expert panel, Table S3: Supplementary data for candidate social cognition measures.

Author Contributions: Conceptualization, R.O., S.I., H.O., R.K., N.H., A.T., A.M., Y.S., and Y.Y.; writing—original draft preparation, H.O.; writing—review and editing, R.O. and S.I.; supervision, T.N. and M.M. All authors have read and agreed to the published version of the manuscript.

Funding: This research was funded by AMED, grant number JP20dk0307092.

Institutional Review Board Statement: The study was conducted according to the guidelines of the Declaration of Helsinki, and approved by the Institutional Review Board of National Center of Neurology and Psychiatry Hospital (B2020-107; 7 December 2020).

Informed Consent Statement: Informed consent was obtained from all subjects involved in the study.

Data Availability Statement: None.

Acknowledgments: We would like to thank the expert panel members for their participation: Akiko Kikuchi, Toshiya Murai, Shinichi Niwa, Tomiki Sumiyoshi, Tatsuya Koeda, Motomu Suga, Daisuke Haga, and Jun Tayama. We would also like to thank Kazuyuki Nakagome for his role in selecting the panel members and reviewing this article.

Conflicts of Interest: The authors declare no conflict of interest.

References

1. Green, M.F.; Penn, D.L.; Bentall, R.; Carpenter, W.T.; Gaebel, W.; Gur, R.C.; Kring, A.M.; Park, S.; Silverstein, S.M.; Heinssen, R. Social cognition in schizophrenia: An NIMH workshop on definitions, assessment, and research opportunities. *Schizophr. Bull.* **2008**, *34*, 1211–1220. [CrossRef] [PubMed]
2. Pinkham, A.E.; Penn, D.L. Neurocognitive and social cognitive predictors of interpersonal skill in schizophrenia. *Psychiatry Res.* **2006**, *143*, 167–178. [CrossRef] [PubMed]
3. Pinkham, A.E.; Penn, D.L.; Green, M.F.; Buck, B.; Healey, K.; Harvey, P.D. The social cognition psychometric evaluation study: Results of the expert survey and RAND panel. *Schizophr. Bull.* **2014**, *40*, 813–823. [CrossRef] [PubMed]
4. Pinkham, A.E.; Penn, D.L.; Green, M.F.; Harvey, P.D. Social Cognition Psychometric Evaluation: Results of the Initial Psychometric Study. *Schizophr. Bull.* **2016**, *42*, 494–504. [CrossRef] [PubMed]
5. Pinkham, A.E.; Harvey, P.D.; Penn, D.L. Social Cognition Psychometric Evaluation: Results of the Final Validation Study. *Schizophr. Bull.* **2018**, *44*, 737–748. [CrossRef]

6. Corcoran, R.; Mercer, G.; Frith, C.D. Schizophrenia, symptomatology and social inference: Investigating "theory of mind" in people with schizophrenia. *Schizophr. Res.* **1995**, *17*, 5–13. [CrossRef]
7. Bryson, G.; Bell, M.; Lysaker, P. Affect recognition in schizophrenia: A function of global impairment or a specific cognitive deficit. *Psychiatry Res.* **1997**, *71*, 105–113. [CrossRef]
8. Kohler, C.G.; Turner, T.H.; Bilker, W.B.; Brensinger, C.M.; Siegel, S.J.; Kanes, S.J.; Gur, R.E.; Gur, R.C. Facial emotion recognition in schizophrenia: Intensity effects and error pattern. *Am. J. Psychiatry* **2003**, *160*, 1768–1774. [CrossRef]
9. Hajdúk, M.; Achim, A.M.; Brunet-Gouet, E.; Mehta, U.M.; Pinkham, A.E. How to move forward in social cognition research? Put it into an international perspective. *Schizophr. Res.* **2020**, *215*, 463–464. [CrossRef]
10. Wu, S.; Keysar, B. The effect of culture on perspective taking. *Psychol. Sci.* **2007**, *18*, 600–606. [CrossRef]
11. Mehta, U.M.; Thirthalli, J.; Gangadhar, B.N.; Keshavan, M.S. Need for culture specific tools to assess social cognition in schizophrenia. *Schizophr. Res.* **2011**, *133*, 255–256. [CrossRef]
12. Chen, K.W.; Lee, S.C.; Chiang, H.Y.; Syu, Y.C.; Yu, X.X.; Hsieh, C.L. Psychometric properties of three measures assessing advanced theory of mind: Evidence from people with schizophrenia. *Psychiatry Res.* **2017**, *257*, 490–496. [CrossRef] [PubMed]
13. Lee, H.S.; Corbera, S.; Poltorak, A.; Park, K.; Assaf, M.; Bell, M.D.; Wexler, B.E.; Cho, Y.I.; Jung, S.; Brocke, S.; et al. Measuring theory of mind in schizophrenia research: Cross-cultural validation. *Schizophr. Res.* **2018**, *201*, 187–195. [CrossRef]
14. Mehta, U.M.; Thirthalli, J.; Naveen Kumar, C.; Mahadevaiah, M.; Rao, K.; Subbakrishna, D.K.; Gangadhar, B.N.; Keshavan, M.S. Validation of Social Cognition Rating Tools in Indian Setting (SOCRATIS): A new test-battery to assess social cognition. *Asian J. Psychiatry* **2011**, *4*, 203–209. [CrossRef] [PubMed]
15. Lim, K.; Lee, S.A.; Pinkham, A.E.; Lam, M.; Lee, J. Evaluation of social cognitive measures in an Asian schizophrenia sample. *Schizophr. Res. Cogn.* **2020**, *20*, 100169. [CrossRef] [PubMed]
16. Kerr, S.L.; Neale, J.M. Emotion perception in schizophrenia: Specific deficit or further evidence of generalized poor performance? *J. Abnorm. Psychol.* **1993**, *102*, 312–318. [CrossRef] [PubMed]
17. Minoshita, S.; Morita, N.; Yamashita, T.; Yoshikawa, M.; Kikuchi, T.; Satoh, S. Recognition of affect in facial expression using the Noh Mask Test: Comparison of individuals with schizophrenia and normal controls. *Psychiatry Clin. Neurosci.* **2005**, *59*, 4–10. [CrossRef]
18. Stone, V.E.; Baron-Cohen, S.; Knight, R.T. Frontal lobe contributions to theory of mind. *J. Cogn. Neurosci.* **1998**, *10*, 640–656. [CrossRef] [PubMed]
19. Adachi, T.; Koeda, T.; Hirabayashi, S.; Maeoka, Y.; Shiota, M.; Wright, E.C.; Wada, A. The metaphor and sarcasm scenario test: A new instrument to help differentiate high functioning pervasive developmental disorder from attention deficit/hyperactivity disorder. *Brain Dev.* **2004**, *26*, 301–306. [CrossRef]
20. Baron-Cohen, S.; Wheelwright, S.; Hill, J.; Raste, Y.; Plumb, I. The "Reading the Mind in the Eyes" Test revised version: A study with normal adults, and adults with Asperger syndrome or high-functioning autism. *J. Child Psychol. Psychiatry* **2001**, *42*, 241–251. [CrossRef]
21. McDonald, S.; Flanagan, S.; Rollins, J.; Kinch, J. TASIT: A new clinical tool for assessing social perception after traumatic brain injury. *J. Head Trauma Rehabil.* **2003**, *18*, 219–238. [CrossRef] [PubMed]
22. Combs, D.R.; Penn, D.L.; Wicher, M.; Waldheter, E. The Ambiguous Intentions Hostility Questionnaire (AIHQ): A new measure for evaluating hostile social-cognitive biases in paranoia. *Cogn. Neuropsychiatry* **2007**, *12*, 128–143. [CrossRef] [PubMed]
23. Rosset, E. It's no accident: Our bias for intentional explanations. *Cognition* **2008**, *108*, 771–780. [CrossRef]
24. Roberts, D.L.; Fiszdon, J.; Tek, C. Initial validity of the Social Cognition Screening Questionnaire (SCSQ). *Schizophr. Bull.* **2011**, *37* (Suppl. 1), 280.
25. Hashimoto, N.; Toyomaki, A.; Hirai, M.; Miyamoto, T.; Narita, H.; Okubo, R.; Kusumi, I. Absent activation in medial prefrontal cortex and temporoparietal junction but not superior temporal sulcus during the perception of biological motion in schizophrenia: A functional MRI study. *Neuropsychiatry Dis. Treat.* **2014**, *10*, 2221–2230. [CrossRef] [PubMed]
26. Bell, M.D.; Fiszdon, J.M.; Greig, T.C.; Wexler, B.E. Social attribution test–multiple choice (SAT-MC) in schizophrenia: Comparison with community sample and relationship to neurocognitive, social cognitive and symptom measures. *Schizophr. Res.* **2010**, *122*, 164–171. [CrossRef]
27. Corrigan, P.W.; Green, M.F. *The Situational Feature Recognition Test: A Measure of Schema Comprehension for Schizophrenia*; John Wiley & Sons: Hoboken, NJ, USA, 1993; pp. 29–35.
28. Fitch, K.; Bernstein, S.J.; Aguilar, M.D.; Burnand, B.; LaCalle, J.R.; Lazaro, P.; van het Loo, M.; McDonnell, J.; Vader, J.; Kahan, J.P. *The RAND/UCLA Appropriateness Method User's Manual*; RAND Corporation: Santa Monica, CA, USA, 2001.
29. Hasson, F.; Keeney, S.; McKenna, H. Research guidelines for the Delphi survey technique. *J. Adv. Nurs.* **2000**, *32*, 1008–1015.
30. Marder, S.R.; Fenton, W. Measurement and Treatment Research to Improve Cognition in Schizophrenia: NIMH MATRICS initiative to support the development of agents for improving cognition in schizophrenia. *Schizophr. Res.* **2004**, *72*, 5–9. [CrossRef]
31. Leifker, F.R.; Patterson, T.L.; Heaton, R.K.; Harvey, P.D. Validating measures of real-world outcome: The results of the VALERO expert survey and RAND panel. *Schizophr. Bull.* **2011**, *37*, 334–343. [CrossRef]
32. Green, B.; Jones, M.; Hughes, D.; Williams, A. Applying the Delphi technique in a study of GPs' information requirements. *Health Soc. Care Community* **1999**, *7*, 198–205. [CrossRef]

33. Kern, R.S.; Penn, D.L.; Lee, J.; Horan, W.P.; Reise, S.P.; Ochsner, K.N.; Marder, S.R.; Green, M.F. Adapting social neuroscience measures for schizophrenia clinical trials, Part 2: Trolling the depths of psychometric properties. *Schizophr. Bull.* **2013**, *39*, 1201–1210. [CrossRef] [PubMed]
34. Olbert, C.M.; Penn, D.L.; Kern, R.S.; Lee, J.; Horan, W.P.; Reise, S.P.; Ochsner, K.N.; Marder, S.R.; Green, M.F. Adapting social neuroscience measures for schizophrenia clinical trials, part 3: Fathoming external validity. *Schizophr. Bull.* **2013**, *39*, 1211–1218. [CrossRef] [PubMed]
35. Buck, B.; Iwanski, C.; Healey, K.M.; Green, M.F.; Horan, W.P.; Kern, R.S.; Lee, J.; Marder, S.R.; Reise, S.P.; Penn, D.L. Improving measurement of attributional style in schizophrenia; A psychometric evaluation of the Ambiguous Intentions Hostility Questionnaire (AIHQ). *J. Psychiatry Res.* **2017**, *89*, 48–54. [CrossRef] [PubMed]
36. Horan, W.P.; Nuechterlein, K.H.; Wynn, J.K.; Lee, J.; Castelli, F.; Green, M.F. Disturbances in the spontaneous attribution of social meaning in schizophrenia. *Psychol. Med.* **2009**, *39*, 635–643. [CrossRef] [PubMed]
37. Johannesen, J.K.; Lurie, J.B.; Fiszdon, J.M.; Bell, M.D. The Social Attribution Task-Multiple Choice (SAT-MC): A Psychometric and Equivalence Study of an Alternate Form. *ISRN Psychiatry* **2013**, *2013*, 830825. [CrossRef]

Article

Study Protocol: The Evaluation Study for Social Cognition Measures in Japan (ESCoM)

Ryotaro Kubota [1], Ryo Okubo [1,2,*], Hisashi Akiyama [3], Hiroki Okano [1], Satoru Ikezawa [4], Akane Miyazaki [3], Atsuhito Toyomaki [3], Yohei Sasaki [2], Yuji Yamada [1], Takashi Uchino [5], Takahiro Nemoto [5], Tomiki Sumiyoshi [1,6], Naoki Yoshimura [1] and Naoki Hashimoto [3,*]

1. Department of Psychiatry, National Center of Neurology and Psychiatry Hospital, Tokyo 187-8551, Japan; kubotar@ncnp.go.jp (R.K.); hokano@ncnp.go.jp (H.O.); yujiyamada@ncnp.go.jp (Y.Y.); sumiyot@ncnp.go.jp (T.S.); naoyoshi@ncnp.go.jp (N.Y.)
2. Department of Clinical Epidemiology, Translational Medical Center, National Center of Neurology and Psychiatry, Tokyo 187-8551, Japan; ysasaki@ncnp.go.jp
3. Department of Psychiatry, Hokkaido University Graduate School of Medicine, Sapporo 060-8638, Japan; hakiyama203@gmail.com (H.A.); a-miyazaki@med.hokudai.ac.jp (A.M.); toyomaki@gmail.com (A.T.)
4. Endowed Institute for Empowering Gifted Minds, University of Tokyo Graduate School of Arts and Sciences, Tokyo 153-0041, Japan; satoru-ikezawa@g.ecc.u-tokyo.ac.jp
5. Department of Neuropsychiatry, Toho University Faculty of Medicine, Tokyo 143-8541, Japan; takashi.uchino@med.toho-u.ac.jp (T.U.); takahiro.nemoto@med.toho-u.ac.jp (T.N.)
6. National Center of Neurology and Psychiatry, Department of Preventive Intervention for Psychiatric Disorders, National Institute of Mental Health, Tokyo 187-8553, Japan
* Correspondence: ryo-okubo@ncnp.go.jp (R.O.); hashinao@med.hokudai.ac.jp (N.H.)

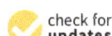

Citation: Kubota, R.; Okubo, R.; Akiyama, H.; Okano, H.; Ikezawa, S.; Miyazaki, A.; Toyomaki, A.; Sasaki, Y.; Yamada, Y.; Uchino, T.; et al. Study Protocol: The Evaluation Study for Social Cognition Measures in Japan (ESCoM). *J. Pers. Med.* **2021**, *11*, 667. https://doi.org/10.3390/jpm11070667

Academic Editor: Rajendra D Badgaiyan

Received: 14 June 2021
Accepted: 14 July 2021
Published: 16 July 2021

Publisher's Note: MDPI stays neutral with regard to jurisdictional claims in published maps and institutional affiliations.

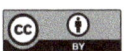

Copyright: © 2021 by the authors. Licensee MDPI, Basel, Switzerland. This article is an open access article distributed under the terms and conditions of the Creative Commons Attribution (CC BY) license (https:// creativecommons.org/licenses/by/ 4.0/).

Abstract: In schizophrenia, social cognitive impairment is considered one of the greatest obstacles to social participation. Although numerous measures have been developed to assess social cognition, only a limited number of them have become available in Japan. We are therefore planning this evaluation study for social cognition measures in Japan (ESCoM) to confirm their psychometric characteristics and to promote research focused on social cognition. Participants in the cross-sectional observational study will be 140 patients with schizophrenia recruited from three Japanese facilities and 70 healthy individuals. In our primary analysis, we will calculate several psychometric indicators with a focus on whether they can independently predict social functioning. In secondary analyses, we will assess the reliability and validity of the Japanese translations of each measure and conduct an exploratory investigation of patient background, psychiatric symptoms, defeatist performance belief, and gut microbiota as determinants of social cognition. The protocol for this study is registered in UMIN-CTR, unique ID UMIN000043777.

Keywords: mental disorders; schizophrenia; developmental disorders; social cognition; social functioning; facial expression recognition; test battery; quality of life

1. Introduction

Schizophrenia is a severe mental disorder for which complete recovery is difficult to achieve by conventional therapies. As a result, patients with schizophrenia continue to have impaired social functioning. Although the prevalence of schizophrenia is a relatively low 1% [1], it is one of the top 15 causes of disability worldwide [2].

Social cognition is defined as "the mental operations that underlie social interactions, including perceiving, interpreting, and generating responses to the intentions, dispositions, and behaviors of others" [3]. In patients with schizophrenia or other mental disorders, social cognitive impairment is considered one of the greatest obstacles to social participation, such as interpersonal relationships, education, and employment [4].

Social cognition has become a major area of schizophrenia research, and the number of publications on this topic has increased remarkably in the past 20 years [3,5]. Measures for assessing social cognitive impairment have been developed from various perspectives. However, many of these measures are based on original theories, and reliability and validity have not been sufficiently examined for some of them [5]. To address this problem, the Social Cognition Psychometric Evaluation (SCOPE) study was conducted in the United States from 2012 to 2017. Through voting and discussion by an expert panel and two observational studies, six measures from a pool of 108 candidates were ultimately recommended for assessing social cognitive impairment in schizophrenia and other mental disorders [5–7]. The SCOPE study made significant advances in the assessment of social cognitive impairment, contributing a provisional test battery and serving as a foundation for future work. However, the results were based on data collected in only the United States, so the generalizability to other cultural contexts remains unclear. Notably, social cognition tasks are more sensitive than neurocognitive tasks to differences in language and culture [8].

In fact, there has been little effort to test the reliability and validity of the measures recommended by the SCOPE study in languages other than English or in cultural areas outside of the United States. A 2020 study of reliability and validity in Singapore by Lim et al. found that even among people who use English as a common language, reliability and validity results may differ by cultural area [9]. Going forward, as therapies are developed for social cognition, it will be absolutely paramount to examine the effects of cultural differences in the underlying assessments of social cognition.

In Japan, some researchers have been working on developing a social cognition test battery for Japanese patients with schizophrenia [10], and validity studies have been conducted for social cognition measures such as the widely used Japanese versions of the Facial Emotion Selection Test (FEST) and Social Cognition Screening Questionnaire (SCSQ) [11,12]. However, reliability and validity have been assessed for only one of the Japanese versions of the six measures recommended by the SCOPE study. In addition, the reliability and validity of some social cognition measures currently used in Japan, including measures unique to Japan, have not been sufficiently assessed. Therefore, in order to prepare for future international clinical trials, it is necessary to assess not only the six measures recommended by the SCOPE study, but also the measures unique to Japan.

Considering the above, we previously recruited a panel of Japanese experts on social cognition who discussed whether social cognition measures developed in the United States could be introduced in Japan, and the panel selected nine promising measures of social cognition in Japanese patients using a modified Delphi method [13]. Accordingly, the main objectives of the present study are to assess these measures selected by the domestic expert panel simultaneously in the same patients and to examine the relative merits of these social cognition measures by calculating psychometric indicators. Another objective is to hold an expert panel discussion of these psychometric indicators to produce recommendations on social cognition measures for Japanese patients.

To date, there have been studies examining cultural differences in social cognition measures between Asian and western countries [14] or attempting to establish new social cognition test batteries suited to their own specific study purposes [15,16]. However, this is the first study that will comprehensively evaluate the psychometric properties of social cognition measures in a non-English context using the framework of the SCOPE study.

We will also examine clinical backgrounds, psychiatric symptoms, and defeatist performance belief as determinants of social cognition. Furthermore, based on the recent focus on the relation between the gut microbiome and schizophrenia [17], we will also measure gut microbiota in an exploratory investigation of social cognitive impairment, for which an effective treatment method has not yet been established. According to an experiment using germ-free mice, the gut microbiome plays an important role in cognition and social behavior [18]. When the gut microbiota of patients with schizophrenia were transplanted into germ-free mice, these animals demonstrated reduced functioning related to memory, learning, and social behavior compared with those receiving transplants of gut microbiota from healthy humans [19]. To date, five studies have been conducted on the gut microbiota in patients with schizophrenia. These studies have shown that the composition of the gut microbiota in patients is different from that in healthy individuals [20] and that gut microbiota composition is associated with symptoms of mental illness [21] and depression [22]. However, no study has yet examined the relation between social cognition and the gut microbiota in patients with schizophrenia. Therefore, in secondary analyses, we will assess the reliability and validity of the Japanese translations of the abovementioned measures and conduct an exploratory investigation of patient background, psychiatric symptoms, defeatist performance belief, and gut microbiota as determinants of social cognition.

2. Methods and Analysis

2.1. Study Participants and Data Collection

This is a cross-sectional study. Patients with schizophrenia will be recruited from the National Center of Neurology and Psychiatry, Hokkaido University Hospital, and Toho University Omori Medical Center. Staff at each facility will screen patients based on their medical records and select eligible patients. Next, these patients will be examined by their attending physicians, who will confirm whether the patients meet the eligibility criteria. Healthy individuals will be recruited by methods such as flyers posted or distributed at the study facilities and e-mails about the study posted on mailing lists. Individuals who volunteer to participate will be interviewed by staff at the participating facilities, who will confirm the individuals' eligibility. Individuals who meet the inclusion criteria will be given a written explanation of the study by staff at the participating facilities, who will then obtain written informed consent. The staff will assess measures with individuals who provide written consent. Anyone involved in the research agrees to participate and agrees to have details the results of the research about them published.

Of the nine tests recommended by the panel, the Penn Emotion Recognition Task (ER-40) [23] was excluded from the present study because a similar task, FEST, which measures cognitive functions related to facial expressions, is already available in Japanese. In addition, it requires the use of a unique interface and is difficult to administer compared with other measures in the same environment.

The study period for this cross-sectional study is from institutional review board (IRB) approval until 31 March 2023. Each measure will be conducted either once or twice. For healthy individuals, all assessments will be completed on the day that informed consent is obtained or within 1 week. For patients with schizophrenia, the initial assessment will be performed on the day that informed consent is obtained (day 0) or within 1 week (Table 1). In consideration of fatigue in participants, measures may be assessed over multiple days. In general, however, all measures are scheduled to be completed within several days.

Table 1. Testing schedule.

	Day 0–7	Day 0–7 (All Measures Below to Be Completed within 2 Days)	Day 14–42
Informed consent (patients, healthy individuals)	○		
Background information (patients, healthy individuals)	○		
M.I.N.I. (patients, healthy individuals)	○		
JART-25 (patients, healthy individuals)	○		
PANSS (patients)		○	

Table 1. Cont.

	Day 0–7	Day 0–7 (All Measures Below to Be Completed within 2 Days)	Day 14–42
BNSS (patients)		○	
DPB (patients *)		○	
BACS-J (patients *)		○	
UPSA-B (patients *)		○	
SLOF (patients *)		○	
Japanese versions of social cognition measures (patients *, healthy individuals)		○	○
Scale of subjective difficulty of social cognition measures (patients *, healthy individuals)		○	
Gut microbiota (patients, healthy individuals)	□		
Duration (min)	40	180 (Healthy individuals: 80)	70

○: mandatory, □: optional. * Measures with an asterisk next to "patients" are conducted with patients for the purposes of this study, while measures without an asterisk are conducted as part of standard clinical practice. BACS-J, Brief Assessment of Cognition for Schizophrenia, Japanese Version; BNSS, Brief Negative Symptom Scale; DPB, Defeatist Performance Beliefs; JART-25, Japanese Adult Reading Test-25; M.I.N.I., Mini-International Neuropsychiatric Interview; PANSS, Positive and Negative Syndrome Scale; SLOF, Specific Levels of Functioning Scale; UPSA-B, University of California, San Diego Performance-based Skill Assessment—Brief.

2.2. Inclusion and Exclusion Criteria

Inclusion criteria for patients with schizophrenia are as follows: (1) primary diagnosis of schizophrenia based on the Diagnostic and Statistical Manual of Mental Disorders (DSM-5) at the time of assessment; (2) no hospitalization in the previous 2 months, no changes in prescriptions in the past 6 weeks, and no changes in prescription dosage in the past 2 weeks; (3) age 20–59 years at the time of obtaining informed consent; and (4) written informed consent to participate in the study based on an understanding of its objective and content (capacity to consent).

The inclusion criteria for healthy individuals are as follows: (1) age 20–59 years at the time of study participation; (2) confirmation of no diagnoses of mental disorders at the time of study participation; and (3) written informed consent to participate in the study.

For both patients with schizophrenia and healthy individuals, the exclusion criteria are as follows: (1) physical/mental disorders that prevent implementation of measures during study participation; (2) insufficient Japanese language ability to respond to self-reported psychological measures based on a sufficient understanding of the questions; and (3) being deemed ineligible to participate for any other reason by an attending physician or study staff.

2.3. Candidate Measures for Social Cognition

2.3.1. Attributional Style Bias

- Ambiguous Intentions and Hostility Questionnaire (AIHQ)

  The participant responds to questions about five situations with negative outcomes, such as questions on the cause of the situation, whether they feel the other person's actions are intentional, and how they would respond to the situation. We obtained permission from the original authors to modify the existing Japanese version of the questionnaire by expanding the number of self-report items and removing rater-scored items, as suggested by Buck et al. [24]. The format was changed to address the limitations presented in the SCOPE study [5–7]. The estimated time required is 6 min [25].

- Intentionality Bias Task (IBT)

The participant responds to 24 short sentences describing human actions within a time limit and indicates whether those actions are intentional or accidental. A Japanese version of the IBT was newly prepared for this study. The 24-question version used in the SCOPE study [7] was first translated into Japanese, and then back-translated to English for revision by the original author. In addition, modifications were made to the time conditions to account for differences in grammatical structure and average reading speed between English and Japanese. The estimated time required is 5 min [26].

2.3.2. Emotion Processing

- Bell Lysaker Emotion Recognition Task (BLERT)

The participant views videos of actors and, using the actor's facial expression, tone of voice, vocal timbre, and upper body movement as clues, responds to multiple-choice questions asking which emotion was being expressed. A new Japanese version, refilmed with a Japanese actor and a translated script, was prepared with permission from the original author. The estimated time required is 7 min [27].

- Facial Emotion Selection Test (FEST)

The participant views photos of Japanese faces of different genders and ages and selects the emotion that most closely matches the expression in the photo from 7 choices (Ekman's six basic emotions and emotionless). This test was created in Japan with reference to the Facial Emotion Identification Task (FEIT) [28]. The estimated time required is 10 min [11].

2.3.3. Social Perception

- Social Attribution Task-Multiple Choice (SAT-MC)

The participant views animations of moving geometric figures and responds to questions about the meaning and motive of the figures' movement. Japanese versions of both the SAT-MC I and II were newly prepared. The original English texts were translated to Japanese and then back-translated to English. The back-translations were reviewed by the original author and modifications were made to the Japanese translation as deemed necessary. The estimated time required is 10 min [29].

- Biological Motion Task (BM)

The BM consists of two tasks that measure the ability to distinguish biological motion. In the first task, the participant distinguishes between human movement and scrambled (nonbiological) motion represented by point-lights. In the second task, scattered moving point-lights are projected onto human movement and scrambled motion, and the participant is asked to distinguish between them. The number of scattered moving point-lights varies depending on the movement in each trial. The estimated time required is 10 min [30].

2.3.4. Theory of Mind

- Hinting Task (Hinting)

The participant reads and hears a dialogue between two characters and identifies the true intention behind one character's indirect speech. A new Japanese version was prepared with permission from the original author. In this new version, in order for the participant to take the test by themselves on a computer, they answer each question twice, first without a hint, and then with a hint. The participant answers the questions aloud and these answers are recorded. Based on the recording, 2 points are given for correct answers in the no-hint phase, 1 point for correct answers in the hint phase, and

0 points for not answering any of the questions correctly. The estimated time required is 6 min [31].

- Metaphor and Sarcasm Scenario Test (MSST)

The participant reads 10 passages involving metaphors and sarcasm and chooses the answer that most accurately describes the passage. The estimated time required is 8 min [32].

2.4. Other Measurements

- Background information

Information such as sex, age, educational background, medical history, treatment history, primary disease, history of allergies, and history of side effects will be collected from medical records or interviews with participants.

- Mini-International Neuropsychiatric Interview (M.I.N.I.)

The M.I.N.I is a structured interview designed to diagnose mental disorders. The present study uses the version of the M.I.N.I adapted to the DSM-V. The M.I.N.I will be conducted after obtaining informed consent to confirm history of mental disorders in healthy participants. For participants with schizophrenia, the M.I.N.I. will be performed after obtaining consent to determine whether they meet the inclusion criteria. The interview will take roughly 30 min [33,34].

- Japanese Adult Reading Test-25 (JART-25)

The JART-25, a measure of verbal IQ, consists of 25 two-character kanji compound words that participants are asked to read aloud. In patients with schizophrenia, the JART-25 is considered to reflect premorbid verbal IQ. The estimated time required is 5 min [35].

- Positive and Negative Syndrome Scale (PANSS)

The PANSS assesses overall psychiatric symptoms in schizophrenia via interview. The scale is composed of 30 items: 7 items on positive symptoms, 7 items on negative symptoms, and 16 items on general psychopathology symptoms. This study will use the Japanese version of the PANSS, which was translated by the Japan Young Psychiatrists Organization. The estimated time required is 30 min. Assessment by an informant (estimated time required: 10 min) is also performed [36,37].

- Brief Negative Symptom Scale (BNSS)

The BNSS is a 13-item scale that assesses negative symptoms in schizophrenia via interview. The estimated time required is 15 min [38,39].

- Defeatist Performance Beliefs (DPB) Scale

The DPB Scale is a self-administered scale for assessing negative beliefs about oneself. The estimated time required is 5 min [40,41].

- General Causality Orientations Scale (GCOS)

The GCOS is a self-administered scale that assesses individual tendencies regarding three different motivational orientations (autonomy, control, and impersonal, which correspond to intrinsic motivation, extrinsic motivation, and amotivation, respectively). The estimated time required is 10 min [42].

- Self-Assessment of Social Cognition Impairments (ACSo)

The ACSo is a 12-item self-administered questionnaire that examines subjective complaints regarding four different domains of social cognitive impairment. The estimated time required is 5 min [43,44]. The original French text was translated to Japanese and then back-translated to French. The back-translation was reviewed by the original authors and modifications were made to the Japanese translation as deemed necessary.

- Observable Social Cognition Rating Scale (OSCARS)

The OSCARS is an 8-item scale that comprehensively examines subjective complaints regarding social cognitive impairment. The scale involves a self-report and an objective assessment from an informant close to the participant. The estimated time required is 5 min [45,46]. The original English text was translated to Japanese and then back-translated to English. The back-translations were reviewed by the original authors and modifications were made to the Japanese translation as deemed necessary.

- Brief Assessment of Cognition for Schizophrenia, Japanese Version (BACS-J)

The BACS, which is a standardized test battery for which validity has been examined, was developed to assess cognitive impairment in schizophrenia. The assessment, which is currently widely used for psychiatric disorders, consists of verbal memory, working memory, motor speed, attention, verbal fluency, and executive functions. The estimated time required is 30 min [47,48].

- University of California, San Diego Performance-based Skill Assessment—Brief (UPSA-B)

The UPSA-B measures functioning in two domains: financial management and communication (by telephone), in a role-playing scenario that models daily living. The estimated time required is 10 min [49,50].

- Specific Levels of Functioning Scale (SLOF)

The SLOF objectively assesses social functioning by integrating the results of interviews with the participant and a close informant with results from a self-administered questionnaire. The estimated time required is 10 min [51,52].

- Gut microbiota

Using a specialized gut microbiota measurement kit, we will measure gut microbiota as described previously [53,54]. Based on reference sequences, we will categorize bacteria into operational taxonomic units and calculate the occupancy rate (the percentage of the gut microbiome occupied by a given bacterium) of each bacterium at the genus level.

2.5. Sample Size Calculation

The present study aims to simultaneously assess measures of social cognition and quantitatively determine which measures are psychometrically superior. We will calculate various psychometric indicators with an emphasis on whether they can independently predict social functioning; specifically, we will emphasize the incremental validity of social functioning (defined as a significant increase in the coefficient of determination when social functioning testing is added after neurocognitive function testing has been included in advance as an independent variable) as determined by hierarchical multiple regression analysis. Sample size was calculated based on hierarchical multiple regression analysis.

In multiple regression analysis, f^2 indicates effect size. According to Cohen [55], f^2 values of 0.02, 0.15, and 0.35 represent small, moderate, and large effect sizes, respectively. In the present study, Model 1 uses the six cognitive domains assessed by the BACS-J (verbal memory, working memory, motor speed, attention, verbal fluency, and executive function) as explanatory variables and social functioning (SLOF and UPSA) as the response variable. In Model 2, each of the social cognition measures is added one at a time. Based on a previous study [7], the effect size of Model 1 is assumed to be 0.25, which is halfway between moderate and large. The present study requires a sample size sufficient to give an increase in the effect size of Model 2 to large (0.35), that is, to detect social cognition measures that, when added, boost the predictive ability of social functioning from halfway between moderate and large. The sample size necessary for detection with $\alpha = 0.05$ and $\beta = 0.2$ is 99 participants (SAS 9.4). To conduct this analysis, all measures must be completed. In view of the high dropout rate of 40% in a previous study [7], we assumed a dropout rate (dropping out at any time before the final analysis) of 30% in the present study; therefore, we set the target sample size at 140 participants.

The purpose of recruiting healthy individuals for this study is to estimate reference values for social cognition measures in the general population in an exploratory fashion.

We will recruit 8 participants in each of eight classifications (men and women in their 20s, 30s, 40s, and 50s). In consideration of dropouts, we set the target sample size at 70 participants.

2.6. Statistical Methods

For participants' background information, we will calculate summary statistics separately for the patient group and the healthy group and compare them between groups. To examine the relative merits of social cognition measures, we will calculate the following psychometric indicators. For reliability, in addition to performing correlation analysis and assessing test–retest reliability, we will calculate Cronbach's alpha to assess internal consistency. For changes from the initial test to the retest (learning effect), we will calculate Cohen's d and state the respective frequencies of floor/ceiling effects. In addition to performing simple correlation analysis for each social cognition test and social functioning, we will perform multiple regression analysis to determine the overall extent to which each of the social cognition measures predicts social functioning. For each social cognition measure, we will also examine the incremental validity of social functioning (defined as a significant increase in the coefficient of determination when social functioning testing is added after neurocognitive function testing has been included in advance as an independent variable) as determined by hierarchical multiple regression analysis. Furthermore, we will calculate the means and standard deviations (SDs) for the time required for each social cognition measure and participants' subjective assessments of each measure separately for the patient group and the healthy group. We will also calculate means and SDs of results for each social cognition measure separately for the patient group and the healthy group, compare means between the two groups, and note Cohen's d.

The details of the above statistical analysis will be shown separately in a statistical analysis protocol that will be drafted by the time final data entry is closed. Interim analysis will not be conducted. For missing data, we are considering listwise deletion as the first option. However, if listwise deletion results in a high percentage of missing data, we will consider statistical analysis that imputes missing data.

3. Ethics and Data Management

3.1. Ethical Considerations

The written explanation and consent form, which have been approved by an IRB, will be handed to participants. Following thorough written and oral explanations, we will obtain informed consent from participants based on their own free will. In the event that information is obtained or changes to the study protocol are made that might affect a participant's consent, we will provide this information to the participant promptly. We will then confirm the participant's willingness to participate in the study, revise the explanation form and consent form with IRB approval, and obtain the participant's informed consent once again. The protocol for this study is registered in the UMIN Clinical Trials Registry (UMIN-CTR), unique ID UMIN000043777.

In terms of possible harm, this is a cross-sectional observational study that does not involve any intervention and is therefore presumed not to inflict any burden related to invasiveness. However, participants will be burdened financially by transportation expenses. The measures take 6 h to complete, meaning that we cannot rule out the possibility of fatigue. In the event of fatigue or any other situation that may make continued testing inappropriate, we will include breaks, readjust the testing schedule, or take any other measures necessary to improve the situation. In addition, the principal investigator or co-investigators will promptly conduct appropriate examination and treatment.

3.2. Patient and Public Involvement

Ken Udagawa of the Community Mental Health & Welfare Bonding Organization (COMHBO) participated in the research team and joined study group meetings. He gave us various forms of advice, such as revising expressions in measures and questionnaires to make them easier for patients with schizophrenia to understand. In addition, Daisuke Haga of One More (managed by the Japan Learning Association) performed assessment of the social cognition measures with 5 patients with schizophrenia in his organization and gave us information regarding the measures' usability.

3.3. Data Management and Monitoring and Auditing

Participants' personal information will be managed by a personal information manager. All samples and information collected during the study will be anonymized at the time of collection by an anonymization manager to prevent identification of participants by sample or information. We will anonymize information by assigning a number unique to the study to each participant's consent form (which contains personally identifiable information such as name and address) and test results and then create a correspondence table. We will store original copies of test forms and data after deleting information that can be used to identify individual participants (name, address, date of birth, etc.). All paper materials relating to individuals will be stored in locked document storage cabinets in the facilities where the research is being conducted (National Center of Neuropsychiatry: locked cabinet in the Translational Medical Center; Hokkaido University: locked cabinet in the Department of Psychiatry; Toho University: locked cabinet in the Department of Neuropsychiatry). The key will be kept by the personal data manager, and the area where personal data are handled will be within the relevant facility, and the data will always be stored in a locked cabinet after use.

Electronic data will be stored using flash memory devices that require mandatory encryption and password authentication. Only the principal investigators at each institution (National Center of Neurology and Psychiatry: Ryo Okubo, Hokkaido University: Naoki Hashimoto, Toho University: Takahiro Nemoto) will have access to the stored flash memory. Access may be granted temporarily to persons approved by the principal investigator as necessary to carry out the research (e.g., data entry and analysis). Measurement of gut microbiota will be outsourced to a testing company called Cykinso, where samples will be managed with numbers unique to the study assigned by the study secretariat. Thorough caution will be taken so that names and other personally identifiable information will not be given to Cykinso. DNA extract from stool-derived gut bacteria will be disposed of after analysis is completed.

Because the present study has no intervention, we will not conduct monitoring or auditing.

4. Discussion

4.1. Dissemination: Process for Final Recommendation

With reference to the results of this study, we will assign all indicators one of three grades based on criteria that were determined in advance through a vote by an expert panel. The grades are "appropriate," "appropriate with reservation," and "use with caution." The appropriateness of each measure depends on its purpose of use, such as for clinical research (observational studies and interventional studies) or for only clinical purposes such as screening and rehabilitation assessment. Therefore, when recommendations are finalized, we will grade the measures according to their intended use and list advantages and points of caution for each.

The members of the expert panel will grade each measure based on the assessment criteria determined by an expert panel in 2020 and with reference to the results of a validity study conducted in 2021 for psychometric assessments. The panel members will vote on which grade best applies to each measure, with additional rounds of discussion and voting conducted until a consensus of $\geq 80\%$ (at least 8 of 9 members) is reached. The number of members who object to the final vote and their reasons for objecting will be recorded and appended to the grading results when they are published.

Good practicality is defined as each social cognition domain taking less than 15 min to administer, while good tolerability is defined as the test having a small burden based on subjective assessment by the participants. For test–retest reliability, a correlation coefficient of ≥ 0.6 is defined as "appropriate." For utility as a repeated measure, we will place importance on the absence of a floor effect in both the first and second measurements. However, in order to use measures as outcomes in interventional studies, we will place importance on the absence of both a floor effect and a ceiling effect in both the first and second measurements.

For validity, we will place importance on a pronounced difference between patients with schizophrenia and healthy individuals and on a strong correlation with social functioning. We will also examine incremental validity, that is, a further increase in the power to predict social functioning resulting from the addition of social cognition performance to neurocognitive performance. For the sake of international comparisons, we will prioritize the six measures recommended by the SCOPE study (BLERT, Hinting, ER-40, and IBT) conducted in the United States when they are equally applicable in Japanese clinical practice.

At a point between the completion of the data analysis and the conclusion of the research project, the results will be linked to anonymized data and presented at relevant academic conferences and in academic journals without revealing identification of participants.

4.2. Prospects for the Future

Generating recommendations for standard measures of social cognition for Japanese patients may lead to (1) the promotion of education/employment support tailored to social cognitive impairment, and (2) greater participation by Japanese researchers in international collaborations on social cognitive impairment and identification of factors in mental disorders in general which worsen social function.

Furthermore, through subsequent research using these social cognition measures, we aim to (1) determine the needs of not only patients with social cognitive impairment but also healthcare workers, (2) identify social cognitive impairments that prominently affect forms of social participation such as employment and education, and (3) support the development of intervention programs to treat social cognitive impairment effectively.

We also hope that our research will help to identify differences in social cognition between countries and ethnic groups, and inform future efforts to examine social cognitive impairment in patients with schizophrenia across populations with various biological and cultural characteristics.

Author Contributions: Conceptualization, all authors (R.K., R.O., H.A., H.O., S.I., A.M., A.T., Y.S., Y.Y., T.U., T.N., T.S., N.Y. and N.H.); writing—original draft preparation, R.K., R.O., H.O., S.I., T.S., and N.H.; writing—review and editing, all authors (R.K., R.O., H.A., H.O., S.I., A.M., A.T., Y.S., Y.Y., T.U., T.N., T.S., N.Y. and N.H.); supervision, T.N., S.I., T.S., N.H. and R.O. All authors have read and agreed to the published version of the manuscript.

Funding: The study is supported by a grant from the Japan Agency for Medical Research and Development (AMED)'s Research and Development Grants for Comprehensive Research for Persons with Disabilities (in the field of mental disorders) "The Evaluation study for Social Cognition Measures in Japan" (principal investigator: Ryo Okubo; period: 1 April 2020–31 March 2023; grant number JP20dk0307092).

Institutional Review Board Statement: The study has been approved by the Institutional Review Board of the National Center of Neurology and Psychiatry Hospital (B2020-107; 7 December 2020) and will be conducted in accordance with the guidelines of the Declaration of Helsinki.

Informed Consent Statement: Informed consent will be obtained from all participants involved in the study.

Data Availability Statement: Not applicable.

Conflicts of Interest: None of the investigators associated with the present study nor their spouses or other family members have any financial interest or employment relationship whatsoever with the funding organization. Therefore, the investigators have planned and will conduct the study independent of the funding organization. All researchers and other personnel involved with the present study have undergone a review by a Conflict-of-Interest Management Committee and have been confirmed to have no conflicts of interest.

References

1. Kahn, R.S.; Sommer, I.E.; Murray, R.M.; Meyer-Lindenberg, A.; Weinberger, D.R.; Cannon, T.D.; O'Donovan, M.; Correll, C.U.; Kane, J.M.; van Os, J.; et al. Schizophrenia. *Nat. Rev. Dis. Primers* **2015**, *1*, 15067. [CrossRef] [PubMed]
2. GBD 2016 Disease and Injury Incidence and Prevalence Collaborators. Global, regional, and national incidence, prevalence, and years lived with disability for 328 diseases and injuries for 195 countries, 1990–2016: A systematic analysis for the Global Burden of Disease Study 2016. *Lancet* **2017**, *390*, 1211–1259. [CrossRef]
3. Green, M.F.; Leitman, D.I. Social cognition in schizophrenia. *Schizophr. Bull.* **2008**, *34*, 670–672. [CrossRef] [PubMed]
4. Green, M.F.; Hellemann, G.; Horan, W.P.; Lee, J.; Wynn, J.K. From perception to functional outcome in schizophrenia: Modeling the role of ability and motivation. *Arch. Gen. Psychiatry* **2012**, *69*, 1216–1224. [CrossRef]
5. Pinkham, A.E.; Penn, D.L.; Green, M.F.; Buck, B.; Healey, K.; Harvey, P.D. The social cognition psychometric evaluation study: Results of the expert survey and RAND panel. *Schizophr. Bull.* **2014**, *40*, 813–823. [CrossRef]
6. Pinkham, A.E.; Penn, D.L.; Green, M.F.; Harvey, P.D. Social Cognition Psychometric Evaluation: Results of the Initial Psychometric Study. *Schizophr. Bull.* **2016**, *42*, 494–504. [CrossRef]
7. Pinkham, A.E.; Harvey, P.D.; Penn, D.L. Social Cognition Psychometric Evaluation: Results of the Final Validation Study. *Schizophr. Bull.* **2018**, *44*, 737–748. [CrossRef]
8. Hajduk, M.; Achim, A.M.; Brunet-Gouet, E.; Mehta, U.M.; Pinkham, A.E. How to move forward in social cognition research? Put it into an international perspective. *Schizophr. Res.* **2020**, *215*, 463–464. [CrossRef]
9. Lim, K.; Lee, S.A.; Pinkham, A.E.; Lam, M.; Lee, J. Evaluation of social cognitive measures in an Asian schizophrenia sample. *Schizophr. Res. Cogn.* **2020**, *20*, 100169. [CrossRef] [PubMed]
10. Kunii, Y.; Hoshino, H.; Niwa, S. Relationship between performance on the ABCD comprehensive test of social cognitive functioning battery and social functioning in schizophrenia. In Proceedings of the 17th Study Group on Mental Illness and Cognitive Function, Tokyo, Japan, November 2017.
11. Hagiya, K.; Sumiyoshi, T.; Kanie, A.; Pu, S.; Kaneko, K.; Mogami, T.; Oshima, S.; Niwa, S.; Inagaki, A.; Ikebuchi, E.; et al. Facial expression perception correlates with verbal working memory function in schizophrenia. *Psychiatry Clin. Neurosci.* **2015**, *69*, 773–781. [CrossRef]
12. Kanie, A.; Hagiya, K.; Ashida, S.; Pu, S.; Kaneko, K.; Mogami, T.; Oshima, S.; Motoya, M.; Niwa, S.; Inagaki, A.; et al. New instrument for measuring multiple domains of social cognition: Construct validity of the Social Cognition Screening Questionnaire (Japanese version). *Psychiatry Clin. Neurosci.* **2014**, *68*, 701–711. [CrossRef] [PubMed]
13. Okano, H.; Kubota, R.; Okubo, R.; Hashimoto, N.; Ikezawa, S.; Toyomaki, A.; Miyazaki, A.; Sasaki, Y.; Yamada, Y.; Nemoto, T.; et al. Evaluation of Social Cognition Measures for Japanese Patients with Schizophrenia Using an Expert Panel and Modified Delphi Method. *J. Pers. Med.* **2021**, *11*, 275. [CrossRef]
14. Lee, H.S.; Corbera, S.; Poltorak, A.; Park, K.; Assaf, M.; Bell, M.D.; Wexler, B.E.; Cho, Y.I.; Jung, S.; Brocke, S.; et al. Measuring theory of mind in schizophrenia research: Cross-cultural validation. *Schizophr. Res.* **2018**, *201*, 187–195. [CrossRef] [PubMed]
15. Social Cognitive Assessment in Autism and Schizophrenia (ClaCoS). Available online: https://www.clinicaltrials.gov/ct2/show/NCT02660775 (accessed on 6 July 2021).
16. Peyroux, E.; Prost, Z.; Danset-Alexandre, C.; Brenugat-Herne, L.; Carteau-Martin, I.; Gaudelus, B.; Jantac, C.; Attali, D.; Amado, I.; Graux, J.; et al. From "under" to "over" social cognition in schizophrenia: Is there distinct profiles of impairments according to negative and positive symptoms? *Schizophr. Res. Cogn.* **2019**, *15*, 21–29. [CrossRef] [PubMed]
17. Kelly, J.R.; Minuto, C.; Cryan, J.F.; Clarke, G.; Dinan, T.G. The role of the gut microbiome in the development of schizophrenia. *Schizophr. Res.* **2020**. [CrossRef] [PubMed]
18. Sarkar, A.; Harty, S.; Lehto, S.M.; Moeller, A.H.; Dinan, T.G.; Dunbar, R.I.M.; Cryan, J.F.; Burnet, P.W.J. The Microbiome in Psychology and Cognitive Neuroscience. *Trends Cogn. Sci.* **2018**, *22*, 611–636. [CrossRef]
19. Zhu, F.; Guo, R.; Wang, W.; Ju, Y.; Wang, Q.; Ma, Q.; Sun, Q.; Fan, Y.; Xie, Y.; Yang, Z.; et al. Transplantation of microbiota from drug-free patients with schizophrenia causes schizophrenia-like abnormal behaviors and dysregulated kynurenine metabolism in mice. *Mol. Psychiatry* **2020**, *25*, 2905–2918. [CrossRef] [PubMed]
20. Nguyen, T.T.; Hathaway, H.; Kosciolek, T.; Knight, R.; Jeste, D.V. Gut microbiome in serious mental illnesses: A systematic review and critical evaluation. *Schizophr. Res.* **2019**. [CrossRef]
21. Zheng, P.; Zeng, B.; Liu, M.; Chen, J.; Pan, J.; Han, Y.; Liu, Y.; Cheng, K.; Zhou, C.; Wang, H.; et al. The gut microbiome from patients with schizophrenia modulates the glutamate-glutamine-GABA cycle and schizophrenia-relevant behaviors in mice. *Sci. Adv.* **2019**, *5*, eaau8317. [CrossRef]
22. Nguyen, T.T.; Kosciolek, T.; Maldonado, Y.; Daly, R.E.; Martin, A.S.; McDonald, D.; Knight, R.; Jeste, D.V. Differences in gut microbiome composition between persons with chronic schizophrenia and healthy comparison subjects. *Schizophr. Res.* **2019**, *204*, 23–29. [CrossRef]

23. Kohler, C.G.; Turner, T.H.; Bilker, W.B.; Brensinger, C.M.; Siegel, S.J.; Kanes, S.J.; Gur, R.E.; Gur, R.C. Facial emotion recognition in schizophrenia: Intensity effects and error pattern. *Am. J. Psychiatry* **2003**, *160*, 1768–1774. [CrossRef] [PubMed]
24. Buck, B.; Iwanski, C.; Healey, K.M.; Green, M.F.; Horan, W.P.; Kern, R.S.; Lee, J.; Marder, S.R.; Reise, S.P.; Penn, D.L. Improving measurement of attributional style in schizophrenia; A psychometric evaluation of the Ambiguous Intentions Hostility Questionnaire (AIHQ). *J. Psychiatr. Res.* **2017**, *89*, 48–54. [CrossRef] [PubMed]
25. Combs, D.R.; Penn, D.L.; Wicher, M.; Waldheter, E. The Ambiguous Intentions Hostility Questionnaire (AIHQ): A new measure for evaluating hostile social-cognitive biases in paranoia. *Cogn. Neuropsychiatry* **2007**, *12*, 128–143. [CrossRef] [PubMed]
26. Peyroux, E.; Strickland, B.; Tapiero, I.; Franck, N. The intentionality bias in schizophrenia. *Psychiatry Res.* **2014**, *219*, 426–430. [CrossRef] [PubMed]
27. Bell, M.; Bryson, G.; Lysaker, P. Positive and negative affect recognition in schizophrenia: A comparison with substance abuse and normal control subjects. *Psychiatry Res.* **1997**, *73*, 73–82. [CrossRef]
28. Kerr, S.L.; Neale, J.M. Emotion perception in schizophrenia: Specific deficit or further evidence of generalized poor performance? *J. Abnorm. Psychol.* **1993**, *102*, 312–318. [CrossRef] [PubMed]
29. Bell, M.D.; Fiszdon, J.M.; Greig, T.C.; Wexler, B.E. Social attribution test–multiple choice (SAT-MC) in schizophrenia: Comparison with community sample and relationship to neurocognitive, social cognitive and symptom measures. *Schizophr. Res.* **2010**, *122*, 164–171. [CrossRef]
30. Grossman, E.D.; Blake, R.; Kim, C.Y. Learning to see biological motion: Brain activity parallels behavior. *J. Cogn. Neurosci.* **2004**, *16*, 1669–1679. [CrossRef]
31. Corcoran, R.; Mercer, G.; Frith, C.D. Schizophrenia, symptomatology and social inference: Investigating "theory of mind" in people with schizophrenia. *Schizophr. Res.* **1995**, *17*, 5–13. [CrossRef]
32. Adachi, T.; Koeda, T.; Hirabayashi, S.; Maeoka, Y.; Shiota, M.; Wright, E.C.; Wada, A. The metaphor and sarcasm scenario test: A new instrument to help differentiate high functioning pervasive developmental disorder from attention deficit/hyperactivity disorder. *Brain Dev.* **2004**, *26*, 301–306. [CrossRef]
33. Sheehan, D.V.; Lecrubier, Y.; Sheehan, K.H.; Amorim, P.; Janavs, J.; Weiller, E.; Hergueta, T.; Baker, R.; Dunbar, G.C. The Mini-International Neuropsychiatric Interview (M.I.N.I.): The development and validation of a structured diagnostic psychiatric interview for DSM-IV and ICD-10. *J. Clin. Psychiatry* **1998**, *59* (Suppl. 20), 22–33; quiz 34–57.
34. Otsubo, T.; Tanaka, K.; Koda, R.; Shinoda, J.; Sano, N.; Tanaka, S.; Aoyama, H.; Mimura, M.; Kamijima, K. Reliability and validity of Japanese version of the Mini-International Neuropsychiatric Interview. *Psychiatry Clin. Neurosci.* **2005**, *59*, 517–526. [CrossRef]
35. Matsuoka, K.; Uno, M.; Kasai, K.; Koyama, K.; Kim, Y. Estimation of premorbid IQ in individuals with Alzheimer's disease using Japanese ideographic script (Kanji) compound words: Japanese version of National Adult Reading Test. *Psychiatry Clin. Neurosci.* **2006**, *60*, 332–339. [CrossRef]
36. Kay, S.R.; Fiszbein, A.; Opler, L.A. The positive and negative syndrome scale (PANSS) for schizophrenia. *Schizophr. Bull.* **1987**, *13*, 261–276. [CrossRef]
37. Hashimoto, N.; Takahashi, K.; Fujisawa, D.; Aoyama, K.; Nakagawa, A.; Okamura, N.; Toyomaki, A.; Oka, M.; Takanobu, K.; Okubo, R.; et al. A pilot validation study of the Japanese translation of the Positive and Negative Syndrome Scale (PANSS). *Asian J. Psychiatry* **2020**, *54*, 102210. [CrossRef]
38. Kirkpatrick, B.; Strauss, G.P.; Nguyen, L.; Fischer, B.A.; Daniel, D.G.; Cienfuegos, A.; Marder, S.R. The brief negative symptom scale: Psychometric properties. *Schizophr. Bull.* **2011**, *37*, 300–305. [CrossRef] [PubMed]
39. Hashimoto, N.; Toyomaki, A.; Oka, M.; Takanobu, K.; Okubo, R.; Narita, H.; Kitagawa, K.; Udo, N.; Maeda, T.; Watanabe, S.; et al. Pilot Validation Study of the Japanese Translation of the Brief Negative Symptoms Scale (BNSS). *Neuropsychiatr. Dis. Treat.* **2019**, *15*, 3511–3518. [CrossRef] [PubMed]
40. Grant, P.M.; Beck, A.T. Defeatist beliefs as a mediator of cognitive impairment, negative symptoms, and functioning in schizophrenia. *Schizophr. Bull.* **2009**, *35*, 798–806. [CrossRef]
41. Tajima, M.; Akiyama, T.; Numa, H.; Kawamura, Y.; Okada, Y.; Sakai, Y.; Miyake, Y.; Ono, Y.; Power, M.J. Reliability and validity of the Japanese version of the 24-item Dysfunctional Attitude Scale. *Acta Neuropsychiatr.* **2007**, *19*, 362–367. [CrossRef] [PubMed]
42. Tobe, M.; Nemoto, T.; Tsujino, N.; Yamaguchi, T.; Katagiri, N.; Fujii, C.; Mizuno, M. Characteristics of motivation and their impacts on the functional outcomes in patients with schizophrenia. *Compr. Psychiatry* **2016**, *65*, 103–109. [CrossRef] [PubMed]
43. Graux, J.; Thillay, A.; Morlec, V.; Sarron, P.Y.; Roux, S.; Gaudelus, B.; Prost, Z.; Brenugat-Herne, L.; Amado, I.; Morel-Kohlmeyer, S.; et al. A Transnosographic Self-Assessment of Social Cognitive Impairments (ACSO): First Data. *Front. Psychiatry* **2019**, *10*, 847. [CrossRef]
44. Jones, M.T.; Deckler, E.; Laurrari, C.; Jarskog, L.F.; Penn, D.L.; Pinkham, A.E.; Harvey, P.D. Confidence, performance, and accuracy of self-assessment of social cognition: A comparison of schizophrenia patients and healthy controls. *Schizophr. Res. Cogn.* **2020**, *19*, 100133. [CrossRef]
45. Healey, K.M.; Combs, D.R.; Gibson, C.M.; Keefe, R.S.; Roberts, D.L.; Penn, D.L. Observable Social Cognition–A Rating Scale: An interview-based assessment for schizophrenia. *Cogn. Neuropsychiatry* **2015**, *20*, 198–221. [CrossRef] [PubMed]
46. Halverson, T.F.; Hajduk, M.; Pinkham, A.E.; Harvey, P.D.; Jarskog, L.F.; Nye, L.; Penn, D.L. Psychometric properties of the Observable Social Cognition Rating Scale (OSCARS): Self-report and informant-rated social cognitive abilities in schizophrenia. *Psychiatry Res.* **2020**, *286*, 112891. [CrossRef] [PubMed]

47. Keefe, R.S.; Goldberg, T.E.; Harvey, P.D.; Gold, J.M.; Poe, M.P.; Coughenour, L. The Brief Assessment of Cognition in Schizophrenia: Reliability, sensitivity, and comparison with a standard neurocognitive battery. *Schizophr. Res.* **2004**, *68*, 283–297. [CrossRef]
48. Kaneda, Y.; Sumiyoshi, T.; Keefe, R.; Ishimoto, Y.; Numata, S.; Ohmori, T. Brief assessment of cognition in schizophrenia: Validation of the Japanese version. *Psychiatry Clin. Neurosci.* **2007**, *61*, 602–609. [CrossRef]
49. Mausbach, B.T.; Harvey, P.D.; Goldman, S.R.; Jeste, D.V.; Patterson, T.L. Development of a brief scale of everyday functioning in persons with serious mental illness. *Schizophr. Bull.* **2007**, *33*, 1364–1372. [CrossRef] [PubMed]
50. Sumiyoshi, C.; Takaki, M.; Okahisa, Y.; Patterson, T.L.; Harvey, P.D.; Sumiyoshi, T. Utility of the UCSD Performance-based Skills Assessment-Brief Japanese version: Discriminative ability and relation to neurocognition. *Schizophr. Res. Cogn.* **2014**, *1*, 137–143. [CrossRef]
51. Schneider, L.C.; Struening, E.L. SLOF: A behavioral rating scale for assessing the mentally ill. *Soc. Work Res. Abstr.* **1983**, *19*, 9–21. [CrossRef] [PubMed]
52. Sumiyoshi, T.; Nishida, K.; Niimura, H.; Toyomaki, A.; Morimoto, T.; Tani, M.; Inada, K.; Ninomiya, T.; Hori, H.; Manabe, J.; et al. Cognitive insight and functional outcome in schizophrenia; a multi-center collaborative study with the specific level of functioning scale-Japanese version. *Schizophr. Res. Cogn.* **2016**, *6*, 9–14. [CrossRef]
53. Okubo, R.; Kinoshita, T.; Katsumata, N.; Uezono, Y.; Xiao, J.; Matsuoka, Y.J. Impact of chemotherapy on the association between fear of cancer recurrence and the gut microbiota in breast cancer survivors. *Brain Behav. Immun.* **2019**. [CrossRef] [PubMed]
54. Okubo, R.; Koga, M.; Katsumata, N.; Odamaki, T.; Matsuyama, S.; Oka, M.; Narita, H.; Hashimoto, N.; Kusumi, I.; Xiao, J.; et al. Effect of Bifidobacterium breve A-1 on anxiety and depressive symptoms in schizophrenia: A proof-of-concept study. *J. Affect. Disord.* **2019**, *245*, 377–385. [CrossRef] [PubMed]
55. Cohen, J. A power primer. *Psychol. Bull.* **1992**, *112*, 155–159. [CrossRef] [PubMed]

Study Protocol

Efficacy and Safety of Multi-Session Transcranial Direct Current Stimulation on Social Cognition in Schizophrenia: A Study Protocol for an Open-Label, Single-Arm Trial

Yuji Yamada [1], Takuma Inagawa [1], Yuma Yokoi [1], Aya Shirama [2], Kazuki Sueyoshi [2], Ayumu Wada [1], Naotsugu Hirabayashi [1], Hideki Oi [3] and Tomiki Sumiyoshi [2,*]

[1] National Center of Neurology and Psychiatry, Department of Psychiatry, National Center Hospital, 4-1-1 Ogawahigashi-cho, Kodaira, Tokyo 187-8551, Japan; iki.witty.mind@gmail.com (Y.Y.); tinagawa@ncnp.go.jp (T.I.); yyokoi@ncnp.go.jp (Y.Y.); a.wada@ncnp.go.jp (A.W.); hirabaya@ncnp.go.jp (N.H.)
[2] National Center of Neurology and Psychiatry, Department of Preventive Intervention for Psychiatric Disorders, National Institute of Mental Health, 4-1-1 Ogawahigashi-cho, Kodaira, Tokyo 187-8551, Japan; shirama@ncnp.go.jp (A.S.); skzskz1000@gmail.com (K.S.)
[3] Translational Medical Center, National Center of Neurology and Psychiatry, Department of Clinical Epidemiology, 4-1-1 Ogawahigashi-cho, Kodaira, Tokyo 187-8551, Japan; oih@ncnp.go.jp
* Correspondence: sumiyot@ncnp.go.jp; Tel.: +81-42-341-2711; Fax: +81-42-346-1979

Abstract: Backgrounds: Social cognition is defined as the mental operations underlying social behavior. Patients with schizophrenia elicit impairments of social cognition, which is linked to poor real-world functional outcomes. In a previous study, transcranial direct current stimulation (tDCS) improved emotional recognition, a domain of social cognition, in patients with schizophrenia. However, since social cognition was only minimally improved by tDCS when administered on frontal brain areas, investigations on the effect of tDCS on other cortical sites more directly related to social cognition are needed. Therefore, we present a study protocol to determine whether multi-session tDCS on superior temporal sulcus (STS) would improve social cognition deficits of schizophrenia. Methods: This is an open-label, single-arm trial, whose objective is to investigate the efficacy and safety of multi-session tDCS over the left STS to improve social cognition in patients with schizophrenia. The primary outcome measure will be the Social Cognition Screening Questionnaire. Neurocognition, functional capacity, and psychotic symptoms will also be evaluated by the Brief Assessment of Cognition in Schizophrenia, UCSD Performance-Based Skills Assessment-Brief, and Positive and Negative Syndrome Scale, respectively. Data will be collected at baseline, and 4 weeks after the end of intervention. If social cognition is improved in patients with schizophrenia by tDCS based on this protocol, we may plan randomized controlled trial.

Keywords: neuromodulation; transcranial direct current stimulation (tDCS); schizophrenia; social cognition; superior temporal sulcus

1. Introduction

The prevalence of schizophrenia is about 0.7% [1], with positive, negative, mood symptoms, and cognitive dysfunction. The first episode appears after adolescence and follows a chronic course with repeated remission and exacerbation of psychotic symptoms. In this process, cognitive and social function decline [2–4]. As a result, 70% of chronic patients are reported to be unable to find employment [5,6].

Cognitive dysfunction is one of the core symptoms of schizophrenia and exists from the early stage of onset to the chronic stage [7]. Several domains of neurocognition, such as learning memory, working memory, executive functioning, verbal fluency, and attention/information processing, are known to be impaired in schizophrenia [7]. Similarly, it has been noted in recent years that social cognition [8], i.e., mental operations underlying social behavior, is also impaired in schizophrenia. Social cognition consists of the domains of emotion recognition, social perception, theory of mind (ToM), and attributional bias [9], whose neural basis differs from that of neurocognition [10]. Moreover, it has been reported that improvement of social cognition is directly linked to improvement of social function, whereas there is argument that the association between neurocognition and social function is mediated by social cognitive function [11]. Therefore, in recent years, the importance of developing treatments for social cognition has been discussed.

The neural substrates of social cognition may include the orbitofrontal cortex, medial prefrontal cortex (mPFC), superior temporal sulcus (STS), and amygdala; these brain regions show a decrease in functional connectivity in schizophrenia [12]. Among these sites, the amygdala is involved in emotion recognition [13], while the prefrontal cortex governs ToM [14]. On the other hand, the STS is considered to play a role in both domains of social cognition [15] (see Table 1 [12–19]).

Table 1. Neural basis of social cognition [12–19].

Domains of Social Cognition	Neural Basis
Emotion recognition	Amygdala, superior temporal sulcus, medial prefrontal cortex, inferior occipital gyrus, etc.
Theory of mind (ToM)	Superior temporal sulcus, medial prefrontal cortex, middle temporal gyrus, etc.
Attributional bias	Orbitofrontal cortex, insular cortex, striatum, amygdala, superior temporal sulcus, etc.

Neuromodulation is a method of changing nerve activity by applying electrical stimulation or the other agents to a specific nerve site in the body. Neuromodulation ranges from noninvasive approaches, such as transcranial magnetic stimulation, to invasive (implanted) approaches, such as spinal cord stimulation and deep brain stimulation [20]. Among them, transcranial direct current stimulation (tDCS) is a safe, inexpensive, and feasible neuromodulation that modifies nerve activity by providing a weak current of 1–2 mA for about 5–30 min/session [21]. The therapeutic effects of tDCS are thought to be mediated by promotion of cortical excitability through anodal stimulation [22]. In addition, enhanced excitatory synaptic transmission via anodal tDCS may promote glutamate transmissions, and suppress gamma-aminobutyric acid transmissions in the cortex. Moreover, it positively or negatively modulates the activities of dopamine, serotonin, and acetylcholine transmissions in the central nervous system. These neural events may change the balance between excitatory and inhibitory inputs [22,23]. With these mechanisms, tDCS has been suggested to ameliorate symptoms of several psychiatric disorders, e.g., major depressive disorder and schizophrenia.

tDCS has been shown to improve several domains of neurocognitive function, especially working memory, in schizophrenia [24]. On the other hand, only two studies have been conducted to determine the ability of tDCS to improve social cognitive disturbances of schizophrenia [25,26]. So far, only one study reported small facilitative effects of tDCS on emotion recognition with the left dorsolateral prefrontal cortex (DLPFC) as the target site in schizophrenia [25]. It should be noted that these studies used anodal stimulation on the frontal areas, i.e., the left DLPFC [26]. As social cognition may be governed mainly by other brain regions, e.g., the STS [12–19], it is hypothesized that anodal stimulation over this cortical area would be advantageous for treating social cognition disturbances.

These considerations prompt us to determine whether stimulation of skull surface above the STS, e.g., T3 or T4 (mid-temporal) of the International 10–20 electroencephalography system, would enhance social cognition in patients with schizophrenia. Moreover, intervention in the STS may affect hallucinations, as the STS is adjacent to the superior temporal gyrus (STG), and the network of cortical areas containing STGs is involved in hallucinations [27]. Therefore, we present a study protocol for an open-label, single-arm trial designed to evaluate the efficacy and safety of tDCS on the left STS. To our knowledge, this is the first attempt to administer tDCS targeting the STS in patients with schizophrenia.

2. Study Protocol

2.1. Trial Design

This study investigates the efficacy and safety of multi-session tDCS over the left STS to improve social cognition for patients with schizophrenia. This is a single-center trial at National Center of Neurology and Psychiatry, Tokyo, Japan. An open-label, single-arm study will be conducted on 15 participants with a diagnosis of schizophrenia based on the Diagnostic and Statistical Manual of Mental Disorders (DSM-5). We selected an open-label, single-arm design, because there is no precedent for tDCS over the left STS, and the major focus of this study is to verify the tolerability and safety of tDCS over the STS. Participants will receive 10 sessions of active tDCS in 5 consecutive days (twice per day) (see Figure 1). The study design is in accordance with the 2013 Standard Protocol Items: Recommendations for Interventional Trials (SPIRIT) Statement (Table S1) [28]. This study was registered within the Japan Registry of Clinical Trials (Trial ID: jRCTs032180026).

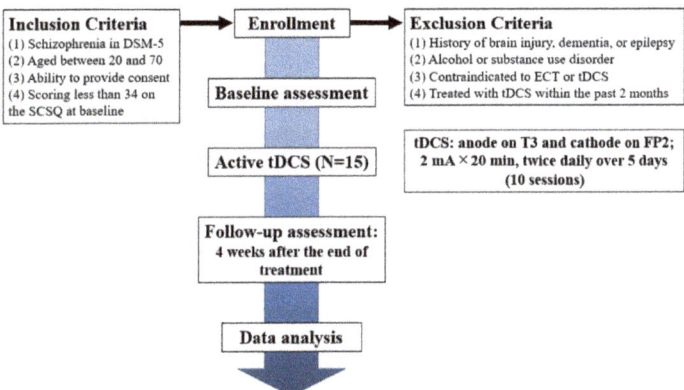

Figure 1. Flowchart summarizing the trial procedure. SCSQ, Social Cognition Screening Questionnaire; ECT, electroconvulsive therapy; tDCS, transcranial direct current stimulation.

2.2. Participants

Inpatients or outpatients treated at National Center Hospital, National Center of Neurology and Psychiatry will be enrolled. Participants will be recruited by referrals from treating psychiatrists. Those psychiatrists will not have any conflicts of interest with the outcomes of this trial. The principal investigator must provide written informed consent before starting the trial. After providing the informed consent, participants will be screened by a treating psychiatrist to establish whether they meet the eligibility criteria. Participants will be given a gift certificate worth JPY 3000 per day as a reimbursement, and a gift certificate worth JPY 21000 in a total of 7 days including each tDCS session, and baseline/follow-up evaluation.

2.3. Inclusion and Exclusion Criteria

Participants must meet the following inclusion criteria:

(1) Diagnosed as schizophrenia in DSM-5.
(2) Aged between 20 and 70.
(3) Being able to understand the objectives and content of the study, and provide consent to participate in it. (The ability to consent to participate in this study will be considered insufficient, when patients' Intelligence Quotient (IQ) is less than 70, or they present with acute psychiatric symptoms. Those patients will be provided with necessary medical care separately from this trial.)

(4) Having Social Cognition Screening Questionnaire (SCSQ) scores of less than 34 points. Therefore, participants whose scores are 34 or more will be excluded from this study.

Patients with any of the following conditions will be excluded from the study:

(1) Present or past history of severe organic lesions in the brain, dementia, or epilepsy.
(2) With alcohol or substance use disorder that was present within 12 months from screening.
(3) Contraindicated against electro convulsive therapy or tDCS, e.g., severe cardiovascular diseases, such as myocardial infarction, or aneurysms at high risk of rupture.
(4) Were treated with tDCS or other neuromodulations within the past 2 months. (We will ask whether participants have any history of tDCS or other neuromodulations.)
(5) Deemed inappropriate to participate judged by the principal investigator, e.g., when participants' psychiatric symptoms are unstable.

The dose of psychotropic drugs will not be changed during the study period. Cognitive rehabilitation will not be performed during the period. Therefore, we will exclude patients who are scheduled for cognitive rehabilitation.

2.4. Sample Size Calculation

Total study sample sizes of $n = 15$ have been recommended by our previous study [29], assuming an estimated mean UCSD Performance-based Skills Assessment-brief (UPSA-B) difference from baseline to follow-up of 10.6, with a standard deviation of 15.5. Under these conditions, the power of the primary analysis was 0.8, so approximately $n = 13$ was estimated (one-sample Student's t-test). Therefore, it was decided to include a total of 15 samples, taking into account the dropouts of the study.

2.5. Intervention

Direct current will be transmitted through 35 cm^2 saline-soaked sponge electrodes, and the intervention will be performed by a 1×1 transcranial direct current low-intensity stimulator (Model 1300 A; Soterix Medical Inc., New York, NY, USA). According to the International 10–20 electroencephalography system, in each session, the tDCS montage will place the anode in the left STS and the cathode in the contralateral supraorbital region, which corresponds to the T3 (mid-temporal) and FP2 (front-polar) regions (see Figure 2). We will apply 10 sessions of direct current of 2 mA for 20 min in 5 consecutive days (twice per day, with an interval of 30 min). The intensity, frequency, and duration of the stimulus are determined based on previous studies [29].

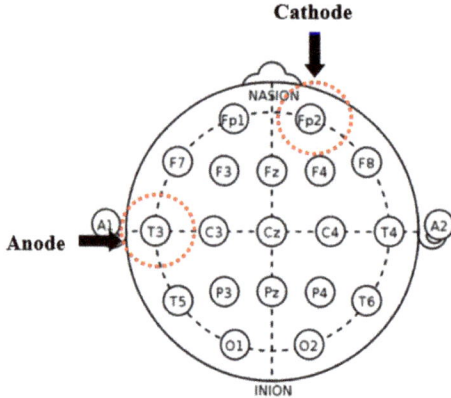

Figure 2. Placement map for the intervention. tDCS montage will place the anode in the left superior temporal sulcus (STS) and the cathode in the contralateral supraorbital region, which corresponds to the T3 (mid-temporal) and FP2 (front-polar) regions in the International 10–20 electroencephalography system.

Trained psychiatrists or researchers will administer tDCS, and they will not evaluate any outcome measures. Neither tDCS-administrants nor participants will be aware of their treatment results until all participants have finished their follow-up evaluations.

2.6. Outcomes

Patients receive a psychological evaluation, including a screening evaluation, after being briefed on the purpose of the study and agreeing to participate in the study. Psychological assessment data will be collected at baseline and 4 weeks after the final stimulus (see Table 2). Baseline and follow-up evaluations will be performed by experienced psychologists who are not blinded. Although the interval between the baseline and follow-up evaluation is more than 5 weeks, which secures adequate washout period, the leaning effect of psychological evaluation will be a possible limitation.

Table 2. Study schedules.

	Study Period				
	Baseline	Intervention			Follow-Up
Time point	Within 2 weeks before the start of intervention	Day 1	Days 2–4	Day 5	4 weeks after the end of the last stimulation
Enrollment					
Eligibility screen	X				
Informed consent	X				
Sociodemographic characteristics	X				
Intervention					
tDCS (twice/day)		X	X	X	
Assessments					
SCSQ	X				X
Hinting Task	X				X
FEST	X				X
False Belief Task	X				X
BACS	X				X
UPSA-B	X				X
PANSS	X				X
AQ	X				X
JART	X				
Adverse events	X	X	X	X	X
Prescribed drugs	X	X	X	X	X

tDCS, transcranial direct current stimulation; SCSQ, Social Cognition Screening Questionnaire; FEST, Facial Emotion Selection Test; BACS, Brief Assessment of Cognition in Schizophrenia; UPSA-B, Brief UCSD Performance-based Skills Assessment; PAMSS, Positive and Negative Syndrome Scale; AQ, Autism-Spectrum Quotient; JART, Japanese Adult Reading Test. The timepoint of follow-up evaluation will be allowed to be up to 7 days off.

2.6.1. Cognition

The primary outcome is scores on the Social Cognition Screening Questionnaire (SCSQ) [30], which includes test of attributional style, and theory of mind (ToM). To evaluate ToM more accurately, we will also use False Belief Task [31], Hinting Task [32], and Autism-Spectrum Quotient (AQ) [33]. To evaluate emotion recognition, we will use the Facial Emotion Selection Test (FEST) [34]. To provide a standard metric for combining test scores into domains and comparing performance over time, Brief Assessment of Cognition in Schizophrenia (BACS) scores will be converted to z-scores, which shows performance relative to healthy people [35]. The premorbid IQ will be also estimated using the Japanese Adult Reading Test (JART) [36] (see Table 3).

Table 3. Primary/secondary outcomes.

Primary/Secondary	Domain	Outcome
Primary outcome	Social cognition (attributional style, theory of mind)	Social Cognition Screening Questionnaire (SCSQ)
Secondary outcome	Social cognition (theory of mind)	Hinting Task
Secondary outcome	Social cognition (theory of mind)	False Belief Task
Secondary outcome	Social cognition (emotion recognition)	Facial Emotion Selection Test (FEST)
Secondary outcome	Cognition	Brief Assessment of Cognition in Schizophrenia (BACS)
Secondary outcome	Cognition	Autism-Spectrum Quotient (AQ)
Secondary outcome	Premorbid intelligence quotient	Japanese Adult Reading Test (JART)
Secondary outcome	Functional capacity (daily-living skills)	UCSD Performance-Based Skills Assessment-Brief (UPSA-B)
Secondary outcome	Global symptoms of schizophrenia	Positive and Negative Syndrome Scale (PANSS)

2.6.2. Functional Capacity (Daily-Living Skills)

The functional capacity will be assessed by the UCSD Performance-Based Skills Assessment-Brief (UPSA-B) [37], which consists of financial and communication skills.

2.6.3. Global Symptoms of Schizophrenia

Global symptoms of schizophrenia will be evaluated by the Positive and Negative Syndrome Scale (PANSS) [38], which consists of positive syndrome, negative syndrome, and general psychopathology subscales.

2.6.4. Adverse Events

Adverse events are defined as unwanted experiences seen during tDCS. Serious adverse events are defined as requiring inpatient treatment, moderate adverse events as requiring therapeutic intervention, and mild adverse events as requiring no therapeutic intervention. The treating physician will record the symptoms, date of onset, severity, treatment given, and association with research interventions. If symptoms are already present at baseline and do not worsen during tDCS intervention, they are not treated as adverse events.

All adverse events will be clinically evaluated and monitored throughout the study period. Previous studies report that the most common adverse events are itching, tingling, headache, burning sensation, and discomfort [39]. An experienced psychiatrist will check the presence and extent of adverse events and their association with tDCS before and after each session and assess safety at all visits during the intervention. We will follow up any unresolved adverse events after trial completion. The principal investigator will be responsible for addressing and explaining serious adverse events in the patient. The sub-investigators will be responsible for reporting any information related to such adverse events to the principal investigator. The principal investigator will have to report any serious adverse events to the Clinical Research Review Board, and to the Ministry of Health, Labor and Welfare. We will cease intervention on a per-patient if we observe severe adverse events and will also cease the whole study if we observe severe adverse events in two patients.

2.6.5. Prescribed Drugs

We will collect information about prescribed drugs throughout the study period. Those drugs will be classified, in principle, into the four categories: antipsychotics, mood stabilizers, antidepressants, and benzodiazepines. Furthermore, the equivalent doses of chlorpromazine, diazepam, and imipramine will be calculated [40].

2.7. Data Collection and Data Management

The assessments will be conducted at baseline and 4 weeks after the end of the last stimulation (Table 2). All evaluations will be conducted by experienced psychologists. The data will initially be recorded in a paper file and each participant will be assigned a code number. These files will be stored in a locked security box. After the follow-up data are collected, all data in the paper files will be transcribed to the Electronic Data Capture system (HOPE eACReSS; Fujitsu, Tokyo, Japan), which is a secure system designed for storage of personal and patient data. The data will be sent to independent data managers to assess whether the data are collected properly, focusing on the status of consent acquisition, eligibility of participants, evaluation items, and confirmation of drop-out/terminated cases. These data managers will also oversee and review the progress of the trial. If a participant withdraws their consent, they will be dismissed from the study. At the same time, we will record the dropout rate, and the number of people with adverse events requiring treatment. We will define a dropout rate of less than 10% as a safety criterion and perform a quantitative assessment of safety. The Efficacy and Safety Assessment Committee, whose members are independent of the research and come from the National Center of Neurology and Psychiatry, will check and assess whether the trial is conducted safely and properly, and will also decide whether to stop the trial if any severe adverse events or protocol violations occur. In addition, an on-site data monitor will conduct monitoring to ensure the trial is performed properly, data is properly recorded, and data reliability is ensured. If we conduct any necessary protocol modifications, we will report them to the Clinical Research Review Board, and to the Ministry of Health, Labor and Welfare for registration in the Japan Registry of Clinical Trials website (https://jrct.niph.go.jp).

2.8. Statistical Analysis

Correlations between baseline values and their changes from baseline of SCSQ, Hinting Task, FEST, BACS, UPSA-B, and PANSS scores, will be evaluated. Correlations will be examined for chlorpromazine equivalent dose of antipsychotics vs. changes from baseline of SCSQ, Hinting Task, FEST, BACS, UPSA-B, and PANSS scores. Correlations will also be examined for the change of UPSA-B scores from baseline and changes of the corresponding scores from baseline.

Statistical analysis will be conducted using STATA 14, created by StataCorp in TX, USA. For continuous variables in the SCSQ, Hinting Task, FEST, BACS, UPSA-B, and PANSS, we will use Student's t-test. Pearson's product moment correlation coefficient will be used for the relationship between clinical variables.

3. Ethics Statement

The study will be performed according to the Declaration of Helsinki and will follow the Clinical Trials Act in Japan. The protocol has been presented for approval by the National Center of Neurology and Psychiatry Clinical Research Review Board (CRB3180006). The principal investigator (TS) will have the ultimate responsibility for providing informed consent to all research participants. All participants must agree to participate in the study. After initial review and approval (September 2018), the institution's clinical research review committee will review the protocol and implementation at least annually. Two annual reviews have proceeded to date (https://jrct.niph.go.jp/re/bulletins/detail/312/22, https://jrct.niph.go.jp/re/bulletins/detail/312/1540). The principal investigator should submit a safety and progress report to the Review Board at least annually, and the researcher should submit the final report within 3 months of the completion of the study.

These reports will include a summary of the total number of enrolled participants, serious/nonserious adverse events that occurred, and safety and monitoring committee reviews [41]. Changes related to the research protocol need to be submitted to the Clinical Research Review Board for review as a protocol modification. If a participant needs to be treated due to a moderate or severe adverse event directly caused by tDCS, the participant will receive the full cost of treatment from clinical trial insurance.

Supplementary Materials: The following are available online at https://www.mdpi.com/article/10.3390/jpm11040317/s1, Table S1. SPIRIT 2013 Checklist.

Author Contributions: Y.Y. (Yuji Yamada) developed the original concept for the trial, and Y.Y. (Yuji Yamada), T.I., T.S. designed it. Y.Y. (Yuma Yokoi) advised on the statistical analysis plan for the original protocol. K.S. advised the outcome measures for the protocol. Y.Y. (Yuji Yamada) established the protocol. A.S. and Y.Y. (Yuji Yamada) will administer tDCS. T.I., A.W., N.H. and T.S. will recruit participants. H.O. will manage the data. Y.Y. (Yuji Yamada) wrote the manuscript, and all other authors reviewed and commented on the subsequent draft. All authors have read and agreed to the published version of the manuscript.

Funding: This study was supported by Japan Society for the Promotion of Science (JSPS) KAKENHI No. 20K16635 and 20H03610, Intramural Research Grant (30-1, 30-8, 2-3, 3-1) for Neurological and Psychiatric Disorders of National Center of Neurology and Psychiatry (NCNP) and JH 2020-B-08, and AMED under Grant Number 0307081 and 0307099.

Institutional Review Board Statement: The study was conducted according to the guidelines of the Declaration of Helsinki and approved by National Center of Neurology and Psychiatry Clinical Research Review Board (CRB3180006) approved this study.

Informed Consent Statement: Informed consent was obtained from all subjects involved in the study.

Data Availability Statement: We registered the protocol information in the Japan Registry of Clinical Trials website (https://jrct.niph.go.jp).

Acknowledgments: We would like to thank DKazuyuki Nakagome, and Shinsuke Kito at National Center of Neurology and Psychiatry for supporting our research activity.

Conflicts of Interest: The authors declared that the research was conducted in the absence of any commercial or financial relationships that could be construed as a potential conflict of interest.

References

1. Macdonald, A.W.; Schulz, S.C. What We Know: Findings That Every Theory of Schizophrenia Should Explain. *Schizophr. Bull.* **2009**, *35*, 493–508. [CrossRef] [PubMed]
2. Yamada, Y.; Inagawa, T.; Sueyoshi, K.; Sugawara, N.; Ueda, N.; Omachi, Y.; Hirabayashi, N.; Matsumoto, M.; Sumiyoshi, T. Social Cognition Deficits as a Target of Early Intervention for Psychoses: A Systematic Review. *Front. Psychiatry* **2019**, *10*. [CrossRef] [PubMed]
3. Andreasen, N.C. Schizophrenia: The fundamental questions. *Brain Res. Rev.* **2000**, *31*, 106–112. [CrossRef]
4. Mueser, K.T.; McGurk, S.R. Schizophrenia. *Lancet* **2004**, *363*, 2063–2072. [CrossRef]
5. Lehman, A.F.; Goldberg, R.; Dixon, L.B.; McNary, S.; Postrado, L.; Hackman, A.; McDonnell, K. Improving employment outcomes for persons with severe mental illnesses. *Arch. Gen. Psychiatry* **2002**, *59*, 165. [CrossRef] [PubMed]
6. Marwaha, S.; Johnson, S. Schizophrenia and employment. *Soc. Psychiatry Psychiatr. Epidemiol.* **2004**, *39*, 337–349. [CrossRef]
7. Fioravanti, M.; Bianchi, V.; Cinti, M.E. Cognitive deficits in schizophrenia: An updated metanalysis of the scientific evidence. *BMC Psychiatry* **2012**, *12*, 64. [CrossRef]
8. Couture, S.M.; Penn, D.L.; Roberts, D.L. The Functional Significance of Social Cognition in Schizophrenia: A Review. *Schizophr. Bull.* **2006**, *32*, S44–S63. [CrossRef]
9. Penn, D.L.; Sanna, L.J.; Roberts, D.L. Social Cognition in Schizophrenia: An Overview. *Schizophr. Bull.* **2007**, *34*, 408–411. [CrossRef]
10. Pinkham, A.E.; Penn, D.L.; Perkins, D.O.; Lieberman, J. Implications for the Neural Basis of Social Cognition for the Study of Schizophrenia. *Am. J. Psychiatry* **2003**, *160*, 815–824. [CrossRef]
11. Brekke, J.; Kay, D.D.; Lee, K.S.; Green, M.F. Biosocial pathways to functional outcome in schizophrenia. *Schizophr. Res.* **2005**, *80*, 213–225. [CrossRef]
12. Frith, C.D.; Frith, U. Social Cognition in Humans. *Curr. Biol.* **2007**, *17*, R724–R732. [CrossRef]

13. Adolphs, R.; Tranel, D. Amygdala damage impairs emotion recognition from scenes only when they contain facial expressions. *Neuropsychologia* **2003**, *41*, 1281–1289. [CrossRef]
14. Baron-Cohen, S.; Ring, H.; Moriarty, J.; Schmitz, B.; Costa, D.C.; Ell, P. Recognition of Mental State Terms. *Br. J. Psychiatry* **1994**, *165*, 640–649. [CrossRef]
15. Brunet-Gouet, E.; Decety, J. Social brain dysfunctions in schizophrenia: A review of neuroimaging studies. *Psychiatry Res. Neuroimaging* **2006**, *148*, 75–92. [CrossRef]
16. Phan, K.L.; Wager, T.; Taylor, S.F.; Liberzon, I. Functional Neuroanatomy of Emotion: A Meta-Analysis of Emotion Activation Studies in PET and fMRI. *NeuroImage* **2002**, *16*, 331–348. [CrossRef]
17. Hirao, K.; Miyata, J.; Fujiwara, H.; Yamada, M.; Namiki, C.; Shimizu, M.; Sawamoto, N.; Fukuyama, H.; Hayashi, T.; Murai, T. Theory of mind and frontal lobe pathology in schizophrenia: A voxel-based morphometry study. *Schizophr. Res.* **2008**, *105*, 165–174. [CrossRef]
18. Kawada, R.; Yoshizumi, M.; Hirao, K.; Fujiwara, H.; Miyata, J.; Shimizu, M.; Namiki, C.; Sawamoto, N.; Fukuyama, H.; Hayashi, T.; et al. Brain volume and dysexecutive behavior in schizophrenia. *Prog. Neuro-Psychopharmacol. Biol. Psychiatry* **2009**, *33*, 1255–1260. [CrossRef]
19. Sasamoto, A.; Miyata, J.; Hirao, K.; Fujiwara, H.; Kawada, R.; Fujimoto, S.; Tanaka, Y.; Kubota, M.; Sawamoto, N.; Fukuyama, H.; et al. Social impairment in schizophrenia revealed by Autism-Spectrum Quotient correlated with gray matter reduction. *Soc. Neurosci.* **2011**, *6*, 548–558. [CrossRef]
20. Narita, Z.; Inagawa, T.; Maruo, K.; Sueyoshi, K.; Sumiyoshi, T. Effect of Transcranial Direct Current Stimulation on Functional Capacity in Schizophrenia: A Study Protocol for a Randomized Controlled Trial. *Front. Psychiatry* **2017**, *8*. [CrossRef]
21. Yokoi, Y.; Narita, Z.; Sumiyoshi, T. Transcranial Direct Current Stimulation in Depression and Psychosis: A Systematic Review. *Clin. EEG Neurosci.* **2017**, *49*, 93–102. [CrossRef]
22. Yamada, Y.; Sumiyoshi, T. Neurobiological Mechanisms of Transcranial Direct Current Stimulation for Psychiatric Disorders; Neurophysiological, Chemical, and Anatomical Considerations. *Front. Hum. Neurosci.* **2021**, *15*. [CrossRef]
23. Yamada, Y.; Matsumoto, M.; Iijima, K.; Sumiyoshi, T. Specificity and Continuity of Schizophrenia and Bipolar Disorder: Relation to Biomarkers. *Curr. Pharm. Des.* **2020**, *26*, 191–200. [CrossRef]
24. Narita, Z.; Stickley, A.; DeVylder, J.; Yokoi, Y.; Inagawa, T.; Yamada, Y.; Maruo, K.; Koyanagi, A.; Oh, H.; Sawa, A.; et al. Effect of multi-session prefrontal transcranial direct current stimulation on cognition in schizophrenia: A systematic review and meta-analysis. *Schizophr. Res.* **2020**, *216*, 367–373. [CrossRef]
25. Rassovsky, Y.; Dunn, W.; Wynn, J.; Wu, A.D.; Iacoboni, M.; Hellemann, G.; Green, M.F. The effect of transcranial direct current stimulation on social cognition in schizophrenia: A preliminary study. *Schizophr. Res.* **2015**, *165*, 171–174. [CrossRef]
26. Yamada, Y.; Inagawa, T.; Hirabayashi, N.; Sumiyoshi, T. Emotion Recognition Deficits in Psychiatric Disorders as a Target of Non-invasive Neuromodulation: A Systematic Review. *Clin. EEG Neurosci.* **2021**, *15*. [CrossRef]
27. Moseley, P.; Fernyhough, C.; Ellison, A. The role of the superior temporal lobe in auditory false perceptions: A transcranial direct current stimulation study. *Neuropsychologia* **2014**, *62*, 202–208. [CrossRef]
28. Chan, A.-W.; Tetzlaff, J.M.; Altman, D.G.; Laupacis, A.; Gøtzsche, P.C.; Krleža-Jerić, K.; Hróbjartsson, A.; Mann, H.; Dickersin, K.; Berlin, J.A.; et al. SPIRIT 2013 Statement: Defining Standard Protocol Items for Clinical Trials. *Ann. Intern. Med.* **2013**, *158*, 200–207. [CrossRef]
29. Narita, Z.; Inagawa, T.; Sueyoshi, K.; Lin, C.; Sumiyoshi, T. Possible Facilitative Effects of Repeated Anodal Transcranial Direct Current Stimulation on Functional Outcome 1 Month Later in Schizophrenia: An Open Trial. *Front. Psychiatry* **2017**, *8*. [CrossRef]
30. Kanie, A.; Hagiya, K.; Ashida, S.; Pu, S.; Kaneko, K.; Mogami, T.; Oshima, S.; Motoya, M.; Niwa, S.-I.; Inagaki, A.; et al. New instrument for measuring multiple domains of social cognition: Construct validity of the Social Cognition Screening Questionnaire (Japanese version). *Psychiatry Clin. Neurosci.* **2014**, *68*, 701–711. [CrossRef]
31. Baron-Cohen, S.; Leslie, A.M.; Frith, U. Does the autistic child have a "theory of mind"? *Cognition* **1985**, *21*, 37–46. [CrossRef]
32. Corcoran, R.; Mercer, G.; Frith, C.D. Schizophrenia, symptomatology and social inference: Investigating "theory of mind" in people with schizophrenia. *Schizophr. Res.* **1995**, *17*, 5–13. [CrossRef]
33. Baron-Cohen, S.; Wheelwright, S.; Skinner, R.; Martin, J.; Clubley, E. The Autism-Spectrum Quotient (AQ): Evidence from Asperger Syndrome/High-Functioning Autism, Malesand Females, Scientists and Mathematicians. *J. Autism Dev. Disord.* **2001**, *31*, 5–17. [CrossRef] [PubMed]
34. Young, A.; Perrett, D.; Calder, A.; Sprengelmeyer, R.; Ekman, P. *Facial Expressions of Emotion: Stimuli and Tests (FEEST)*; Thames Valley Test Company: Edmunds, UK, 2002.
35. Saykin, A.J.; Gur, R.C.; Gur, R.E.; Mozley, P.D.; Mozley, L.H.; Resnick, S.M.; Kester, D.B.; Stafiniak, P. Neuropsychological function in schizophrenia. Selective impairment in memory and learning. *Arch. Gen. Psychiatr.* **1991**, *48*, 618–624. [CrossRef]
36. Matsuoka, K.; Uno, M.; Kasai, K.; Koyama, K.; Kim, Y. Estimation of premorbid IQ in individuals with Alzheimer's disease using Japanese ideographic script (Kanji) compound words: Japanese version of National Adult Reading Test. *Psychiatry Clin. Neurosci.* **2006**, *60*, 332–339. [CrossRef]
37. Sumiyoshi, C.; Takaki, M.; Okahisa, Y.; Patterson, T.L.; Harvey, P.D.; Sumiyoshi, T. Utility of the UCSD Performance-based Skills Assessment-Brief Japanese version: Discriminative ability and relation to neurocognition. *Schizophr. Res. Cogn.* **2014**, *1*, 137–143. [CrossRef]

38. Kay, S.R.; Opler, L.A.; Lindenmayer, J.-P. Reliability and validity of the positive and negative syndrome scale for schizophrenics. *Psychiatry Res.* **1988**, *23*, 99–110. [CrossRef]
39. Brunoni, A.R.; Amadera, J.; Berbel, B.; Volz, M.S.; Rizzerio, B.G.; Fregni, F. A systematic review on reporting and assessment of adverse effects associated with transcranial direct current stimulation. *Int. J. Neuropsychopharmacol.* **2011**, *14*, 1133–1145. [CrossRef]
40. Inada, T.; Inagaki, A. Psychotropic dose equivalence in Japan. *Psychiatry Clin. Neurosci.* **2015**, *69*, 440–447. [CrossRef]
41. Inagawa, T.; Yokoi, Y.; Yamada, Y.; Miyagawa, N.; Otsuka, T.; Yasuma, N.; Omachi, Y.; Tsukamoto, T.; Takano, H.; Sakata, M.; et al. Effects of multisession transcranial direct current stimulation as an augmentation to cognitive tasks in patients with neurocognitive disorders in Japan: A study protocol for a randomised controlled trial. *BMJ Open* **2020**, *10*, e037654. [CrossRef]

MDPI
St. Alban-Anlage 66
4052 Basel
Switzerland
Tel. +41 61 683 77 34
Fax +41 61 302 89 18
www.mdpi.com

Journal of Personalized Medicine Editorial Office
E-mail: jpm@mdpi.com
www.mdpi.com/journal/jpm

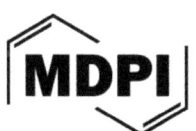

www.ingramcontent.com/pod-product-compliance
Lightning Source LLC
LaVergne TN
LVHW070615100526
838202LV00012B/656